Thieme

Anatomy for Plastic Surgery of the Face, Head, and Neck

Koichi Watanabe, MD, PhD
Assistant Professor
Department of Anatomy
Kurume University School of Medicine
Fukuoka-Prefecture, Japan

Mohammadali M. Shoja, MD
Research Scientist
Section of Pediatric Neurosurgery
Children's Hospital
Birmingham, Alabama, USA

Marios Loukas, MD, PhD
Dean of Basic Sciences
Professor and Chair
Department of Anatomical Sciences
St. George's University
Grenada, West Indies

R. Shane Tubbs, MS, PA-C, PhD
Professor and Chief Scientific Officer
Seattle Science Foundation
Seattle, Washington, USA

269 illustrations

Thieme
New York • Stuttgart • Delhi • Rio de Janeiro

Executive Editor: Timothy Hiscock
Managing Editor: Elizabeth Palumbo
Director, Editorial Services: Mary Jo Casey
Editorial Assistant: Haley Paskalides
Production Editor: Barbara A. Chernow
International Production Director: Andreas Schabert
Vice President, Editorial and E-Product Development: Vera Spillner
International Marketing Director: Fiona Henderson
International Sales Director: Louisa Turrell
Director of Sales, North America: Mike Roseman
Senior Vice President and Chief Operating Officer: Sarah Vanderbilt
President: Brian D. Scanlan
Typesetting by Carol Pierson, Chernow Editorial Services, Inc.

Library of Congress Cataloging-in-Publication Data

Names: Watanabe, Kåoichi, 1968– author. | Shoja, Mohammadali M., author. | Loukas, Marios, author. | Tubbs, R. Shane, author.
Title: Anatomy for plastic surgery of the face, head, and neck / Kåoichi Watanabe, Mohammadali M. Shoja, Marios Loukas, R. Shane Tubbs.
Description: New York : Thieme, [2016] | Includes bibliographical references and index.
Identifiers: LCCN 2015031107| ISBN 9781626230910 (alk. paper) | ISBN 9781626230927 (eISBN)
Subjects: | MESH: Head—anatomy & histology—Atlases. | Neck—anatomy & histology—Atlases. | Reconstructive Surgical Procedures—Atlases.
Classification: LCC RD119 | NLM WE 17 | DDC 617.9/52—dc23
LC record available at http://lccn.loc.gov/2015031107

Thieme Publishers New York
333 Seventh Avenue, New York, NY 10001
USA +1 800 782 3488, customerservice@thieme.com

Thieme Publishers Stuttgart
Rüdigerstrasse 14, 70469 Stuttgart, Germany
+49 [0]711 8931 421, customerservice@thieme.de

Thieme Publishers Delhi
A-12, Second Floor, Sector-2, Noida-201301
Uttar Pradesh, India
+91 120 45 566 00, customerservice@thieme.in

Thieme Publishers Rio de Janeiro, Thieme Publicações Ltda.
Edifício Rodolpho de Paoli, 25º andar
Av. Nilo Peçanha, 50 – Sala 2508
Rio de Janeiro 20020-906, Brasil
+55 21 3172 2297

Printed in India by Manipal Technologies Ltd., Manipal

ISBN 978-1-62623-091-0

Also available as an e-book:
eISBN 978-1-62623-092-7

Contents

List of Videos

Preface

This book was planned as a head and neck surgical anatomy book for plastic surgeons, head and neck surgeons, and surgeons who practice in related fields. Unfortunately, few surgical textbooks emphasize anatomy, especially textbooks in the field of plastic surgery. In most surgical textbooks, the procedures are described only in minute detail. Conversely, traditional anatomical textbooks do not provide adequate information on the regional anatomy, preventing surgeons from obtaining the knowledge necessary to expertly perform various surgical procedures. One reason for this is that although the basic anatomy of the human body was almost completely described more than 100 years ago, the anatomy in the head and neck region, especially that applicable to plastic surgery, is still developing. Additionally, anatomical textbooks often do not provide the most up-to-date information. Therefore, we have attempted to include the latest anatomical understanding of the head and neck anatomy from a plastic surgeon's perspective.

In writing this preface, I (KW) discussed head and neck anatomy with my mentors in two specialties: gross anatomy and plastic surgery. This allowed me to consider anatomy from two different viewpoints.

First, my mentor in gross anatomy made the following observations: The anatomy of the head and neck is extremely complicated and the details differ among individuals and during different stages of life. These differences include the thickness of the tissues, their changes in response to aging, and even anatomical variations in vessels, nerves, and muscles. Each organ in the head and neck region has a very distinct function. Consequently, pathologies involving the head that require surgery will be operated on by surgeons specializing in neurosurgery, otorhinopharyngolaryngology, ophthalmology, dental medicine, and plastic surgery. While in-depth knowledge in the anatomical area of specialization is extremely important in treating patients, the surgeon as well as the medical staff must also be highly familiar with not just related regions of the body but also with unrelated regions. In medical education, unfortunately, the importance of anatomical education has been downplayed globally in recent years. This may be because nowadays medical students have less time to study anatomy, given the many new fields of medicine that they are expected to be familiar with. Apparently, some medical schools no longer offer anatomical dissection. Thus, not surprisingly, the number of anatomists, especially gross anatomists, is decreasing. This tendency has critical, negative implications for surgery. Gross anatomy is the basis of knowledge for every surgeon. Surgeons must be experts in gross anatomy if they hope to acquire the surgical skills to become experts in surgery.

My second mentor, a specialist in plastic surgery, offered the following: The most important aspect of performing plastic surgery is knowledge of three-dimensional regional anatomy. For example, each nerve and blood vessel takes up space three dimensionally. It is important to recognize how these structures travel on the surface plane, but it is more important for the success of the actual surgery to know which tissue layers these structures run through. Anatomical atlases and textbooks provide detailed images of these structures, but the knowledge gained from them is two-dimensional. Novice surgeons typically memorize the two-dimensional image of their surgical field. Because of this, surgical results are sometimes unsatisfactory, or unexpected surgical complications may occur. To perform surgeries with a high degree of difficulty, a surgeon has to be able to vividly visualize the three-dimensional regional anatomy of the surgical field. Plastic surgery residents have to study the regional anatomy in anatomical atlases and textbooks, and confirm their anatomical knowledge in practical operations. By repeating this pattern many times, a resident is able to establish and practice three-dimensional anatomical knowledge. By having surgical training based on accurate anatomical knowledge, a surgeon will be better equipped to perform high-degree operations.

We hope that our textbook will not only help to improve the surgical skill of individual surgeons, but will also promote the development of head and neck surgery. I would like to thank Dr. Koh-ichi Yamaki, Professor of Anatomy, and Dr. Kensuke Kiyokawa, Professor of Plastic Surgery, for kindly contributing the above comments to the preface.

Contributors

Toomas Arusoo, MS
Medical Student, Year 2
Michigan State University College of Human Medicine
Grand Rapids, Michigan, USA

Jenny C. Barker, MD, PhD
Resident
Department of Plastic Surgery
Ohio State University Wexner Medical Center
Columbus, Ohio, USA

Servet Celik, MD
Assistant Professor
Department of Anatomy
Faculty of Medicine
Ege University
Izmir, Turkey

Philip R. Chapman, MD
Chief, Neuroradiology
Associate Professor, Neuroradiology Section
University of Alabama at Birmingham School of Medicine
Birmingham, Alabama, USA

Junichi Fukushima, MD, PhD
Department of Otorhinolaryngology
Graduate School of Medical Science
Kyushu University
Fukuoka, Japan

Figen Govsa, MD
Professor
Department of Anatomy
Ege University, Faculty of Medicine
Izmir, Turkey

Orlando Guntinas-Lichius, MD
Professor and Chairman
ENT Department
Jena University Hospital
Dean of Students
Medical Faculty
Friedrich-Schiller University
Jena, Germany

Kyung-Seok Hu, DDS, PhD
Associate Professor
Department of Oral Biology
Division in Anatomy & Developmental Biology
Yonsei University College of Dentistry
Seoul, Republic of Korea

Nobuaki Imanishi, MD
Associate Professor
Department of Anatomy
School of Medicine, Keio University
Tokyo, Japan

Lucian Ion, FRCS(Plast)
Consultant Plastic Surgeon
Director, Aesthetic Plastic Surgery Ltd
London, UK
Honorary Consultant
Chelsea and Westminster Hospital
London, UK

Joe Iwanaga, DDS
Assistant Professor
Department of Anatomy
Kurume University School of Medicine
Fukuoka, Japan

Jeffrey E. Janis, MD, FACS
Professor and Executive Vice Chairman
Chief of Plastic Surgery
University Hospitals
Department of Plastic Surgery
Ohio State University Wexner Medical Center
Columbus, Ohio, USA

David Kahn, MD
Clinical Associate Professor Plastic Surgery
Section Chief, Cosmetic Surgery
Division of Plastic Surgery
Stanford University
Palo Alto, California, USA

Ibrahim Khansa, MD
Resident
Department of Plastic Surgery
Ohio State University Wexner Medical Center
Columbus, Ohio, USA

Hee-Jin Kim, DDS, PhD
Professor
Division in Anatomy & Developmental Biology
Department of Oral Biology
Yonsei University College of Dentistry
Seoul, Korea

Kensuke Kiyokawa, MD, PhD
Professor and Chairman
Department of Plastic & Reconstructive Surgery & Maxillofacial Surgery
Kurume University School of Medicine
Fukuoka, Japan

Noriyuki Koga, MD, PhD
Assistant Professor
Department of Plastic Surgery, Reconstructive and Maxillofacial Surgery
Kurume University School of Medicine
Kurume, Japan

Noritaka Komune, MD, PhD
Fellow
Department of Otorhinolaryngology and Head and Neck Surgery
Kyushu University Hospital
Fukuoka-ken, Japan

Catherine Y. Liu, MD, PhD
Resident, Ophthalmology
Gavin Herbert Eye Institute
University of California, Irvine
Irvine, California, USA

Marios Loukas, MD, PhD
Dean of Basic Sciences
Professor and Chair
Department of Anatomical Sciences
St. George's University
Grenada, West Indies

Shinya Mikushi, DDS, PhD
Nagasaki University Hospital
Department of Special Care Dentistry
Clinic for Oral Care and Dysphagia Rehabilitation
Nagasaki, Japan

Yang Hun Mu, DDS, PhD
Assistant Professor
Department of Anatomy College of Medicine
Dankook University
Chungnam, Korea

Yelda Atamaz Pinar, MD
Professor
Department of Anatomy
Faculty of Medicine
EGE University, Faculty of Medicine
Izmir, Turkey

Sherine S. Raveendran, FRCSEd, EBOPRAS, MSc, MS, MBBS
Director
Toronto Medical Aesthetics
Markham, Ontario, Canada

Albert L. Rhoton, Jr., MD
R. D. Keene Family Professor and Chairman Emeritus
Department of Neurological Surgery
University of Florida
Gainesville, Florida, USA

Hideaki Rikimaru, MD, PhD
Department of Plastic Reconstructive Surgery and Maxillofacial Surgery
Kurume University School of Medicine
Fukuoka, Japan

Tsuyoshi Saga, PhD
Associate Professor
Department of Anatomy
Kurume University School of Medicine
Fukuoka, Japan

Yusuke Shimizu, MD, PhD
Associate Professor
Department of Plastic and Reconstructive Surgery
Keio University, School of Medicine
Tokyo, Japan

Mohammadali M. Shoja, MD
Research Scientist
Section of Pediatric Neurosurgery
Children's Hospital
Birmingham, Alabama, USA

Yoko Tabira, PhD
Research Associate
Department of Anatomy
Kurume University School of Medicine
Kurume, Japan

Jeremiah P. Tao, MD, FACS
Chief, Oculoplastic & Orbital Surgery
American Society of Ophthalmic Plastic and Reconstructive Surgery Fellowship Director
Ophthalmology Residency Director
Associate Professor
Gavin Herbert Eye Institute
University of California, Irvine
Irvine, California, USA

Haruka Tohara, DDS, PhD
Gerodontology and Oral Rehabilitation,
Department of Gerontology and Gerodontology
Graduate School of Medical and Dental Sciences
Tokyo Medical and Dental University
Yushima, Bunkyo
Tokyo, Japan

Andrew P. Trussler, MD, FACS
Plastic Surgeon, Private Practice
Austin, Texas, USA

R. Shane Tubbs, MS, PA-C, PhD
Professor and Chief Scientific Officer
Seattle Science Foundation
Seattle, Washington, USA

Surjith Vattoth, MD, FRCR
Senior Consutant, Neuroradiologist
Hamad Medical Corporation
Doha, Qatar

Swapna Vemuri, MD
Fellow, Oculoplastic and Orbital Surgery
Gavin Herbert Eye Institute
University of California, Irvine
Irvine, California, USA

Koichi Watanabe, MD, PhD
Assistant Professor
Department of Anatomy
Kurume University School of Medicine
Fukuoka-Prefecture, Japan

Eric J. Wright, MD
Chief Resident
Division of Plastic & Reconstructive Surgery
Stanford University Medical Center
Palo Alto, California, USA

Koh-ichi Yamaki, MD, PhD
Professor and Chair
Department of Anatomy
Kurume University School of Medicine
Kurume, Japan

1 Neurocranium and Facial Skeleton

David Kahn, Toomas Arusoo, and Eric J. Wright

Introduction

The skull can be divided into two parts: the *neurocranium*, which forms a protective case around the brain, and the *viscerocranium*, which forms the skeleton of the face. This chapter details the viscerocranium and bones of the neurocranium that pertain to the viscerocranium.

Neurocranium

The neurocranium in adults is formed by a series of eight bones: the singular frontal, ethmoid, sphenoid, occipital bones centered on the midline, and the temporal and parietal bones occurring as bilateral pairs.[1] The primarily flat frontal, parietal, and occipital bones form the calvaria (skullcap) by intramembranous ossification of head mesenchyme derived from the neural crest. The primarily irregular, yet considerably flat, sphenoid and temporal bones contribute to the cranial base via endochondral ossification of cartilage or from more than one type of ossification. The irregular ethmoid bone slightly contributes to the neurocranium but is primarily part of the viscerocranium. In reality, the flat bones and flat portions of the bones forming the neurocranium consist of convex external and concave internal curved surfaces.[1]

Fibrous interlocking sutures unite most calvarial bones in adulthood, although during childhood, the sphenoid and occipital bones are unified by synchondroses.[2] Some sutures, comprising narrow closures of connective tissue at birth, remain open until adulthood. The sagittal suture is derived from neural crest cells and the coronal suture from paraxial mesoderm.[2] The newborn skull contains *fontanels*, the most prominent being the anterior fontanel, which are widened sutures at points where more than two bones meet. The anterior fontanel, found where the two parietal and frontal bones meet, closes in most cases by 18 months of age, and the posterior fontanel closes by 1 to 2 months of age.[2]

Two primary centers of ossification traverse the frontal (metopic) suture in the second year, dividing the frontal bone into halves. Usually, the frontal suture disappears by age 6 years, when the halves fuse, but it can persist into adulthood as a metopic suture either totally, running from the midline of the glabella to the bregma, or partially.[2] The *glabella* is a smooth anterior projecting prominence on the frontal bone superior to the root of the nose, and the *bregma* is the junction of the coronal and sagittal sutures.

The maxillae and mandible provide the sockets and supporting bone for the maxillary and mandibular teeth. The maxillae contribute the greatest part of the upper facial skeleton, forming the skeleton of the upper jaw, which is fixed to the cranial base. (The mandible is detailed in Chapter 19.)

On the lateral aspect of the skull is the thin pterion. The pterion, located two finger breadths superior to the zygomatic arch and a thumb's breadth posterior to the frontal process of the zygomatic bone, is formed by the articulations of the frontal, parietal, sphenoid, and temporal bones.[1] The pterion overlies the anterior branch of the middle meningeal artery. Therefore, an injury to this region can damage the vessel, producing an epidural hematoma.[1]

The air-filled paranasal sinuses, including the maxillary, frontal, and ethmoidal sinuses, are discussed. The sphenoidal sinuses are discussed in Chapters 2 and 16. The bony articulations of the neurocranium and viscerocranium are described in **Table 1.1**, and the general processes of ossification are displayed in **Table 1.2**.

Frontal Bone

The frontal bone forms the forehead via its squamous, orbital, and nasal parts and two cavities, the frontal sinuses.

Squamous Part

The flat squamous part is the largest part of the frontal bone forming most of the forehead.[3] The supraorbital margin of the frontal bone is the angular boundary between the squamous and the orbital parts (**Fig. 1.1**).[4]

On the external surface of the squamous part, about 3 cm above the midpoint of this margin, are the frontal tuberosities.[4] These tubercles are more prominent in children and adult women. Ventrally, a shallow groove separates the frontal tuberosities from the paired and curved superciliary arches.[4] These arches extend laterally from the medially located, smooth, and elevated glabella and are more prominent in males. Partly dependent on frontal sinus size, supercilliary arch prominence is occasionally associated with small sinuses.[4]

The supraorbital notch (or foramen), which transmits the supraorbital vessels and nerve, lies at the junction between the sharp, lateral two-thirds and the rounded medial third of the supraorbital margin.[4] The variably occurring frontal notch (or foramen) occurs medial to the supraorbital notch in 50% of skulls.[4]

Surgical Annotation

Recent interest in the surgical treatment of migraines has led to numerous anatomical studies identifying areas of nerve compression. The supraorbital nerve, as it emerges from the

Table 1.1 Neurocranium and viscerocranium articulations

Bone	Single	Paired	Articulates with
Frontal	X		Parietal, sphenoid, zygomatic, maxilla, ethmoid, nasal, lacrimal
Ethmoid	X		Frontal, sphenoid, maxilla, palatine, vomer, nasal, lacrimal, inferior nasal concha
Temporal		X	Parietal, occipital, sphenoid, zygomatic, mandible
Nasal		X	Frontal, maxilla, nasal
Vomer	X		Sphenoid, maxilla, ethmoid, palatine
Inferior nasal concha		X	Maxilla, ethmoid, palatine, lacrimal
Maxilla		X	Frontal, sphenoid, zygomatic, maxilla, ethmoid, palatine, vomer, nasal, lacrimal, inferior nasal concha
Palatine		X	Sphenoid, maxilla, ethmoid, palatine, vomer, inferior nasal concha
Zygomatic		X	Frontal, temporal, maxilla, sphenoid
Lacrimal		X	Frontal, maxilla, ethmoid, inferior nasal concha

Source: Data from Norton NS. Netter's Head and Neck Anatomy for Dentistry. 1st ed. Philadelphia, PA: Elsevier Saunders; 2006.

supraorbital foramen or notch, has been identified as a migraine trigger area.[5] The supraorbital nerve can have compression from both a foramen as well as a notch as a result of the associated fascial bands. In addition to the soft tissue procedure, a supraorbital foraminotomy or fascial band release has been shown to improve postoperative outcomes.[6] A transpalpebral incision can be used to access the supraorbital nerves to perform the decompression. An incision is made in the upper tarsal crease, with subsequent dissection identifying the supraorbital nerve. Muscles such as the corrugator supercilii are resected, and the foraminotomy is performed. Endoscopic techniques have also been described.[7] With the use of the endoscopic technique, release of the zygomaticotemporal branch can also be performed.

The supraorbital margin extends laterally, forming the prominent zygomatic process, which articulates with the zygomatic bone. A posterosuperiorly curving line, which continues onto the squamous part of the temporal bone, divides into superior and inferior temporal lines.[4] The temporal surface of the frontal bone is inferior and posterior relative to these temporal lines. The anterior surface of the temporal surface forms the anterior part of the temporal fossa. The rough inferior surface of the posterior margin of the squamous part articulates with the greater wing of the sphenoid.[4]

The nasal part of the frontal bone is discussed in the *Nasal Bone: Nasal Bridge and Bony Septum* section of this chapter. The interior surface of the frontal bone is detailed in Chapter 2.

Orbital Parts of the Frontal Bone

The two orbital parts of the frontal bone are thin, curved, and triangular laminae, consisting entirely of compact bone (**Fig. 1.2**).[4] Forming the largest part of the orbital roofs, the orbital parts are separated by a wide, quadrilateral ethmoidal notch that is occupied by the cribriform plate of the ethmoid bone.[4] The labyrinths of the ethmoid bone, which contain the ethmoidal air cells, articulate with the inferior surface of the lateral margins of the ethmoidal notch. This articulation converts two transverse grooves across each margin into anterior and posterior ethmoidal canals. These canals transmit the anterior and posterior ethmoidal nerves and vessels into the medial orbit.[4]

The posterolaterally ascending frontal sinuses open anterior to the ethmoidal notch and lateral to the nasal spine (**Fig. 1.3**). Deflecting from the median plane, these rarely symmetrical sinuses ascend between the frontal laminae and are separated by a thin septum.[4] Each sinus communicates with the ipsilateral nasal cavity's middle meatus via the frontonasal canal.[4]

Table 1.2 Neurocranium and viscerocranium ossification patterns

Bone	Parts	Ossification
Frontal	Squamous, orbital, nasal portions	Intramembranous
Ethmoid	Perpendicular plate, cribriform plate, ethmoid labyrinth	Endochondral
Temporal	Squamous part, tympanic part	Intramembranous
	petromastoid part, styloid process	Endochondral
Nasal		Intramembranous
Vomer		Intramembranous
Inferior Nasal Concha		Endochondral
Maxilla	Body; frontal, zygomatic, palatine, alveolar processes	Intramembranous
Palatine	Perpendicular plate, horizontal plate, pyramidal process	Intramembranous
Zygomatic	Frontal, temporal, maxillary processes	Intramembranous
Lacrimal		Intramembranous

Source: Data from Norton NS. Netter's Head and Neck Anatomy for Dentistry. 1st ed. Philadelphia, PA: Elsevier Saunders; 2006.

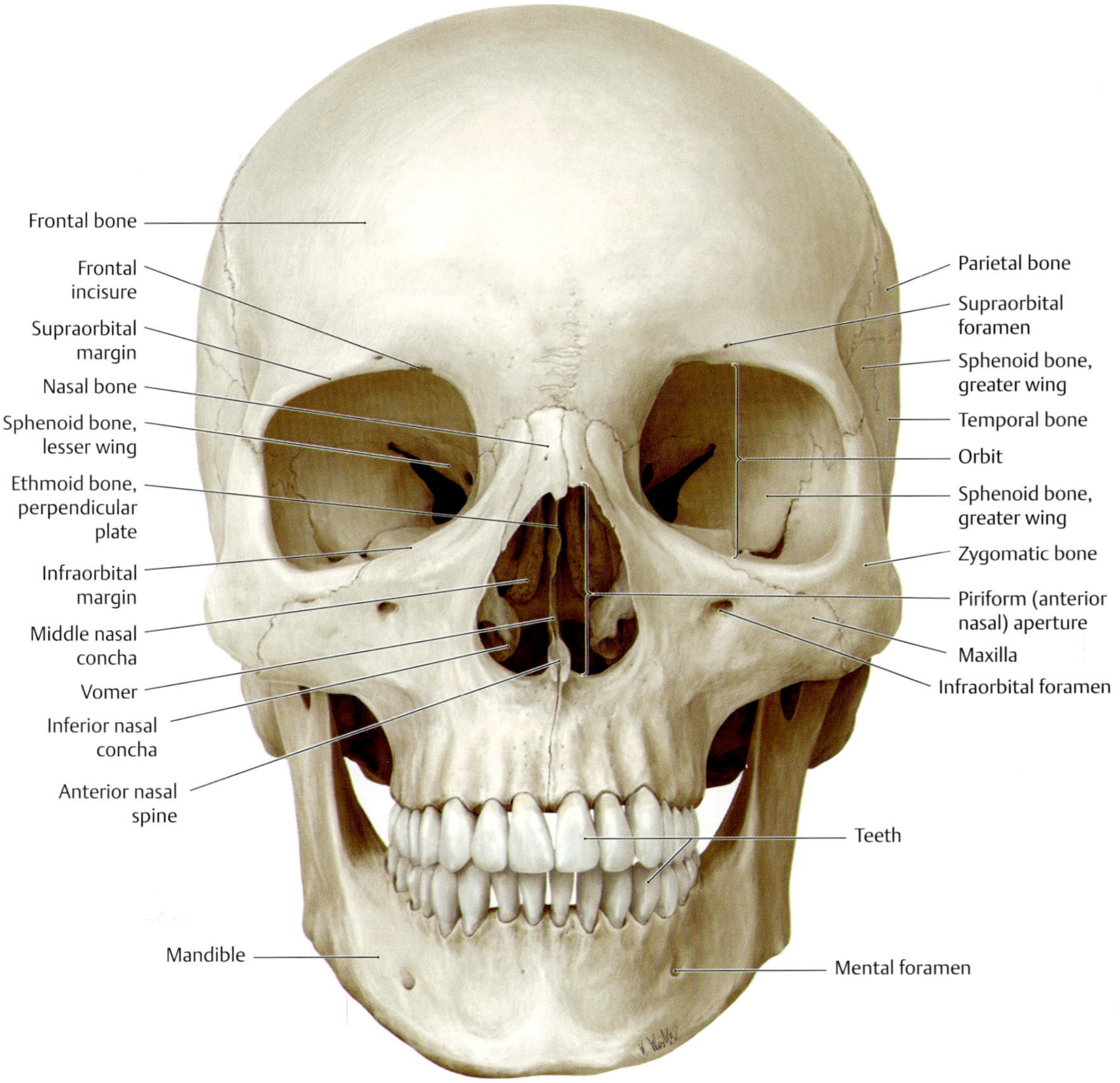

Fig. 1.1 Anterior view of the skull. The boundaries of the viscerocranium in relation to the neurocranium can be appreciated in this view. Visible features include the anterior nasal aperture, marking the start of the bony respiratory tract; a metopic suture projects superiorly from the nasion; and the supraorbital foramen, infraorbital foramen, and mental foramen through which cutaneous nerves pass, are visible. (Reproduced from THIEME Atlas of Anatomy, General Anatomy and Musculoskeletal System, © Thieme 2005, Illustration by Karl Wesker.)

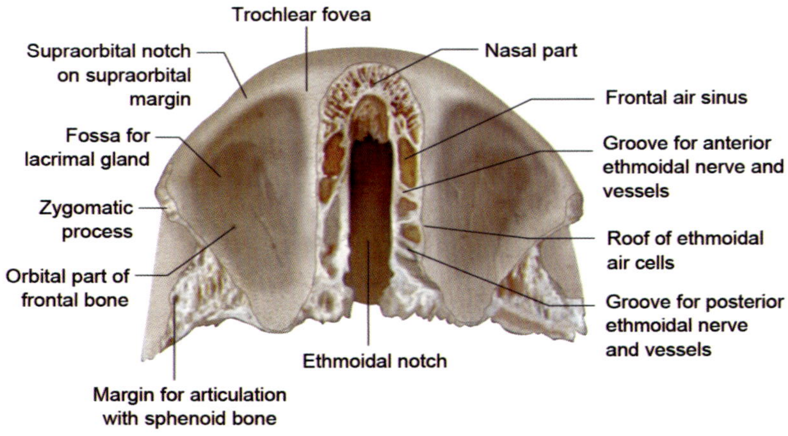

Fig. 1.2 Inferior view of the frontal bone. From this view, the ethmoidal notch and ethmoidal air sinuses can clearly be appreciated. Additional visibility of the orbital part surface features, including the fossa for the lacrimal gland, the sphenoidal articulating surface, and the zygomatic process, is obtained from this view.

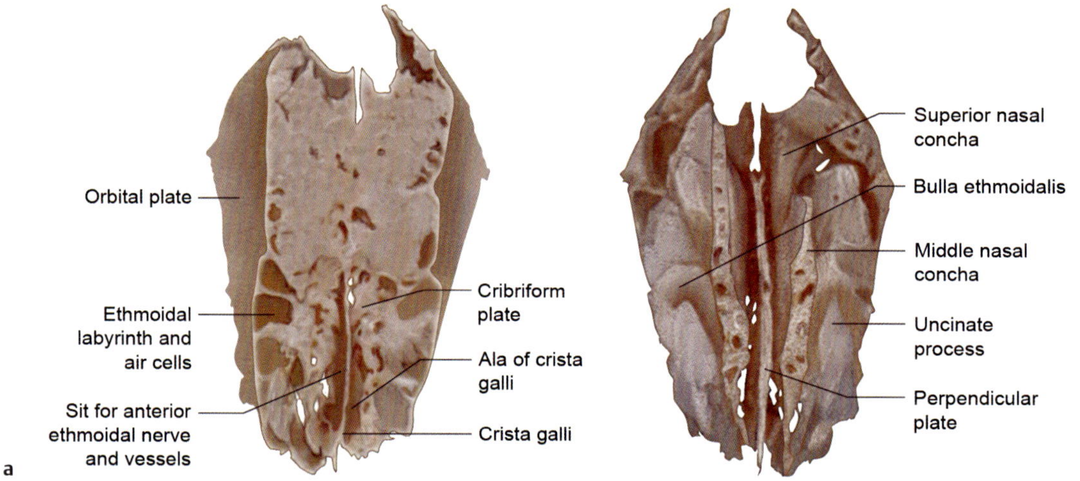

Fig. 1.3 **(a)** Superior view of the ethmoid bone. This view of the ethmoid bone provides a better appreciation for the ethmoidal labyrinth and air cells, the cribriform plate, and the crista galli and its associated alae. **(b)** Inferior view of the ethmoidal bone. Viewing the ethmoid bone from below allows better appreciation of the nasal conchae, uncinate process, and the perpendicular plate.

Frontal Sinus Fractures

Surgical Annotation

Frontal sinus fractures can serve as a source of infection and cosmetic deformity. Approximately 10% of facial fractures involve the frontal sinuses.[8] When outflow of the sinus is blocked as a result of injury to the nasofrontal duct, frontal sinus mucoceles can develop. In accessing the injury, management depends on which wall of the sinus is fractured, the extent of fracture displacement, and the involvement of the nasofrontal duct. Correction of the anterior table of the sinus, which is done mainly to correct the cosmetic deformity, can be performed through an existing laceration or coronal incision. When the posterior table is displaced, the coronal incision allows access to perform a cranialization, which involves removing the posterior wall and allowing for the sinus to be part of the intracranial cavity. The sinus mucosal surface must be removed and the outflow tract and dead space obliterated to prevent postinjury infection.

Different techniques for performing the obliteration have been described.[8] Management of sinus preservation can also be performed with few complications depending on the fracture pattern.[9]

Each smooth and concave orbital surface contains a shallow anterolateral fossa for the lacrimal gland. The posterior border of the orbital plate articulates with the lesser wings of the sphenoid.[4]

Ethmoid Bone

The fragile cuboidal ethmoid bone lies anteriorly in the cranial base, contributing to the medial orbital walls, nasal septum, roof, and lateral walls of the nasal cavity. The ethmoid is composed of a horizontal, perforated cribriform plate, a median perpendicular plate, and the two lateral labyrinths.[3]

Cribriform Plate

As mentioned, the horizontal cribriform plate fills the ethmoidal notch of the frontal bone (**Fig. 1.3a**). Penetrated by numerous foramina that contain olfactory nerve branches, the plate forms a large part of the nasal roof.[3] The triangular and median crista galli projects superiorly from the plate and joins the frontal bone anteriorly via its two alae.[3] Depressions in the cribriform plate on either side of the crista galli exist for the overlying olfactory bulb and gyrus rectus. Antero and lateral to the crista, foramina exist to transmit the anterior ethmoidal nerve and vessels from the nasal cavity to the foramen cecum.[4]

Perpendicular Plate

The perpendicular plate is discussed in the Nasal Bone: Nasal Bridge and Bony Septum section of this chapter.

Ethmoidal Labyrinths

On average, the ethmoidal labyrinths consist of 20 thin-walled air cells arranged as anterior, middle, and posterior groups containing 11, 3, and 6 air cells, respectively.[4] The lateral orbital plate forms part of the medial orbital wall (**Fig. 1.4**). Adjoining articulations, save those that open into the nasal cavity, close all air cells. The air cells of the superior and posterior surfaces are closed by the ethmoidal notch of the frontal bone and both the sphenoidal conchae and orbital process of the palatine bone, respectively.[4]

The orbital plate covers the middle and posterior ethmoidal air cells articulating superiorly with the orbital plate of the frontal bone, anteriorly with the lacrimal bone, inferiorly with the maxilla and orbital process of the palatine bone, and posteriorly with the sphenoid bone.[4] Anterior to the orbital plate, the lacrimal bone and frontal process of the maxilla complete the walls.

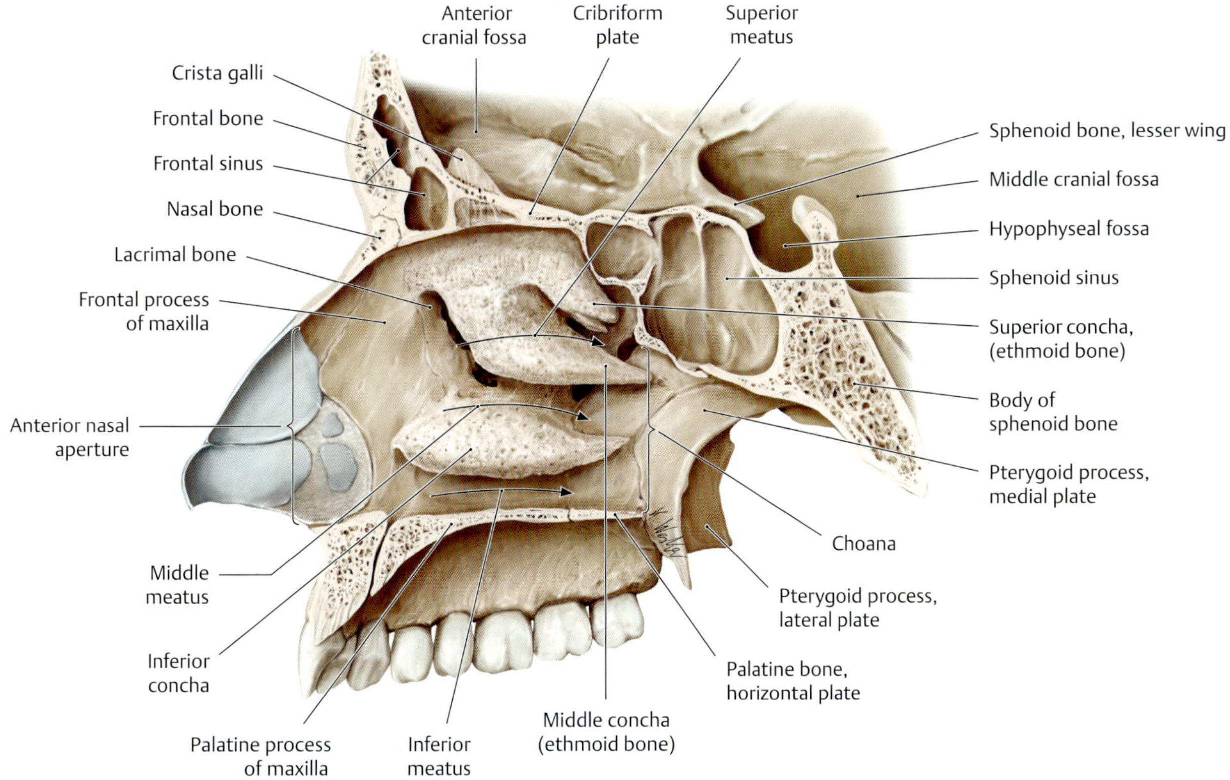

Fig. 1.4 Medial view of the right nasal cavity. This view of the nasal cavity allows better appreciation of the conchae, meatuses, portions of the hard palate, the frontal sinus, ethmoidal contributions to the nasal cavity, and the anterior nasal aperture. (Reproduced from THIEME Atlas of Anatomy, Head and Neuroanatomy, © Thieme 2010, Illustration by Karl Wesker.)

Projecting posteroinferiorly from the labyrinth, the thin uncinate process crosses the ostium of the maxillary sinus to join the ethmoidal process of the inferior nasal concha.[4]

Descending from the inferior surface of the cribriform plate, the medial surface of the labyrinth forms part of the lateral nasal wall as the thin, lamellated, and convoluted middle nasal concha (**Fig. 1.3b**). Its anteroninferior lateral surface forms part of the middle meatus (**Fig. 1.4**).[4] On the lateral wall of the middle meatus, middle ethmoidal air cells produce the ethmoidal bulla and open either on the bulla or above it. Posterior ethmoidal air cells open into the superior meatus, which is bounded by the superior nasal concha of the ethmoid.[4] A curved infundibulum extends anteriorly and superiorly from the middle meatus, communicating with the anterior ethmoidal sinuses and in half of skulls continues superiorly as the frontonasal duct, which drains the frontal sinus.[4]

Temporal Bone

The paired temporal bones help form the base and lateral walls of the skull and are discussed in further detail in subsequent chapters (**Fig. 1.1**). The temporal bone houses the auditory and vestibular apparatuses and contains mastoid air cells.[3] Each bone has eight centers of ossification that give rise to the three major centers observed before birth.[2] The temporal bone comprises the squamous, petromastoid, and tympanic parts, as well as the styloid process.[3] The temporal bone also has two associated canals. On its lateral surface, the external acoustic meatus conveys sound waves to the tympanic membrane. On its medial surface, the internal acoustic meatus conveys the facial and vestibulocochlear nerves.[4]

Squamous Part

The largest, squamous part lies anterosuperiorly and contains the thin and largest temporal portion, a zygomatic process and a mandibular fossa (**Fig. 1.5**).[3] Its external temporal surface forms part of the temporal fossa. The concave, internal cerebral surface of the squamous part is grooved by the middle meningeal vessels.[3] The lower border, fused to the anterior petrous part often contains traces of a petrosquamosal suture. Posteriorly, the squamous part fuses with the mastoid part. The anteroinferior border articulates with the greater wing of the sphenoid, and the superior border articulates with the inferior parietal bone at the squamosal suture.[4]

The zygomatic process extends anterolaterally from the squamous portion. It forms the zygomatic arch via an articulation between its obliquely posteroinferiorly sloping, deeply serrated anterior end, and the temporal process of the zygomatic bone.[3] Its inferior surface forms a short articular tubercle, which contacts the articular disc of the temporomandibular joint and forms the anterior limit of the mandibular fossa.[4]

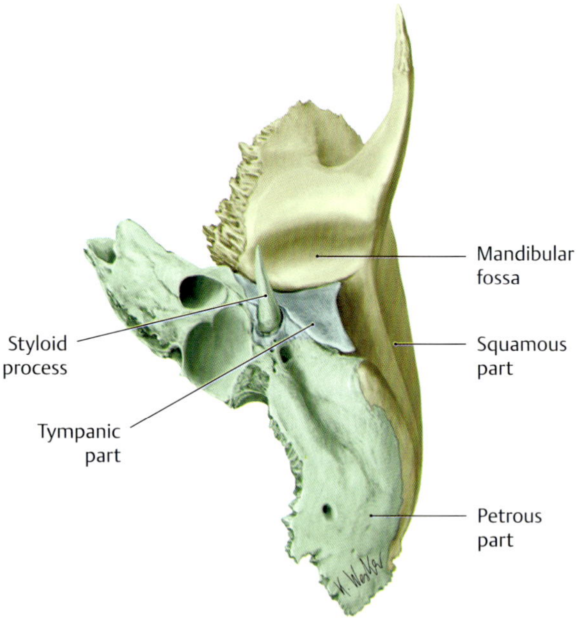

Fig. 1.5 Left temporal bone: inferior view. The squamous part, which bears the mandibular fossa; the petromastoid part, which contains the auditory and vestibular apparatus; and the tympanic part, which forms much of the external auditory canal, are best appreciated from this inferior view. (Reproduced from THIEME Atlas of Anatomy, Head and Neuroanatomy. © Thieme 2010, Illustration by Karl Wesker.)

The mandibular fossa presents an anterior articular area and a posterior nonarticular area, formed by the tympanic element. This smooth, concave articular surface, formed by the squamous part, contacts the mandibular condyle's temporomandibular joint articular disc. The squamotympanic fissure separates the posterior mandibular fossa from the tympanic part.[4]

Petromastoid Part

The petromastoid part is relatively large and better described as two parts. The trabecular mastoid part, which internally contains the mastoid air cells and mastoid antrum, constitutes the posterior region of the temporal bone. The posteriorly projecting mastoid process, which is larger in adult men, attaches the sternocleidomastoid, splenius capitis, and longissimus capitis to its lateral surface and the posterior belly of the digastric on its medial surface.[4]

The petrous part formed of compact bone inclines superiorly and anteromedialy from the cranial base.[4] It houses the auditory and vestibular apparatuses and separates the temporal and occipital lobes of the brain.[3] The mass of the petrous part is wedged between the sphenoid and occipital bones.[4] The petrous part's base, apex, three surfaces, and three borders are described in subsequent chapters.

The petrous potion extends anteriorly and medially, forming the foramen lacerum via sphenoid articulation. On the medial side lies the internal acoustic meatus and superior and inferior petrosal sinus grooves.[3]

The tympanic part is located below the squamous part and anterior to the mastoid process. Internally fused with the petrous part and posteriorly fused with the squamous part and mastoid process, the tympanic part forms a thin, incomplete ring.[4] The posterior surface forms the anterior wall, floor, and posterior wall of the external acoustic meatus. The anterior surface forms the posterior wall of the mandibular fossa.[3] The pointed, slender styloid process projects anteroinferiorly from the inferior surface of the temporal bone. Further explanation of temporal bone relationships is covered in subsequent chapters.

Viscerocranium

The viscerocranium consists of 15 irregular bones. These are the singular midline-centered mandible, ethmoid, and vomer, and the six bilateral pairs of bones, including the maxillae, inferior nasal conchae, and the zygomatic, palatine, nasal, and lacrimal bones.

Nasal Bone: Nasal Bridge and Bony Septum

The nasal bones, placed side by side between the frontal processes of the maxillae, jointly form the nasal bridge and internasal suture. Each small, oblong, and variable bone has external and internal surfaces and superior, inferior, lateral, and medial borders.[4] The transversely convex external surface is centrally perforated by a vein-traversing foramen. A longitudinal groove for the anterior ethmoidal nerve traverses the transversely concave internal surface (**Fig. 1.6**).[4]

The thick, serrated superior border articulates with the nasal part of the frontal bone, forming the frontonasal suture (**Fig. 1.7**).[4] The nasion is a craniometric point on the cranium where the frontonasal and internasal sutures meet. The medial border articulates with the contralateral nasal bone and pro-

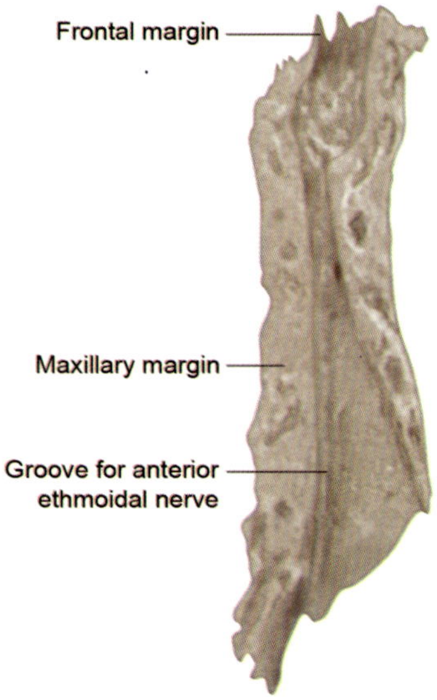

Fig. 1.6 Left nasal bone: internal view. The four articulating borders and the groove for the anterior ethmoidal nerve are appreciated from this view.

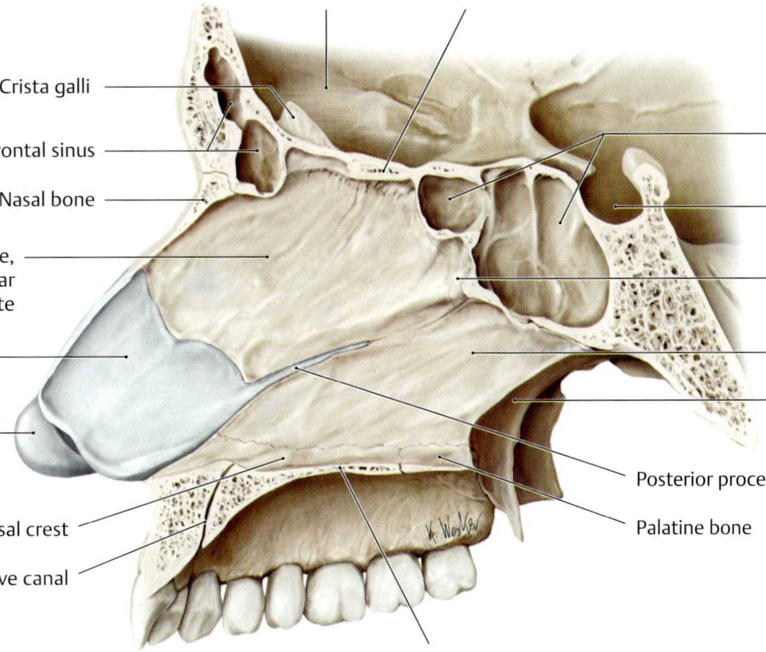

Fig. 1.7 Nasal septum. Parasagittal section viewed form the left side. The lateral wall of the left nasal cavity, including adjacent bones, has been removed. The contributions of the frontal, nasal, vomer, and ethmoid bones to the bony nasal septum can be appreciated from this view. (Reproduced from THIEME Atlas of Anatomy, Head and Neuroanatomy. © Thieme 2010, Illustration by Karl Wesker).

jects caudally as a vertical crest. This crest forms part of the bony nasal septum and further articulates with the nasal spine of the frontal bone dorsally, the perpendicular plate of the ethmoid bone, and the nasal septal cartilage.[4]

Surgical Annotation

Nasoethmoidal orbital fractures involve injury to numerous osseous structures in the upper midface. The frontal process of the maxilla is isolated from the abutting osseous structures. This fracture pattern allows for displacement of the medial canthal tendon, leading to traumatic telecanthus. This type of injury is commonly seen after direct impact to the upper nasal area. The fracture can present a surgical challenge to obtain adequate exposure of the numerous anatomical structures within this area. An existing laceration can be used to obtain access; however, a coronal incision, lower eyelid incision, and gingival buccal incision are needed to allow for access.[10] Re-establishment of the medial canthal tendon position is essential during this procedure and can be accomplished by direct plating or transnasal wiring, depending on the extent of comminution of the area.[11] Use of bone grafting is dependent on the need to re-establish the nasal height. Lacrimal system injury can occur given its close proximity and will require repair.

The notched inferior border is continuous with the upper lateral nasal cartilage at its cephalic margin. The lateral border articulates with the frontal process of the maxilla, forming the nasomaxillary suture lines.

The nasal part of the frontal bone lies between the supraorbital margins. A nasal notch inferiorly articulates with the nasal bones and laterally articulates with the frontal processes of the maxilla and the lacrimal bones.[4] This notch supports the nasal bridge via an anteroinferior projection from its posterior surface. This projection runs behind the nasal bones and the frontal processes of the maxillae, ending in a sharp nasal spine.[4] The nasal spine laterally forms part of the nasal cavity and makes a small contribution to the nasal septum via anterior articulations with the crest of the nasal bone and posterior articulations with the perpendicular plate of the ethmoid.[4]

The flat, median, and quadrilateral perpendicular plate of the ethmoid bone descends from the cribriform plate. This plate usually deviates slightly to form the upper part of the nasal septum. It articulates via its anterior border with the nasal spine of the frontal bone and the crests of the nasal bones.[4] Posteriorly, the plate articulates with the crest of the sphenoid body superiorly and the vomer inferiorly. The broad inferior border attaches to the nasal septal cartilage. The superior surface contains grooves and canals for medial cribriform plate foramina; all other surfaces are smooth.[4]

Vomer

The thin, medially situated vomer bone forms the posterior, inferior part of the nasal septum. Both surfaces of the vomer contain a prominent groove for the nasopalatine nerve and vessels that runs obliquely anteriorly and inferiorly (**Fig. 1.8**).[4]

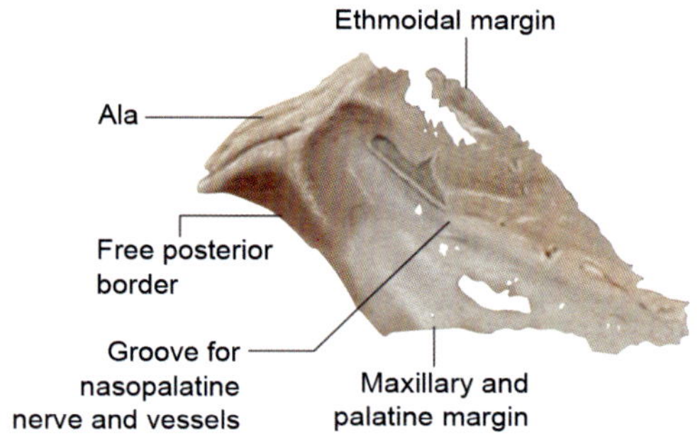

Fig. 1.8 Vomer: lateral border. The four articulating borders and the groove for the nasopalatine nerve and vessels are realized from this view.

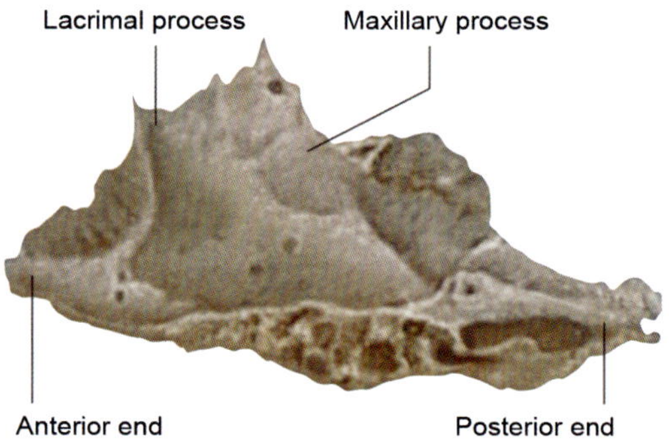

Fig. 1.9 Left inferior nasal concha: lateral view. Forming part of the inferior meatus, the superior border and its three processes and the free inferior border can be appreciated from this view.

The superior border is the thickest of the vomer's four borders. Presenting as a deep furrow, articulating with the rostrum of the body of the sphenoid, it is bound on either side by horizontally projecting alae.[4] The alae articulate with the sphenoidal conchae and with both the sphenoidal processes of the palatine bones and the vaginal processes of the medial pterygoid plates of the sphenoid rostrally and caudally, respectively.[4]

The rostral and inferiorly sloping anterior border fuses with the perpendicular plate of the ethmoid in its upper half. The lower half is grooved to articulate with the inferior margin of the nasal septal cartilage. The anterior extremity descends between the incisive canals, articulating with the posterior margin of the maxillary incisor crest.[4] Median nasal crests of the palatine and maxillae bones articulate with the inferior vomer border. The dorsally bifid, concave posterior border separates the nasal apertures and does not articulate with any other bones.[3]

Inferior Nasal Concha

Consisting of a lamina of cancellous bone, the curved inferior nasal concha forms part of the lateral wall of the nasal cavity. The perforated, convex medial surface includes longitudinal grooves for traversing vessels. The concave lateral surface forms part of the inferior meatus (**Fig. 1.9**).[4] The superior border, divided into three regions, articulates with the conchal crests of the maxilla anteriorly and the palatine posteriorly.[4]

The middle of these three regions comprises three articulating processes. As discussed herein, the rostral lacrimal process helps form the nasolacrimal canal via articulations with the lacrimal bone and maxilla. The ascending ethmoidal process joins the uncinate process of the ethmoid. Intermediately, the ventral and laterally curving maxillary process articulates with the medial maxilla at the opening of the maxillary sinus.[4] The anterior and posterior ends of the inferior nasal concha tapering and the inferior border are free, thick, and cellular.[3]

Maxilla

The maxilla jointly forms most of the upper jaw and face. Each bone forms the bulk of the floor and lateral wall of the nasal cavity and the orbital floor. It also contributes to the infratemporal and pterygopalatine fossae. The maxilla comprises a body and frontal, zygomatic, palatine, and alveolar processes.[3]

Body

Anterior Surface

Enclosing the maxillary sinus, the pyramidal body of the maxilla has anterior, infratemporal (posterior), orbital, and nasal surfaces (**Fig. 1.10a**).[4] The anterolaterally facing anterior surface contains inferior elevations and the alveolar processes dorsal to the roots of teeth. The canine eminence overlies the canine tooth socket and separates the shallow incisive fossa, posterior to the incisors, from the deeper, more lateral canine fossa. Dorsal to the canine fossa lies the infraorbital foramen, which transmits the infraorbital vessels and nerve.[4] The anterior median intermaxillary suture is formed between the two maxillae, the inferior border of the nasal aperture, and the central incisor teeth.

Posterior Surface

The concave posterior (infratemporal) surface forms the anterior wall of the infratemporal and pterygopalatine fossae.[4] Separating the posterior and anterior maxillary body surfaces are the ascending zygomaticoalveolar ridge (jugal crest) and the zygomatic process (**Fig. 1.10b**).[4] Posteroinferiorly located is the maxillary tuberosity, which articulates with the pyramidal process of the palatine bone.[4]

Orbital Surface

The orbital surface forms most of the orbital floor. Along its medial border, the orbital surface articulates with the lacrimal bone, the orbital plate of the ethmoid, and the orbital processes of the palatine bone. It also forms the infraorbital groove, part of the infraorbital canal, and the anterior edge of the inferior orbital fissure.[4]

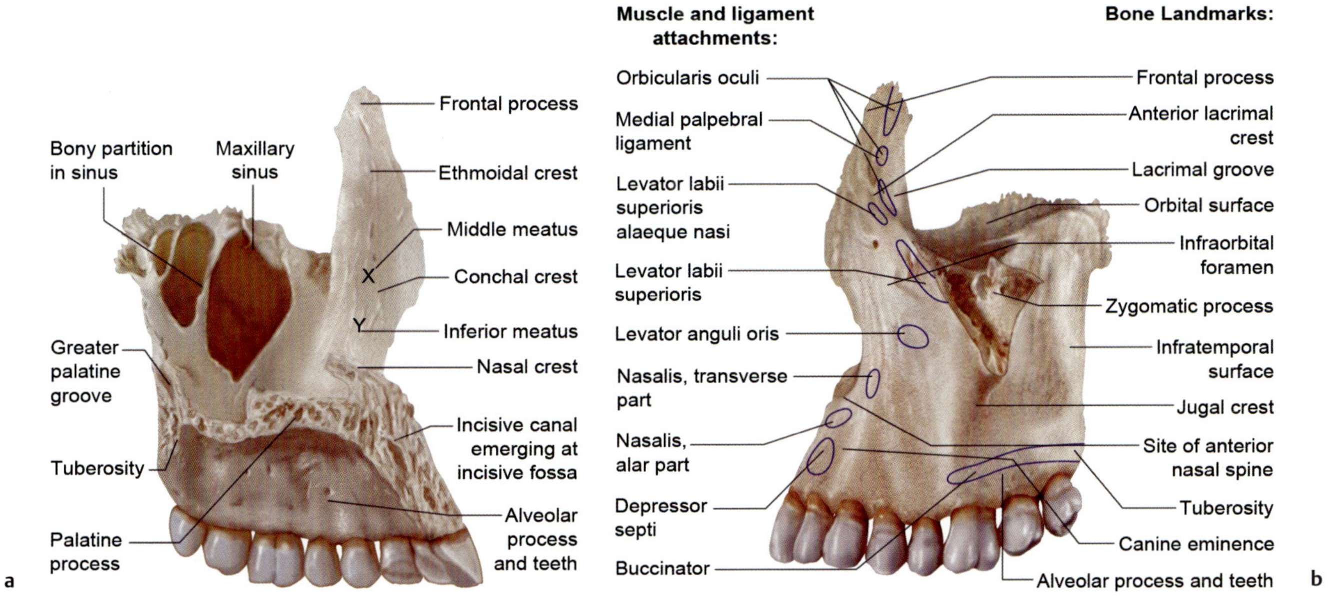

Fig. 1.10 **(a)** Medial view of the left maxilla. Much of the body; the palatine, frontal, and alveolar process; and the maxillary sinus can be realized from this view. Additionally, the emerging incisive canal, greater palatine groove, and the conchal and nasal crests can be appreciated via this medial view. **(b)** Lateral view of the left maxilla. The remainder of the body and its associated jugal crest and orbital and infratemporal surfaces are viewed best laterally. Additionally, the lateral frontal zygomatic process can be appreciated via this lateral view.

Nasal Surface

The large maxillary hiatus, which leads to the maxillary sinus, defines the posterosuperior nasal surface. The aerated sinus is partially closed by ethmoid and lacrimal bone articulations. Inferior to the sinus is part of the inferior meatus and posteriorly a roughened surface for articulation with the perpendicular plate of the palatine bone.[4] Anterior to the hiatus is the nasolacrimal groove, comprising about two-thirds of the circumference of the nasolacrimal canal; the remainder is contributed by the descending part of the lacrimal bone and the lacrimal process of the inferior nasal concha.[4] This canal leads the nasolacrimal duct to the inferior meatus. Anteriorly, the oblique conchal crest articulates with the inferior nasal concha, separating the inferior meatus from the more superior atrium of the middle meatus.[4]

Zygomatic Process

The anterior, infratemporal and orbital surfaces converge at the laterally projecting zygomatic process. This serrated process articulates with the maxillary process of the zygomatic bone. The thick, arched, and inferiorly projecting alveolar process supports the maxillary teeth. These socketed processes vary in depth, width, and septation according to the tooth type.[4]

Frontal Process

The posterosuperiorly projecting frontal process articulates superiorly with the nasal part of the frontal bone, anteriorly with the nasal bone, and posteriorly with the lacrimal bone.[4] The vertical lacrimal crest divides the frontal process; posterior to this crest, vertical grooves of the frontal process and the lacrimal bone combine to complete the lacrimal fossa.[4] The medial surface of the frontal process forms part of the lateral nasal wall. Subapical articulations with the ethmoid close the anterior ethmoidal air cells, and an oblique ethmoidal crest, which forms the superior border of the middle meatus, posteriorly articulates with the middle nasal concha.[4]

Palatine Process

Projecting from the most inferior part of the medial maxilla is the thick, horizontal palatine process. Together, the articulated contralateral palatine processes form most of the nasal floor and three-quarters of the osseous (hard) palate.[4] The horizontal plate of the palatine bone forms the remainder, subsequently forming the transverse palatomaxillary suture. Posterolaterally, two grooves in the palatine process transmit the greater palatine vessels and nerves. These two lateral incisive canals, each ascending into its half of the nasal cavity, open into the infundibular incisive fossa and transmit the terminations of the greater palatine artery and nasopalatine nerve.[4]

Occasionally, the median anterior and posterior incisive foramina are present.[4] The median intermaxillary palatal suture runs posterior to the infundibular incisive fossa.

The thicker anteromedial border articulates with the contralateral palatine process, forming a raised nasal crest that creates a groove for the vomer. Anteriorly, this ridge rises as an incisor crest, which articulates contralaterally with the paired process, forming the anterior nasal spine.[4]

Maxillary Sinus

The pyramidal maxillary sinus, located in the body of the maxilla, is the largest of the paranasal sinuses (**Fig. 1.11**). The medial

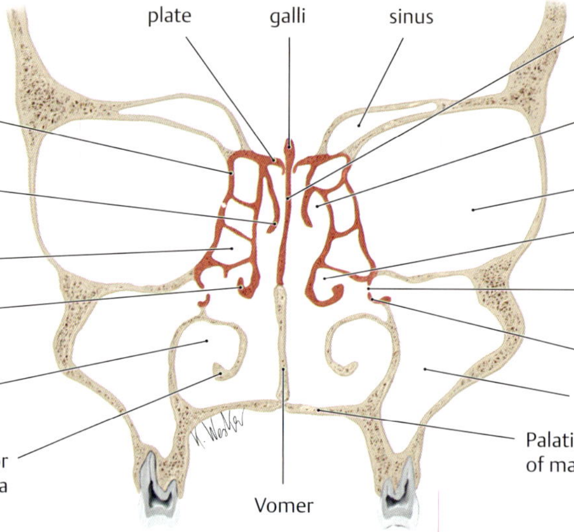

Fig. 1.11 Bony structure of the paranasal sinuses: anterior view. This coronal section elucidates the relationship of the paranasal sinuses with their associated structures to the viscerocranium. (Reproduced from THIEME Atlas of Anatomy, Head and Neuroanatomy. © Thieme 2010, Illustration by Karl Wesker.)

wall forms part of the lateral wall of the nose, and the roof forms the largest portion of the orbital floor. The maxilla forms the floor, anterior wall, and posterior wall of the sinus via its alveolar process and part of the palatine process, the facial surface, and infratemporal surface respectively. The apex of the sinus extends into the zygomatic process of the maxilla.[4]

High on the posterior medial wall of the maxillary sinus is the ostium of the sinus. Portions of the perpendicular plate of the palatine bone, the uncinate process of the ethmoid bone, the inferior nasal concha, the lacrimal bone, and overlying nasal mucosa limit the size of the ostium.[4] The ostium usually opens into the posterior part of the ethmoidal infundibulum, which communicates with the middle meatus, although an accessory ostium is sometimes present posterior to the major ostium.[4]

Palatine Bone

The paired palatine bones each comprise a horizontal and perpendicular plate, arranged as L-shaped pyramidal, orbital, and sphenoidal processes (**Fig. 1.12**).[3] The palatine bones contribute to the floors of the palate, orbit, and nasal cavity; to the lateral wall of the nasal cavity; to the pterygopalatine and pterygoid fossae; and to the inferior orbital fissures. These bones are placed in the posterior nasal cavity between the maxillae and pterygoid processes of the sphenoid bone.[3]

Horizontal Plate

The quadrilateral horizontal plate has nasal and palatine surfaces and anterior, posterior, lateral, and medial borders. The nasal surface transversely forms the posterior nasal floor. The palatine surface forms the posterior quarter of the bony palate via midline articulations with its pair at the medial border and with the palatine process of the maxilla at its anterior border.[4] The midline articulating horizontal plates form the posterior part of the nasal crest, which articulates with the posteroinferior edge of the vomer. The posterior border projects posteriorly as the posterior nasal spine. The lateral border, continuous with the perpendicular plate of the palatine bone, contains the greater palatine foramen.[3]

Perpendicular Plate

The perpendicular plate has nasal and maxillary surfaces and anterior, posterior, superior, and inferior borders.[4] The nasal surface of the perpendicular plate inferiorly contributes to the inferior meatus. Superiorly, a horizontal conchal crest articulates with the inferior concha. Moving superiorly are a depres-

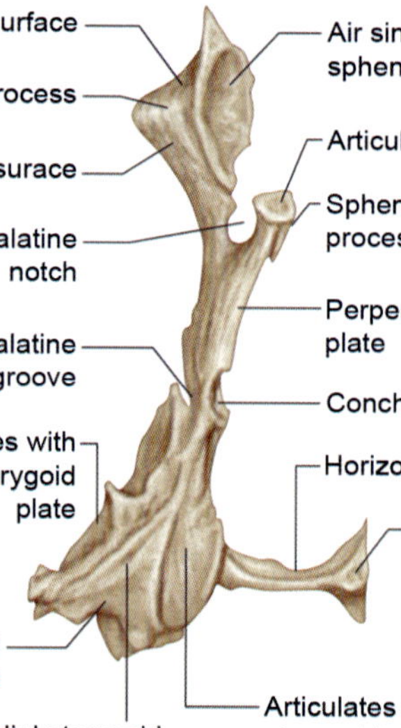

Fig. 1.12 Posterior view of the left palatine bone. The palatine bone, which comprises the horizontal and perpendicular plates, pyramidal, orbital, and sphenoidal processes and some of their articulating surfaces, can be understood from this posterior view.

sion that forms part of the middle meatus, an ethmoidal crest for the middle nasal concha, and a horizontal groove that forms part of the superior meatus.[4]

The maxillary surface articulates with the nasal surface of the maxilla. Posterosuperiorly, it forms a medial wall to the pterygopalatine fossa and anteriorly forms part of the medial wall of the maxillary sinus. The palatine groove (i.e., canal on maxillary articulation) descends posteriorly on the maxillary surface and transmits the greater palatine vessel and nerve.[4]

The anterior border articulates with the maxillary process of the inferior concha, appearing in the medial wall of the maxillary sinus. The posterior border articulates with the medial pterygoid plate. The sphenopalatine foramen is formed by the sphenopalatine notch on the superior border articulating with the body of the sphenoid. This foramen provides connections from the pterygopalatine fossa to the posterior part of the superior meatus.[4]

Pyramidal Process

The pyramidal process extends posterolaterally from the horizontal and perpendicular palatine plate junction to an angle between the pterygoid plates of the sphenoid bone.[3] The posterior surface completes the lower part of the pterygoid fossa, and the anterior lateral surface articulates with the maxillary tuberosity.[4] The inferior surface contains the lesser palatine foramina.[3]

Orbital Process

The orbital process, extending superolaterally from the anterior perpendicular plate, has three articulating and two nonarticulating surfaces. The anterior (maxillary) surface articulates anterolaterally with the maxilla. The posterior (sphenoidal) surface bears the opening of an air sinus that usually communicates with the sphenoid sinus, which is closed by the sphenoidal concha.[4] The medial (ethmoidal) surface articulates with the labyrinth of the ethmoid bone, on which the sinus of the orbital process can form, thus communicating with the posterior ethmoidal air cells. Rarely, the sinus of the orbital process can open on both the ethmoidal and sphenoidal surfaces. Separating the nonarticulating superior (orbital) and lateral surfaces is a rounded border that forms a medial part of the lower margin of the inferior orbital fissure.[4]

Sphenoidal Process

The superior surface of the superomedially projecting sphenoidal process articulates with the sphenoidal concha and contributes to the palatovaginal canal formation. The superior and lateral surfaces and the posterior border of the sphenoidal process articulate with the root of, the medial surface of, and the vaginal process of the medial pterygoid plate, respectively.[4] The medial border of the sphenoidal process articulates with the ala of the vomer, and the inferomedial surface forms part of the roof and lateral wall of the nose.[4]

Zygomatic Bone

The quadrangular zygomatic (zygoma) bones form the prominences of the cheeks and rests on the maxillae. The zygoma forms the anterolateral rims, walls, floor, much of the infraorbital margins of the orbits, and the walls of the temporal and infratemporal fossae.[3] It includes lateral, temporal, and orbital surfaces; two processes, the frontal and temporal; three foramina; and five borders (**Fig. 1.13**).[4]

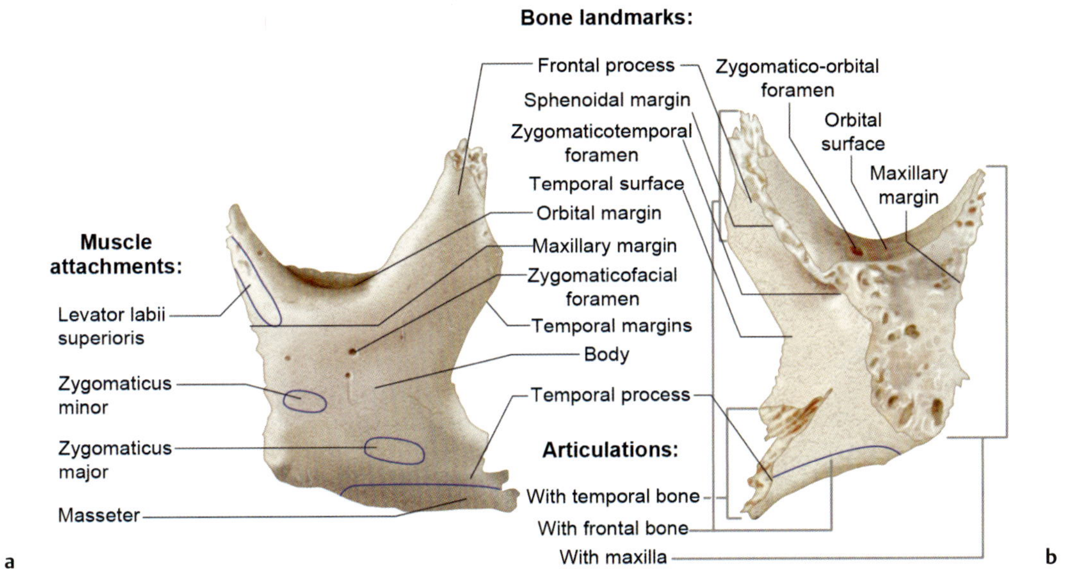

Fig. 1.13 (a) External view of the left zygomatic bone. The facial surface of the zygomatic body displays the zygomaticofacial foramen near the orbital surface. The frontal and temporal processes, as well as the orbital, temporal, and maxillary margins, are visible from this anterior view. **(b)** Internal view of left zygomatic bone. The internal view provides a better appreciation for the serrated maxillary and sphenoidal margins and those surfaces that articulate with the frontal bone, temporal bone, and maxilla. The zygomatico-orbital foramen on the orbital surface is also viewed from this angle.

Surfaces

The convex lateral (facial) surface contains the centrally located zyomaticofacial foramen, allowing passage of the zygomaticofacial nerve and vessels. This foramen is often double and occasionally absent. The zygomaticus minor and major originate inferior to the foramen anteriorly and posteriorly, respectively.[4]

The posteromedial (temporal) surface articulates medially with the zygomatic process of the maxilla. This smooth, concave surface transmits the zygomaticotemporal nerve via the zygomaticotemporal foramen near the base of the frontal process.[4]

The orbital surface extends up on the medial aspect of the frontal process and forms the anterolateral part of the orbital floor and adjoining lateral wall. This smooth, concave surface usually contains the zygomatico-orbital foramina representing canal openings leading to the zygomaticofacial and zygomaticotemporal foramina.[4]

Borders

The anteroinferior (maxillary) border articulates with the maxilla. Its medial end tapers to a point that provides partial attachment for the levator labii superioris muscle. The sinuous posterosuperior (temporal) border is continuous with the posterior border of the frontal process and, thus, the upper border of the zygomatic arch.[4] The temporal fascia attaches to this border. The serrated posteromedial border articulates superiorly with the greater wing of the sphenoid and inferiorly with the orbital surface of the maxilla. This surface usually forms the lateral edge of the inferior orbital fissure by the presence of a non-articulating concave indent.[4] A posteroinferior border, roughened for masseter attachment and the anterosuperior (orbital) border, forms the inferolateral circumference of the orbital opening.[4]

Processes

The thick, serrated frontal process articulates with the zygomatic process of the frontal bone superiorly and with the greater wing of the sphenoid bone posteriorly.[4] Varying in size and form, Whitnall's tubercle is usually present on the orbital aspect, 1 cm below the frontozygomatic suture.[4] The zygomatic arch is formed by articulations between the long, narrow, and serrated temporal process of the zygoma and the zygomatic process of the temporal bone.[3]

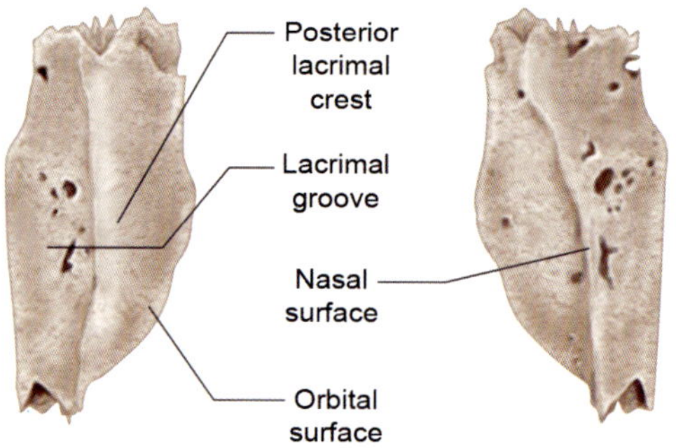

Fig. 1.14 External view of the right lacrimal bone. This view elucidates the orbital surface of the lacrimal bone with its associated lacrimal groove, which lies anterior to the posterior lacrimal crest.

Lacrimal Bone

The paired small, thin, fragile lacrimal bones contribute to the anterior medial wall of the orbit.[3] A vertical posterior lacrimal crest divides the lateral (orbital) surface of the lacrimal bone (**Fig. 1.14**). Rostral to this crest, the rostral edge of a vertical groove meets the posterior border of the frontal process of the maxilla, completing the fossa for the lacrimal sac. The medial wall of this groove joins the nasolacrimal groove of the nasal maxilla and the lacrimal process of the inferior nasal concha, contributing to the formation of the nasolacrimal canal. The upper opening of the nasolacrimal canal is completed by the maxilla and the lacrimal hamulus, caudal and ventral to the posterior lacrimal crest.[4]

The medial (nasal) surface forms part of the middle meatus via its anteroinferior region. The posterosuperior part of the medial surface meets the ethmoid, completing some anterior ethmoidal air cells. The lacrimal bones contain anterior, posterior, superior, and inferior borders. They articulate with the frontal process of the maxilla, the orbital plate of the ethmoid, the frontal bone, and the orbital surface of the maxilla, respectively.[4]

References

1. Moore KL, Dalley AF, Agur AMR. Clinically Oriented Anatomy. 6th ed. Baltimore, MD, and Philadelphia, PA: Lippincott Williams & Wilkins; 2010
2. Sadler TW. Langman's Medical Embrology. 12th ed. New York, NY: Lippincott Williams & Wilkins; 2012
3. Norton NS. Netter's Head and Neck Anatomy for Dentistry. 1st ed. Philadelphia, PA: Elsevier Saunders; 2006
4. Standring S, Gray HFRS. Gray's Anatomy: The Anatomical Basis of Clinical Practice. 39th ed. Philadelphia, PA: Elsevier Churchill Livingstone; 2005
5. Fallucco M, Janis JE, Hagan RR. The anatomical morphology of the supraorbital notch: clinical relevance to the surgical treatment of migraine headaches. Plast Reconstr Surg 2012;130(6):1227–1233
6. Chepla KJ, Oh E, Guyuron B. Clinical outcomes following supraorbital foraminotomy for treatment of frontal migraine headache. Plast Reconstr Surg 2012;129(4):656e–662e
7. Kung TA, Guyuron B, Cederna PS. Migraine surgery: a plastic surgery solution for refractory migraine headache. Plast Reconstr Surg 2011;127(1):181–189
8. Tiwari P, Higuera S, Thornton J, Hollier LH. The management of frontal sinus fractures. J Oral Maxillofac Surg 2005;63(9):1354–1360
9. Bell RB, Dierks EJ, Brar P, Potter JK, Potter BE. A protocol for the management of frontal sinus fractures emphasizing sinus preservation. J Oral Maxillofac Surg 2007;65(5):825–839
10. Pawar SS, Rhee JS. Frontal sinus and naso-orbital-ethmoid fractures. JAMA Facial Plast Surg 2014;16(4):284–289
11. Kochhar A, Byrne PJ. Surgical management of complex midfacial fractures. Otolaryngol Clin North Am 2013;46(5):759–778

2 Anterior Skull Base

Surjith Vattoth and Philip R. Chapman

Introduction

The skull base is traditionally divided into anterior, central, and posterior zones based principally on the appearance of the skull base as viewed from above (**Fig. 2.1**). This approach supports the general delineation of the intracranial compartment into the anterior, middle, and posterior fossae. The anterior skull base forms the broad floor of the anterior cranial fossa, which is filled predominantly with the frontal lobes of the brain. The anterior skull base is traditionally defined as the region of the skull base lying anterior to the lesser wing of sphenoid and planum sphenoidale (**Fig. 2.2**). The lesser wing of the sphenoid spans anterolaterally from the anterior clinoid process. The posterior and superior margins of the lesser wing form a curvilinear ridge that takes on the shape of a wing—hence its name. The lesser wing of the sphenoid bone fuses anteriorly with the posterior margin of the orbital plate of the frontal bone. The planum sphenoidale is the superomedial plate of sphenoid bone seen posterior to the cribriform plate of ethmoid and anterior to the anterior wall of sella turcica (tuberculum sellae). Medially, the anterior skull base forms the roof of the nasal cavity and ethmoid sinus, including the cribriform plate of the ethmoid. Laterally, the orbital plates of the frontal bones form the orbital roof portion of the anterior skull base on either side. Posteriorly, the midline or parasagittal anterior skull base is constituted by the planum sphenoidale and laterally by the lesser wing of the sphenoid bone.[1] The middle or central skull base is separated from the anterior skull base by a horizontal line along the anterior sellar margin extending laterally along the posterior margin of lesser wing of the sphenoid bone bilaterally, which includes the medial anterior clinoid processes.[2]

Midline or Parasagittal Anterior Skull Base Forming the Roof of the Nasal Cavity and Ethmoid Sinuses

The anterior skull base, especially in the region of the nasal vault and ethmoid roof, is only minimally ossified at birth and ossifies gradually from cartilage. The roof of the nasal cavity begins to ossify by around the age of 3 months and is predominantly ossified at 6 months. The crista galli, a midline triangle-shaped, superiorly projecting bony process of the ethmoid bone, begins to ossify from the tip at 3 months and is usually ossified by the first year. The name is derived from the Latin and means crest of the cock (rooster's comb). The crista galli provides attachment to the anteroinferior part of the falx cerebri and should not be confused with the frontal crest, a more anterior midline bony ridge–like portion of the frontal bones, which also provides attachment to the falx cerebri (**Fig. 2.3**). The crista galli is pneumatized in 10 to 15% of patients as identified on computed tomography (CT) scans. Although the crista galli is technically part of the ethmoid bone, pneumatization generally occurs as an extension of the left or right frontal sinus.[3] The perpendicular plate of the ethmoid, which forms the superior portion of the bony nasal septum and is seen directly below the crista galli, begins to ossify at 6 months and fuses with the vomer, which forms the inferior portion of the bony nasal septum by around 2 years of age.[1]

The cribriform plate (lamina cribrosa) of the ethmoid in the adult is a horizontal perforated bony plate at the medial aspect of ethmoid bone, with deep grooves lying on either side of the midline crista galli. It forms part of the roof of the nasal cavity and constitutes the floor of the olfactory fossa lodging the olfactory bulbs (**Fig. 2.4**). The olfactory fossa is the lowest point in the anterior skull base. The perforations and foramina in the middle of the grooves are small and transmit the afferent olfactory nerve fibers from the nasal vault mucosa to the olfactory bulbs intracranially. The larger foramina at the medial aspect of the grooves transmit nerves to the superior nasal septum and those at the lateral aspect to the superior turbinate region. More than two-thirds of the population will have ossified posterior cribriform plates by 1 year of age, and most of the anterior skull base, including the cribriform plates, are ossified after 2 years; however, small gaps can be seen in the nasal roof until early in year 3 of life.

The ethmoid roof is formed by the vertically oriented lateral lamella of the cribriform plate of the ethmoid bone medially and the more horizontal fovea ethmoidalis of the orbital plate of frontal bone superolaterally. The vertical lateral lamella lies just lateral to the horizontal cribriform plate proper. The lateral lamella is 10 times thinner than the fovea ethmoidalis.[4] The skull-base attachment of the middle turbinate of the nasal cavity to the anterior cribriform plate is quite delicate, and its detachment at surgery can damage the dura mater with resultant cerebrospinal fluid leak.

Ethmoid air cells lie inferior to the plane of cribriform plate until 3 months of age. By 6 months, they extend above the horizontal cribriform plate plane, and the more superolateral fovea ethmoidalis portion of ethmoid sinus roof begins to develop from the orbital plate of the frontal bone by 18 months and matures by 2 years of age. Knowledge of this lateral-to-medial slope of the anterior skull base is extremely important during transethmoidal surgical approaches to anterior skull-base lesions. Using the same axial plane of surgical dissection, which is safe along the more lateral ethmoid roof, could injure the brain and dura mater if extended medially to the region of cribriform plate.[5]

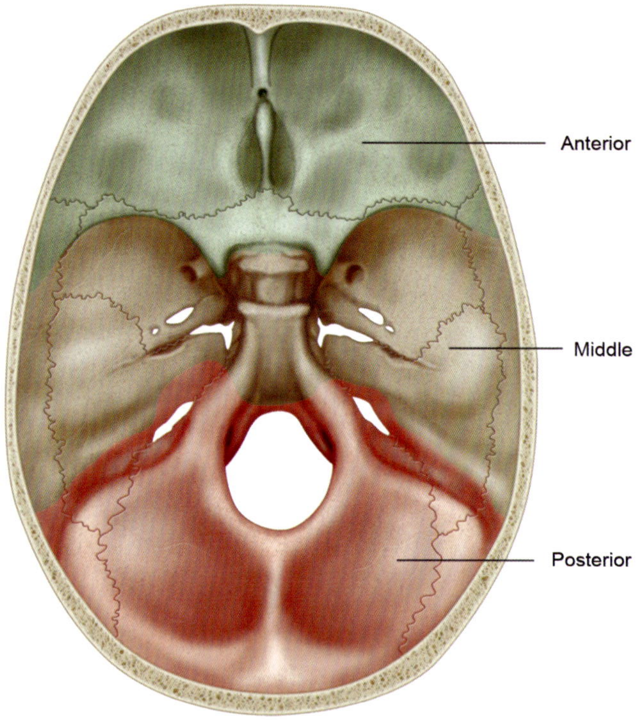

Fig. 2.1 View of the skull base from above. Traditionally, the skull base is divided into anterior, middle, and posterior components.

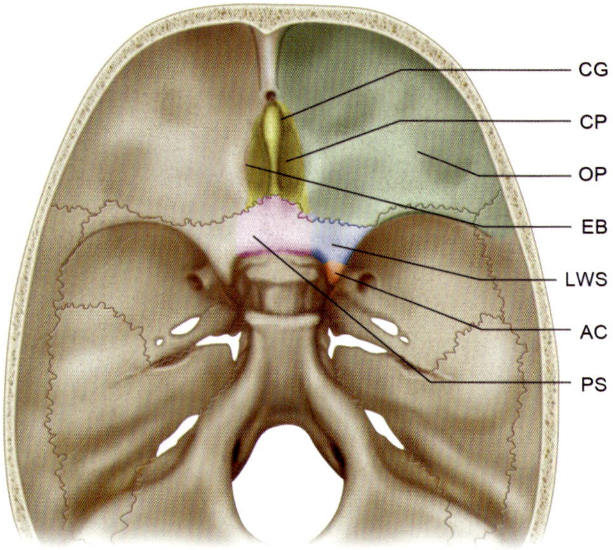

Fig. 2.2 Magnified view of the anterior skull base. The anterior clinoid process (AC) merges anteriorly with the lesser wing of the sphenoid bone (LWS). Medially, the lesser wing of the sphenoid merges with a flat portion of the sphenoid bone that serves as the ventral roof to the sphenoid sinus, the planum sphenoidale (PS). The lesser wing of the sphenoid is joined anteriorly with the orbital plate (OP) of the frontal bone. The orbital plate of the sphenoid bone serves as the roof of the orbit. The ethmoid bone (EB) is in the center of the anterior skull base and contains the cribriform plate (CP) and the crista galli (CG).

A horizontal line drawn along the roof of the ethmoid sinus passes through the orbit superior to the orbital vertical midpoint in most cases (88%), with 10% crossing at the midpoint and only 2% below that plane.[6] Preoperative imaging should be critically reviewed to assess for a low-lying skull base. The safest anatomy is when the horizontal line drawn from the roof of the ethmoid crosses the upper third of the orbit; precautions to avoid injury to the skull base should be taken when the horizontal plane of the ethmoid roof crosses below the vertical midpoint of the orbit.[1]

The skull base also slopes downward in an anterior to posterior direction in the sagittal plane from the frontal recess to the planum sphenoidale along the ethmoid roof. The degree of slope is highly variable and should be assessed by preoperative imaging. During endoscopic sinus surgery, the skull base could be injured while using a front-to-back technique. Skull-base injury can be avoided by early identification using the back-to-front technique of endoscopic surgery whereby the skull base is easily located at the roof of sphenoid sinus after identifying the superior meatus and sphenoid ostium.[7–11]

The Keros classification of the ethmoid roof and olfactory fossa into three types takes into account the vertical height of the lateral lamella of the ethmoid and the resultant depth of the olfactory fossa (**Fig. 2.5**). An olfactory fossa that is only 1 to 3 mm deep because of a nearly nonexistent lateral lamella constitutes a Keros type 1 (12%). The olfactory fossa is 4 to 7 mm deep in Keros type 2 (70%) and 8 to 16 mm deep in type 3 (18%) with progressively increasing vertical height of the lateral lamella.[12] Asymmetry of more than 2 mm is seen in 8% of cases.[13] During endoscopic surgery, Keros type 3 has the largest risk for iatrogenic injury to the lateral lamella. Also, the anterior ethmoidal artery could be iatrogenically injured in the anterior ethmoidal foramen (along with the anterior ethmoidal vein and nerve) (**Fig. 2.6**) lying between the ethmoid and frontal bones just anterolateral to the cribriform plate and cause catastrophic bleeding into the orbit. The posterior ethmoidal foramen containing the posterior ethmoidal artery, vein, and nerve lies between the ethmoid and sphenoid bones, just posterolateral to the cribriform plate of the ethmoid.

More Anterior Portions of Midline/Parasagittal Anterior Skull Base

The foramen cecum is a small midline pit lying between the frontal and ethmoid bones, just anterior to the crista galli of the ethmoid (**Fig. 2.7**). It is close to 4 mm in diameter at birth, and the ossification is usually complete by 2 years but can sometimes be delayed until the age of 5 years.[14] Ossification defects in the region of the foramen cecum, nose, and forehead can lead to the formation of three subtypes of frontoethmoidal (sincipital) cephaloceles: frontonasal (40–60%), nasoethmoidal (30%), and nasoorbital (10%) cephaloceles. Associated ocular or intracranial abnormalities are present in 80% of cases with frontoethmoidal cephaloceles.[15]

During early intrauterine life, a small anterior skull base fontanel at the anterior boundary of the anterior skull base, called

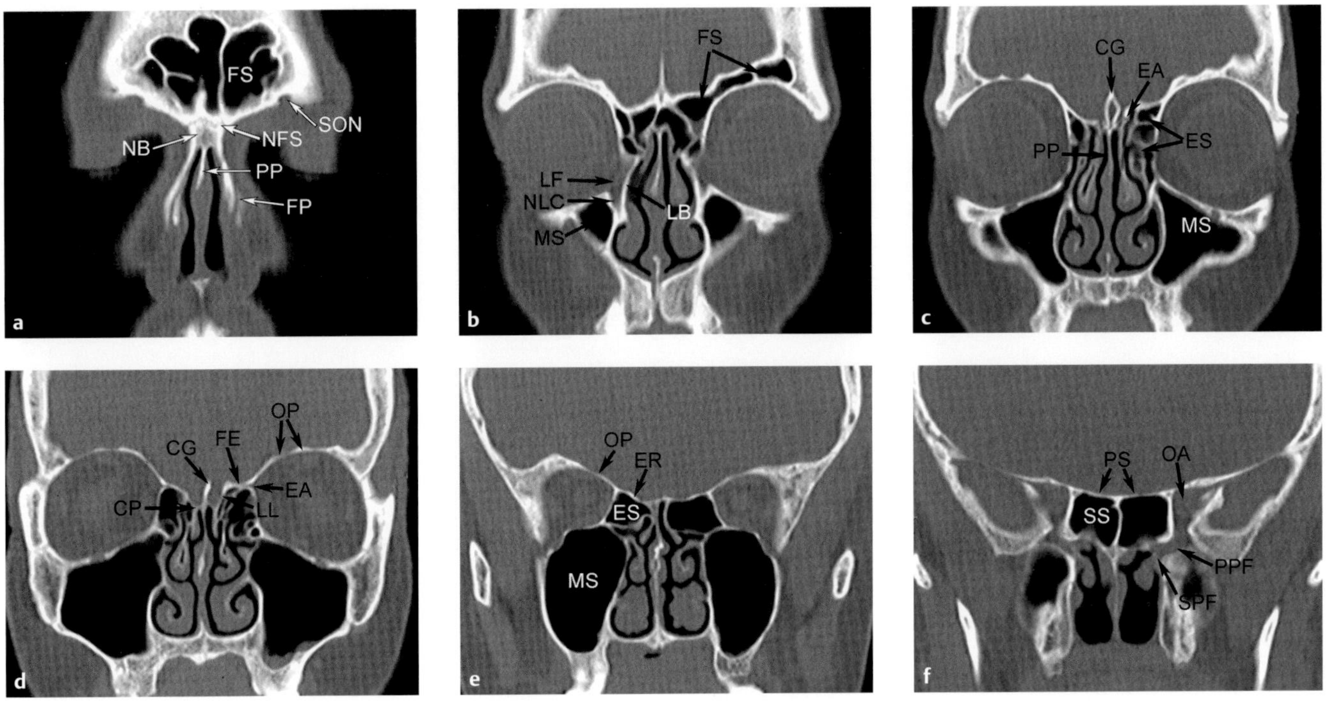

Fig. 2.3 Serial high-resolution computerized tomography (CT) coronal images through the anterior skull base, anterior to posterior. **(a)** Pneumatized frontal sinus (FS) air cells are seen bilaterally. The supraorbital notch (SON) marks the exit of the supraorbital nerve and associated vessels from the orbit to the forehead. The paired nasal bones (NBs) merge anteriorly at the nasal bridge and fuse superiorly at the nasofrontal suture (NFS). The perpendicular plate (PP) of the ethmoid bone forms the bony nasal septum superiorly. The inferior and lateral bony support of the nose is provided by the frontal process (FP) of the maxilla. **(b)** Frontal sinus (FS) air cells extend posteriorly above the orbital roof. There is a depression, the lacrimal fossa (LF), in the inferior and medial orbit that houses the lacrimal sac. The medial wall of the lacrimal fossa is formed by the lacrimal bone (LB).The lacrimal fossa is contiguous with the bony nasolacrimal canal (NLC). **(c)** More posteriorly, the crista galli (CG) is seen as a thin bony protrusion in the sagittal plane. The perpendicular plate (PP) of the ethmoid bone forms the bony nasal septum superiorly. The ethmoid sinus (ES) and maxillary sinus (MS) are seen at this level. A small foramen can be seen at this level as the anterior ethmoid artery (EA) pierces the lateral lamella of the cribriform plate. **(d)** At this level, the anatomy of the cribriform plate and ethmoid roof are well demonstrated. The crista galli (CG) again seen as midline sagittal bone projecting above the cribriform plate (CP). The lateral margin of the cribriform plate is formed by a vertical portion of bone called the lateral lamella (LL) of the cribriform plate. The lateral roof of the ethmoid sinus is formed by a horizontal projection of bone that arises from the medial orbit, called the fovea ethmoidalis (FE). At this level, the proximal anterior ethmoid artery (EA) can be seen leaving the orbit as it extends anteromedially toward the cribriform plate. **(e)** More posteriorly, the cribriform plate and ethmoid roof (ER) flatten. The orbital plate of frontal bone separates the orbit from the frontal fossa. The posterior ethmoid (ES) and maxillary sinuses (MS) are shown. **(f)** More posteriorly, through the orbital apex (OA), the sphenoid sinus (SS) air cells are seen, along with the flat midline bony roof, the planum sphenoidale (PS). At this level, a portion of the pterygopalatine fossa (PPF), as well as the sphenopalatine foramen (SPF), can be seen.

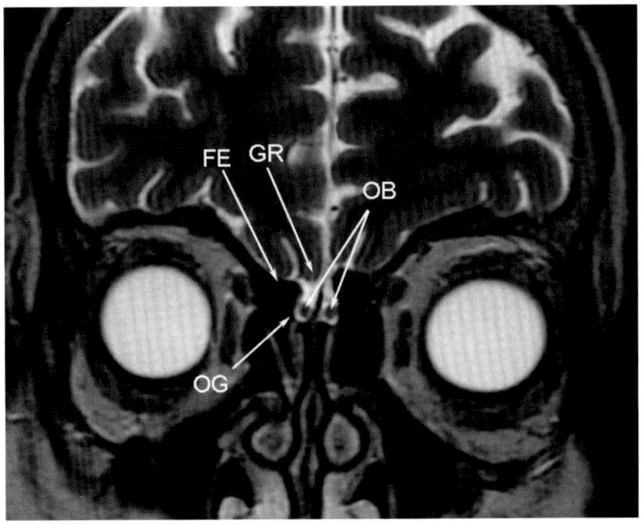

Fig. 2.4 Coronal T2-weighted magnetic resonance imaging through the orbits demonstrates the relationship of the frontal lobes, olfactory bulbs, and olfactory grooves. The olfactory bulbs (OBs) lie inferior to the gyrus rectii (GR) of the frontal lobes. The olfactory grooves (OGs) vary in depth in relationship to the ethmoid roof. The lateral aspect of the ethmoid roof is the fovea ethmoidalis (FE).

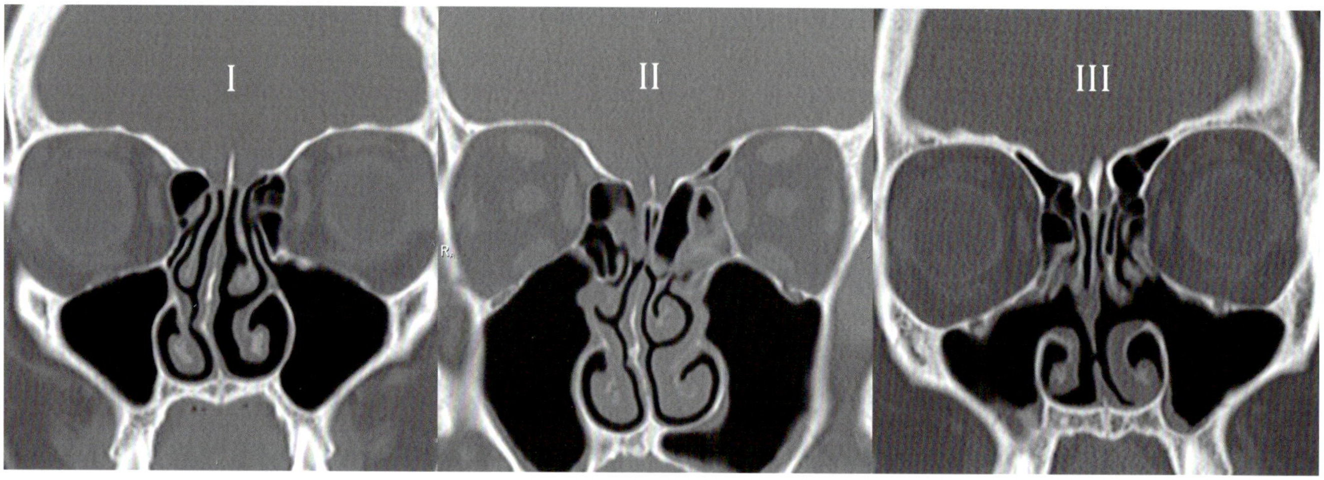

Fig. 2.5 Coronal computed tomography images in three different patients depicts the variable depth of the olfactory fossa, corresponding to the Keros classification, I–III. The image on the left shows a depth of 3 mm (I). The middle image demonstrates a depth of 5 mm (II); the image on the right shows a depth of 8 mm (III).

the fonticulus frontalis, lies between the superior partially ossified frontal bone and inferior nasal bones. At this time, there is also a small space filled with dura just posterior to the developing nasal bones and anterior to the cartilage of the developing nasal capsule, called the prenasal space. When the chondrocranium begins to ossify, the fonticulus frontalis closes, and failure of its closure leads to development of a frontonasal cephalocele. In this condition, a small portion of meninges with (meningoencephalocele) or without (meningocele) brain herniates into the forehead at the region of the glabella or dorsum of the nose through a patent fonticulus frontalis, between the frontal bone superiorly and the nasal bones inferiorly.[16]

As a result of ossification of the chondrocranium of the anterior skull base from posterior to anterior, leaving a small portion of cartilage anteriorly for the nasal capsule and further ossification of nasal bones, the prenasal space lying between these becomes encased in bone and obliterates, leaving a small dural diverticulum called the foramen cecum just anterior to the site of the future crista galli. The foramen cecum can connect anteroinferiorly to the skin of the nasal region transiently through a dura-lined stalk called the anterior neuropore, which later regresses. Defects in regression lead to a nasoethmoidal cephalocele through a midline foramen cecum defect into the prenasal space and nasal cavity. Mass effect by the cephalocele may bow the nasal bones anteriorly. The crista galli lies posterior to the anterior skull base foramen cecum defect and may be bifid or even absent, and an associated cribriform plate defect or absence may be seen.[17] The least common subtype of an frontoethmoidal or sincipital cephalocele, called a naso-orbital cephalocele, develops as a result of defects in the lacrimal bones or frontal process of the maxilla with meninges and brain herniating inferomedially into the orbit.

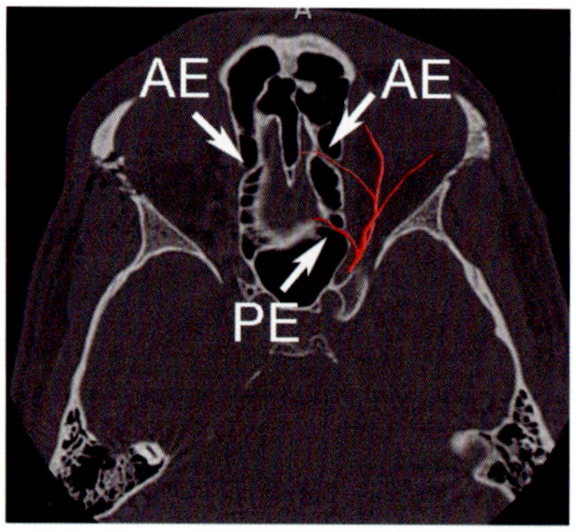

Fig. 2.6 Axial image through the level of the olfactory recess in patient with acute right orbital fracture. The anterior ethmoidal (AE) artery canals are demonstrated bilaterally. Superimposed illustration of the left ophthalmic artery branches also demonstrates the posterior ethmoid artery (PE) travelling more posteriorly.

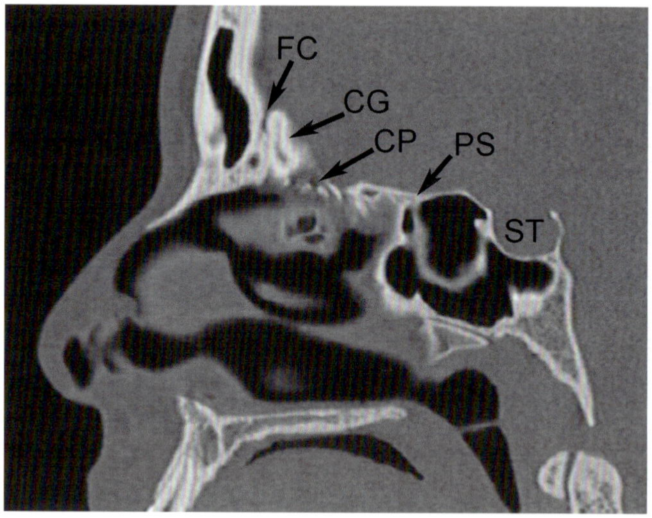

Fig. 2.7 Midline sagittal reformation of CT scan through the sinuses demonstrates midline structures from front to back. The residual foramen cecum (FC) is identified anterior to the crista galli (CG). The perforations along the cribriform plate (CP) can be seen. The planum sphenoidale (PS) is the flat, ventral roof of the sphenoid sinus, anterior to the sella turcica (ST).

Nasal dermal sinus with associated dermoid or epidermoid and nasal cerebral heterotopia (so-called nasal glioma), also present as congenital midline nasal masses, share common embryologic patterns and form the major differential diagnoses for frontoethmoidal cephaloceles. Nasal dermal sinus is lined by epithelial dermis, variably extends intracranially, and may be seen as a small nasal dimple. It does not contain brain or meninges but can be confused with a frontoethmoidal cephalocele when associated with a dermoid or epidermoid cyst somewhere along the tract. Nasal glioma (a misnomer because it contains nonneoplastic tissue) comprises of heterotopic dysplastic glial tissue without any demonstrable intracranial connection. Approximately two-thirds are extranasal and are located along the dorsum of the nose; the rest are under the nasal bones in an intranasal location.[18]

Anatomical Relationships of the Remainder of the Paranasal Sinuses with the Anterior Skull Base

The anatomy of the paranasal sinuses is given in detail in Chapter 17. Only the relevant anatomy of those portions of the paranasal sinuses associated with anterior skull base is discussed in this chapter.

The frontal sinuses are divided by a central septum into two parts, and multiple septa may be seen. The frontal recess, which is the drainage pathway of the frontal sinus, drains into the middle meatus of the nose, where the anterior ethmoid and maxillary sinuses also drain (**Fig. 2.8**). The uncinate process, which is attached inferiorly to the inferior turbinate of the nasal cavity, forms the upper medial wall of maxillary sinus. It also forms the boundary of the ethmoid infundibulum, which is the common drainage pathway of maxillary and anterior ethmoid sinuses into the middle meatus. It may be attached superiorly, orienting laterally to the lamina papyracea (lateral ethmoid wall or medial orbital wall) or orienting medially to the nasal middle turbinate or anterior skull base. If the uncinate process attaches to the middle turbinate of nasal cavity or anterior skull base orienting medially, the frontal recess opens into the ethmoid infundibulum. The clinical importance of this anatomical relationship is that infection in the ethmoid infundibulum can affect the frontal sinus, resulting in combined involvement of the frontal anterior ethmoid and maxillary sinuses. On the other hand, if the uncinate process orients laterally and inserts into the lamina papyracea, the frontal recess has an isolated direct drainage into the anterior aspect of the middle meatus. In this case, the ethmoid infundibulum is closed superiorly by a blind-ending pouch known as the recessus terminalis[19]; hence, ethmoid infundibula inflammation results in anterior ethmoid and maxillary sinusitis without frontal sinus involvement; however, the presence of a recessus terminalis increases the incidence of frontal sinusitis, presumably because of the lack of an anatomical barrier between the frontal recess and middle meatus against the ascent of predisposing factors like allergens, irritants, and infections from the nasal cavity.[20]

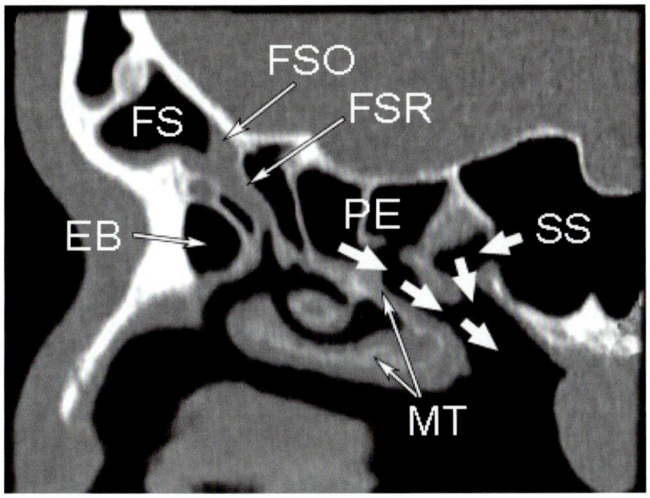

Fig. 2.8 Parasagittal reformation of CT scan through the sinuses demonstrates the frontal sinus (FS), the frontal sinus ostium (FSO), and the frontal sinus recess (FSR). The frontal sinus recess is conical shaped and extends inferiorly into the medial meatus. Also identified is the ethmoid bulla (EB), posterior ethmoid air cells (PE), and the sphenoid sinus (SS).The middle turminate (MT) is labeled.

The posterior limit of the frontal recess is defined by the upward continuation of the bulla ethmoidalis (a prominent anterior ethmoid cell forming the superolateral margin of the ethmoid infundibulum) and the anterior ethmoidal artery, a branch of the ophthalmic artery.[21] The anterior ethmoidal artery travels from the orbit through a canal piercing the lamina papyracea into the anterior ethmoid sinus immediately posterior to the frontal recess, crosses the sinus, and enters the anterior cranial fossa. As stated previously, injury to the anterior ethmoid foramen lying just anterolateral to the cribriform plate of the ethmoid should be avoided during surgery in this location. It gives off an anterior meningeal artery to the dura and also nasal branches, which re-enter the nasal cavity through the cribriform plate.

The frontal recess has a somewhat conical or inverted funnel shape with its superior apex at the frontal ostium.[22] Anterior ethmoid cell pneumatization is variable, and both classic and accessory cells may compress the frontal sinus drainage pathway. The agger nasi cells and Kuhn's frontal recess cell types 1 to 4 occur along the anterior aspect of frontal recess, whereas suprabullar cells and frontal bullar cells are found posteriorly and supraorbital ethmoid cells posterolaterally.[23] Agger nasi (Latin for nasal mound) cells are the most anterior of the anterior ethmoid cells, lie anteroinferior to the frontal recess and inferior to the frontal sinus and are almost always present. These lie posterior to the frontal process of the maxilla, posteromedial to nasal bone, superomedial to the lacrimal bone, and superolateral to the uncinate process. They are seen inferior to the frontal recess and lateral to the middle turbinate on coronal CT scans, form important surgical landmarks, and are opened during endoscopic surgery to gain access to the frontal recess. Agger nasi cell inflammatory disease may obstruct the frontal recess, producing isolated opacification of the frontal sinus without involvement of the anterior ethmoid or maxillary sinuses.[24] There is a strong correlation between agger nasi cells and frontal sinus diseases on CT scans in patients undergoing revision functional endoscopic sinus surgery.[25]

Frontal recess (Kuhn's) cells extend from the anterior ethmoid into the frontal recess, and these are all seen posterosuperior to the agger nasi cells. They are similar to agger nasi cells in that their posterior and superior walls appear as partitions within the frontal recess or within the the frontal sinus in type 3 and 4 cells.[23] A type 1 cell is a single frontal recess cell superior to the agger nasi but below the floor of the frontal sinus. Type 2 cells are multiple cells in the frontal recess above the agger nasi that might extend into the frontal sinus. A type 3 cell is a single large frontal recess air cell that pneumatize superiorly into the frontal sinus. A type 4 cell is a single isolated cell within the frontal sinus. An intersinus cell is seen between the frontal sinuses, arises from the frontal sinus, and can sometimes narrow the frontal recess.[26] Mucosal inflammation is presumed to play a more crucial role than agger nasi cells and frontal recess cells 1–3 in the occurrence of frontal sinusitis.[27]

As noted, accessory air cells along the posterior aspect of frontal recess include the frontal bullar cells, suprabullar cells, and supraorbital ethmoid cells. Frontal bullar cells are formed by anterior skull base pneumatization in the posterior frontal recess and extend through the frontal ostium into the true frontal sinus. Suprabullar cells are seen above the bulla ethmoidalis and are also located in the posterior frontal recess similar to frontal bullar cells, but they do not extend into the frontal sinus. Supraorbital ethmoid cells are seen between the ethmoid roof and medial orbital wall and arise from anterior ethmoid sinus, and they might open into the lateral aspect of frontal recess. They pneumatize the orbital plate of frontal bone posterior to the frontal recess and superolateral to frontal sinus. These cells are found lateral to the frontal sinus in coronal CT scan images, whereas the frontal bullar cells are medial to the sinus.[28] The presence of accessory cells predispose one to a higher incidence of frontal sinusitis by narrowing the frontal sinus drainage pathway. Posteriorly, the suprabullar cells narrow the anteroposterior diameter of the frontal recess, frontal bullar cells narrow the frontal recess and also the more superior frontal ostium, and supraorbital ethmoid cells narrow the frontal ostium.[27]

Another important paranasal sinus structure at the posterior aspect of the anterior skull base is the sphenoethmoid Onodi cell, a posterior ethmoid air cell that extends superior and lateral to the anterior aspect of the sphenoid sinus and abuts the optic nerve. Dehiscence of the adjacent optic canal and carotid canal can be associated with an Onodi cell,[29] which can be seen as a bulge of the optic canal at transnasal endoscopy and should not be breached so as to avoid optic nerve injury.

References

1. Harnsberger HR. Anterior skull base. In: Harnsberger HR, Osborn AG, Macdonald AJ, Ross JS AJ, eds. Diagnostic and Surgical Imaging Anatomy: Brain, Head & Neck, Spine. 1st ed. Philadelphia, PA: Amirsys; 2010:II12–II25
2. Chapman PR, Bag AK, Tubbs RS, Gohlke P. Practical anatomy of the central skull base region. Semin Ultrasound CT MR 2013;34(5): 381–392
3. Som PM, Park EE, Naidich TP, Lawson W. Crista galli pneumatization is an extension of the adjacent frontal sinuses. AJNR Am J Neuroradiol 2009;30(1):31–33
4. Kainz J. Heinz Stammberger. The roof of the anterior ethmoid: a place of least resistance in the skull base. Am J Rhinol. 1989;3: 191–199
5. Nuss DW, O'Malley BW. Surgery of the anterior and middle cranial base. In: Cummings CW, ed. Cummings Otolaryngology Head and Neck Surgery. 4th ed. St Louis, MO: Elsevier Mosby; 2005:3760–3775
6. Meyers RM, Valvassori G. Interpretation of anatomic variations of computed tomography scans of the sinuses: a surgeon's perspective. Laryngoscope 1998;108(3):422–425
7. Stankiewicz JA, Chow JM. The low skull base: an invitation to disaster. Am J Rhinol 2004;18(1):35–40
8. Kim E, Russell PT. Prevention and management of skull base injury. Otolaryngol Clin North Am 2010;43(4):809–816
9. Messerklinger W. [Endoscopy technique of the middle nasal meatus] (author's transl). Arch Otorhinolaryngol 1978;221(4):297–305
10. Wigand ME. Transnasal, endoscopical sinus surgery for chronic sinusitis. II Endonasal ethmoidectomy. HNO 1981;29:287–293
11. Gray ST, Wu AW. Pathophysiology of iatrogenic and traumatic skull base injury. In: Bleier BS, ed. Comprehensive Techniques in CSF Leak Repair and Skull Base Reconstruction. Adv Otorhinolaryngol. 2013;74:12–23
12. Keros P. [On the practical value of differences in the level of the lamina cribrosa of the ethmoid]. Z Laryngol Rhinol Otol 1962;41: 809–813
13. Savvateeva DM, Güldner C, Murthum T, et al. Digital volume tomography (DVT) measurements of the olfactory cleft and olfactory fossa. Acta Otolaryngol 2010;130(3):398–404
14. Osborn AG. Anomalies of the skull and meninges. In: Osborn AG, ed. Osborn's brain: imaging, pathology, and anatomy.1st ed. Salt Lake City, UT: Amirsys; 2013:1187–1208.
15. Hoving EW, Vermeij-Keers C. Frontoethmoidal encephaloceles, a study of their pathogenesis. Pediatr Neurosurg 1997;27(5):246–256
16. Hedlund G. Congenital frontonasal masses: developmental anatomy, malformations, and MR imaging. Pediatr Radiol 2006;36(7): 647–662, quiz 726–727
17. Barkovich AJ. Congenital malformations of the brain and skull. In: Barkovich AJ, ed. *Pediatric Neuroimaging*. 4th ed. Philadelphia: Lippincott Williams & Wilkins; 2005:308–313
18. Barkovich AJ, Vandermarck P, Edwards MS, Cogen PH. Congenital nasal masses: CT and MR imaging features in 16 cases. AJNR Am J Neuroradiol 1991;12(1):105–116
19. McLaughlin RB Jr, Rehl RM, Lanza DC. Clinically relevant frontal sinus anatomy and physiology. Otolaryngol Clin North Am 2001; 34(1):1–22
20. Turgut S, Ercan I, Sayin I, Başak M. The relationship between frontal sinusitis and localization of the frontal sinus outflow tract: a computer-assisted anatomical and clinical study. Arch Otolaryngol Head Neck Surg 2005;131(6):518–522
21. Wormald PJ. Three-dimensional building block approach to understanding the anatomy of the frontal recess and frontal sinus. Oper Tech Otolaryngol–Head Neck Surg 2006;17:2–5
22. Kuhn FA. Chronic frontal sinusitis: the endoscopic frontal recess approach. Oper Tech Otolaryngol–Head Neck Surg 1996;7:222–229

23. Lee WT, Kuhn FA, Citardi MJ. 3D computed tomographic analysis of frontal recess anatomy in patients without frontal sinusitis. Otolaryngol Head Neck Surg 2004;131(3):164–173
24. Vattoth S, Sullivan JC. Face and Neck Anatomy. In: Canon CL, ed. McGraw-Hill Specialty Board Review: Radiology. 1st ed. New York: McGraw-Hill; 2010:99–114
25. Bradley DT, Kountakis SE. The role of agger nasi air cells in patients requiring revision endoscopic frontal sinus surgery. Otolaryngol Head Neck Surg 2004;131(4):525–527
26. Coates MH, Whyte AM, Earwaker JW. Frontal recess air cells: spectrum of CT appearances. Australas Radiol 2003;47(1):4–10
27. Lien CF, Weng HH, Chang YC, Lin YC, Wang WH. Computed tomographic analysis of frontal recess anatomy and its effect on the development of frontal sinusitis. Laryngoscope 2010;120(12): 2521–2527
28. Zhang L, Han D, Ge W, et al. Computed tomographic and endoscopic analysis of supraorbital ethmoid cells. Otolaryngol Head Neck Surg 2007;137(4):562–568
29. Weinberger DG, Anand VK, Al-Rawi M, Cheng HJ, Messina AV. Surgical anatomy and variations of the Onodi cell. Am J Rhinol 1996;10(6):365–370

3 Middle Skull Base

Philip R. Chapman and Surjith Vattoth

Introduction

The middle or central skull base has customarily been delineated from the anterior skull base by a horizontal line along the anterior sellar margin (tuberculum sellae), which extends laterally along the posterior margin of the lesser wing of the sphenoid bone on both sides and includes the medial anterior clinoid processes. The posterior boundary of the middle skull base is formed medially by the dorsum sella and laterally by the petrous ridges. The appearance of the skull base, as viewed from above and through an open calvaria, naturally separates the skull into its three classic anatomical divisions. The anatomical boundaries of the skull base coincide with the boundaries of the proposed intracranial spaces, producing the anterior, middle, and posterior cranial fossae. This archetypical approach does not take into account the practically important, three-dimensional (3D) connections of the middle skull base in the current era of advanced cross-sectional imaging or the availability of sophisticated surgical and radiation treatment methods.[1,2]

The 3D anatomy of the middle skull base should encompass the contiguous anatomical regions of the orbital apex and optic canal, including the optic nerve leading posteriorly to the optic chiasm, the superior orbital fissure, the pterygopalatine fossa, and the sella. In addition, the suprasellar and parasellar structures, including the pituitary gland and stalk, cavernous sinus, internal carotid artery, cranial nerves, Meckel's cave, regional skull-base foramina, sphenoid sinus, clivus, petrous apex, petro-occipital fissure, foramen lacerum, and parts of the nasopharynx should also be incorporated as part of the middle skull base. This region can be conceptualized as having a roughly spherical shape with the optic chiasm at the superior pole, nasopharynx at the inferior pole, pterygopalatine fossa at the anterior pole, and the foramen ovale at the lateral and prepontine cistern at the posterior poles, respectively. Attributing a 3D configuration to the middle skull base allows for compartmentalization of the anatomy, which in turn helps to predict pathology based on the knowledge of intrinsic structures dwelling in the particular location. In addition, it sheds light on the complex anatomical connections and aids in assessing the origin and spread of various trans-spatial disease processes. The lateral aspect of the middle skull base, constituted predominantly by the greater wing of the sphenoid bone, forms the floor of the middle cranial fossa, which houses the temporal lobes of the brain.[1,3]

Center of the Sphere: Sphenoid Bone and Sphenoid Sinus

The sphenoid bone has a central body and is constituted on either side by the lateral greater and lesser wings and the inferior pterygoid process with the medial and lateral pterygoid plates. The body of the sphenoid contains the sella turcica superiorly and the sphenoid sinus inferiorly. Posteriorly, it forms the anterosuperior aspect of the clivus, joining the posteroinferior aspect from occipital bone at the spheno-occipital synchondrosis. The spheno-occipital synchondrosis separates the basisphenoid from the basiocciput (**Fig. 3.1**). Chordomas can arise from notochordal remnants near the synchondrosis, and the presence of vascularized bone marrow predisposes the clivus to pathologies like myeloma and metastasis. The lesser wing of the sphenoid forms the posterior margin of the anterior skull base—harboring the optic canal. The greater wing of sphenoid forms the floor of middle cranial fossa. The superior orbital fissure lies between

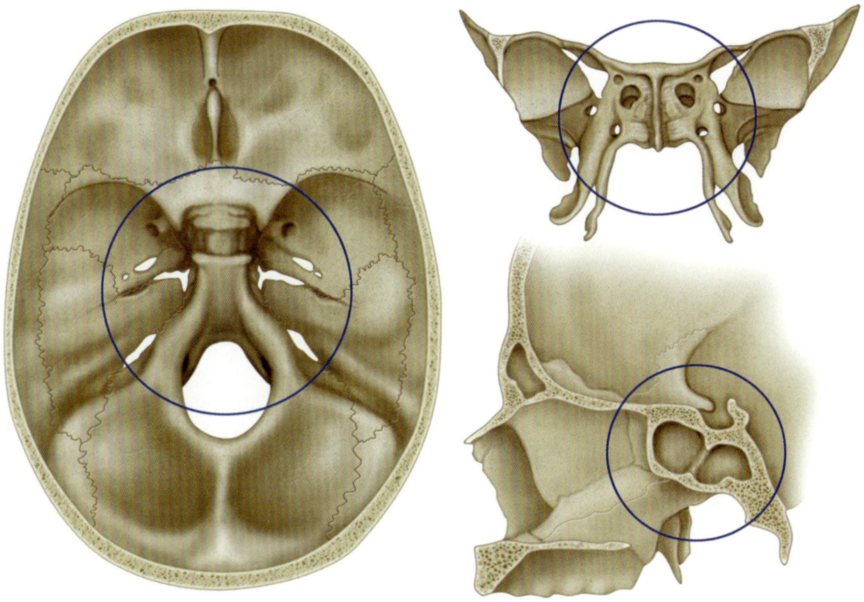

Fig. 3.1 Three-dimensional illustrations of the superior, anterior, and lateral views of the sphenoid bone and the osseous foundation of the central skull base. The outlined spherical region denotes the central skull base region and includes the adjacent endocranial structures including the pituitary gland and the exocranial structures of the neck including the nasopharynx.

the lesser wing of the sphenoid superomedially and the greater wing of the sphenoid inferolaterally, separated by the optic strut, a small bony bridge that projects from the anterior clinoid process of the lesser wing to the sphenoid body.[4,5] The osseous architecture of the sphenoid bone, sphenoid sinus, and associated relationships with adjacent osseous skull base, canals, and foramina is best studied with high-resolution computed tomography (CT) scans using thin slices and bone algorithms (**Fig. 3.2**, **Fig. 3.3**).

The extent of sphenoid sinus pneumatization (or lack thereof) is classified as conchal, presellar, and sellar.[6] In the conchal form, the sphenoid bone is essentially solid without development of an aerated sphenoid sinus. With presellar pneumatization, the sphenoid sinus is pneumatized but does not extend posteriorly to the coronal level of the anterior sellar. With sellar pneumatization, the sphenoid sinus extends posteriorly inferior to the sella and can extend to the posterior clival margin. The anterior wall and floor of sella are quite thin in the latter subtype, measuring less than a millimeter in thickness. Sphenoid sinus pneumatization may extend into the optic strut and anterior clinoid process, resulting in thinning of the boundary with the optic canal and superior orbital fissure. Passage of the vidian canal through the body of sphenoid bone and the foramen rotundum, along the lateral aspect of sphenoid sinus roof, lies in close relation to sphenoid sinus.[7] The sphenoid sinus lies close to the internal carotid arteries (ICAs) and cavernous sinuses. The ICA lies along a shallow groove on the intracranial side of the lateral wall of the sphenoid sinus. The variable intercarotid distance between the ICAs of both sides makes pituitary surgery more risky. Sphenoid sinus septation also varies considerably. Although it is usually single, septation can be multiple with septa deviating laterally, inserting near the carotid artery.[8] Contiguous spread of pathology, bony destruction, and potential for iatrogenic injury to adjacent critical structures during surgery should be carefully estimated during presurgical imaging evaluation of the sphenoid sinus.

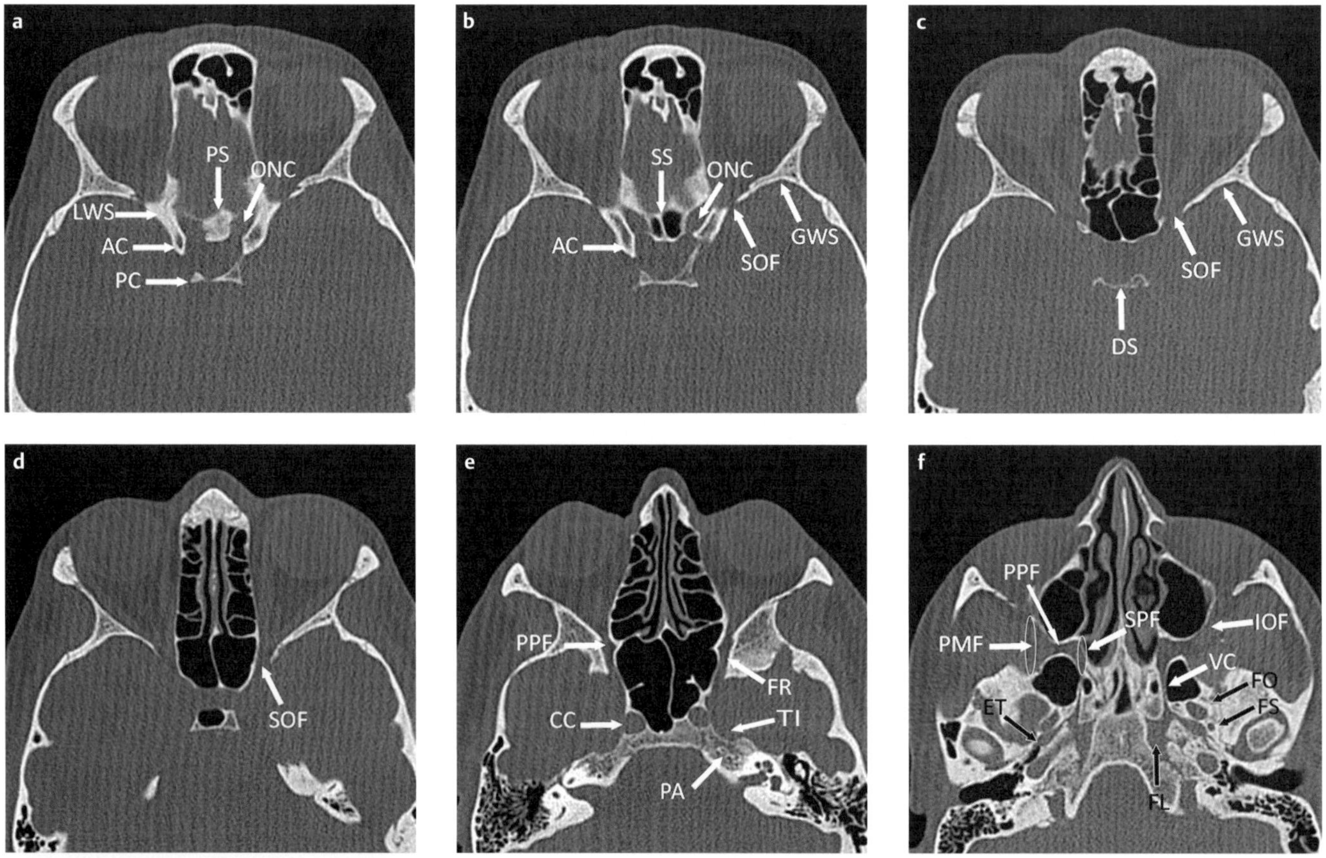

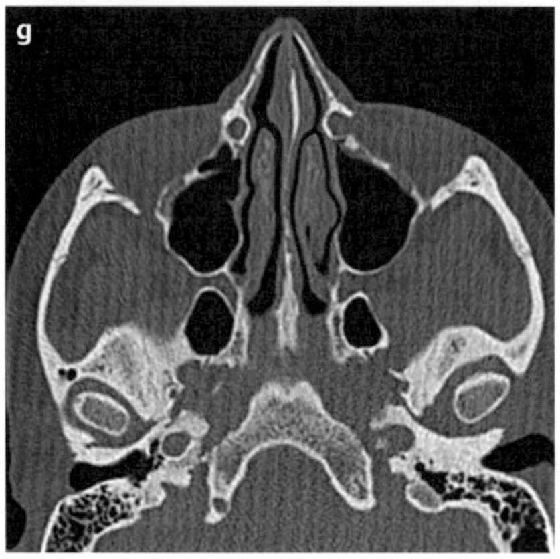

Fig. 3.2 Axial computed tomography (CT) anatomy **(a–g)**. Axial, unenhanced CT images through the skull base, superior to inferior. **(a)** The posterolateral margin of the sella is marked by the posterior clinoid process (PC).The anterior clinoid (AC) is a bony projection along the anterolateral sella that is contiguous with the lesser wing of the sphenoid bone (LWS). Medial-to-the-anterior clinoid process is the optic canal (ONC) that transmits the optic nerve and ophthalmic artery. The planum sphenoidale (PS) is a horizontal segment of bone just anterior to the sella that forms part of the roof of the sphenoid sinus. **(b)** As the axial images move inferiorly, the superior orbital fissure (SOF) becomes more conspicuous. The optic canal (ONC) is intimately related to the sphenoid sinus (SS) medially and bony strut of the anterior clinoid process (AC) laterally. **(c)** The posterior vertical margin of the sella is the dorsum sella (DS). At this level, there is contiguous soft tissue density between the middle cranial fossa (specifically, the cavernous sinus) and the orbital apex through the superior orbital fissure. The SOF transmits the ophthalmic vein; V1 segment of the trigeminal nerve; and cranial nerves III, IV, and VI. Please note the greater wing of sphenoid (GWS). **(d)** In this example, there is a single sagittal septum in the sphenoid sinus. The natural sphenoid ostia are identified on either side of the septum, allowing mucus to drain into the posterior nasal passage. The superior orbital fissure (SOF) is noted (arrow). **(e)** At this level, the petrous apex (PA) can be seen as a pyramidal shaped, medial extension of the temporal bone. Along the superior and medial margin of the petrous apex is a shallow concavity, the trigeminal impression (TI). The medial opening of the carotid canal (CC) is seen, separated from the sphenoid sinus by thin cortical bone. The foramen rotundum (FR) opens into the upper recess of the pterygopalatine fossa (PPF). **(f)** The foramen lacerum (FL) is a triangular shaped, horizontal layer of cartilage between the clivus and petrous apex. The eustachian tube (ET) is seen just lateral to the carotid canal, extending lateral tomedial and superior to inferior. The foramen ovale (FO) and foramen spinosum (FS) are seen in the lateral sphenoid bone. The vidian canal (VC) contains the vidian nerve and travels from a point near the foramen lacerum forward to the pterygopalatine fossa (PPF). The PPF connects with the masticator space laterally through the pterygomaxillary fissure (PMF, large oval) and medially through the sphenopalatine foramen (SPF, small oval) with the nasal cavity. The infraorbital nerve passes from the PPF into the inferior orbital fissure (IOF) on its way to the cheek. **(g)** At this level, soft tissues that form the roof of the nasopharynx begin to show up ventral to the clivus. Note that these soft tissues are directly contiguous with the region of the eustachian tube and foramen lacerum.

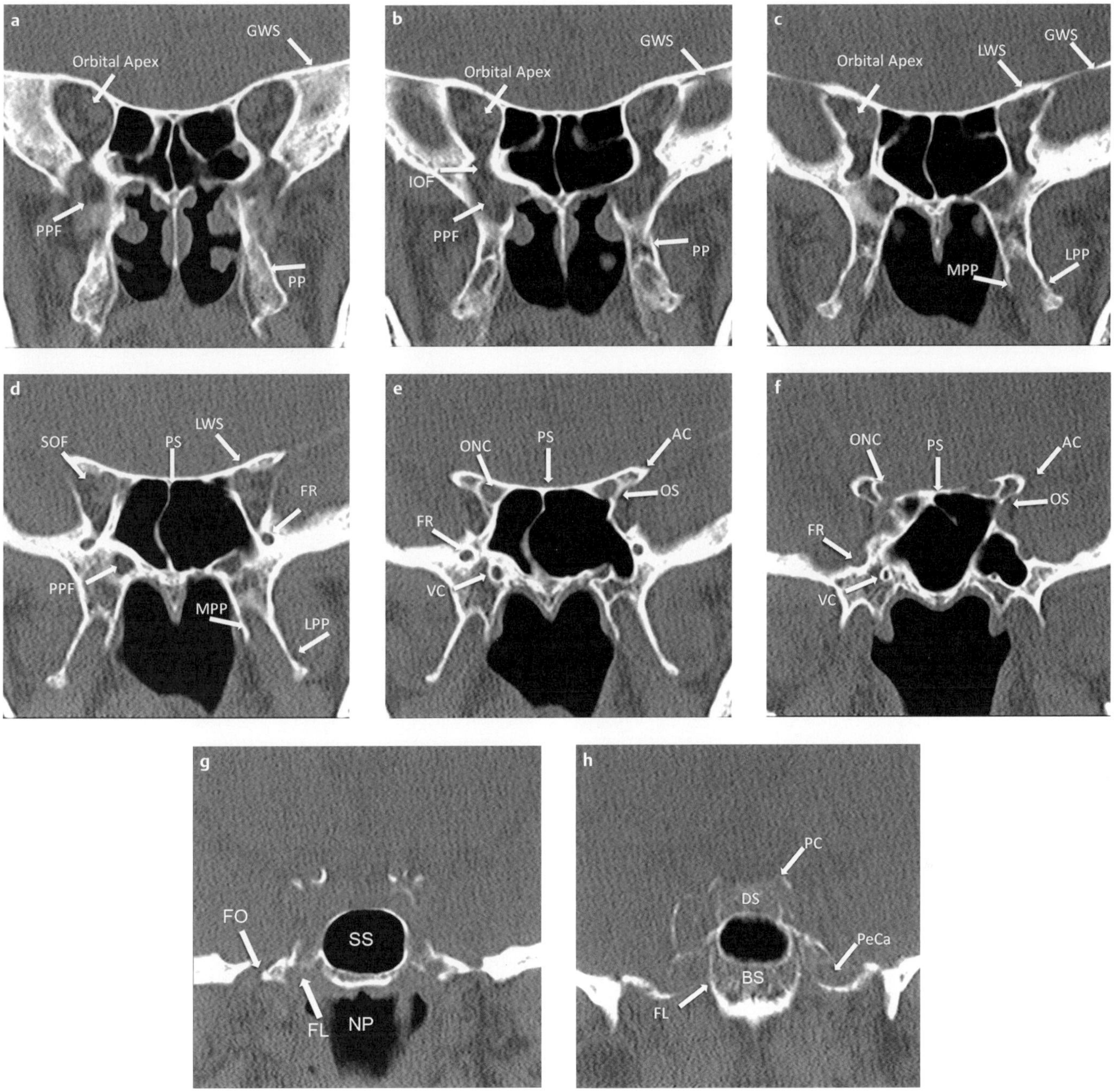

Fig.3.3 Coronal computed tomography (CT) anatomy, anterior to posterior **(a–h)**. Coronal, unenhanced CT images through the central skull base. **(a)** Coronal image through orbital apices at the level of the pterygoid process (PP) demonstrates the relationship between the pterygopalatine fossa and the orbital apex. **(b)** The pterygopalatine fossa (PPF) contains fat, the distal branches of the internal maxillary artery, veins, the pterygopalatine ganglion, and its connections. The PPF is contiguous with the inferior orbital fissure (IOF) and, ultimately, the orbital apex. **(c)** Near the apex, the orbital roof is formed by the lesser wing of the sphenoid bone (LWS). The medial (MPP) and lateral (LPP) pterygoid plates project posteriorly from the pterygoid process (PP). **(d)** Near the apex, there is an obliquely oriented superolateral fissure, the superior orbital fissure (SOF), which transmits the ophthalmic vein; V1 segment of the trigeminal nerve; and cranial nerves III, IV, and VI. **(e)** The foramen rotundum (FR) opens into the upper recess of the pterygopalatine fossa (PPF). In the coronal plane, the foramen rotundum is seen superolateral to the vidian canal (VC). **(f)** Coronal image through the sphenoid sinus demonstrates the relationship between the anterior clinoid process (AC) and the optic canal (ONC). The roof of the sphenoid sinus is flat and is referred to as the planum sphenoidale (PS). The optic strut (OS) is a thin bridge of bone defines the lateral margin of the optic canal. At this level, the foramen rotundum opens into the middle cranial fossa as V2 travels toward the lateral wall of the cavernous sinus. **(g)** Coronal image through sphenoid sinus demonstrates foramen ovale (FO) laterally, which transmits V3 into the masticator space and more poorly defined foramen lacerum (FL) medially. **(h)** Coronal image through the posterior aspect of the sella. The posterior clinoid processes (PC) can be seen as bilateral superolateral projections. The posterior wall of the sella is the dorsum sella (DS). The upper one-half of the clivus is formed from the sphenoid bone and is referred to as the basisphenoid (BS).

Intracranial Structures Superior to Center of the Sphere

Sella Turcica and Suprasellar Region

The sella turcica (Turkish saddle) is a saddle-shaped depression in the body of the sphenoid bone. The seat of the saddle supports the pituitary gland and is known as the hypophyseal fossa (**Fig. 3.4**). Its anterior margin is the tuberculum sella, and its posterior margin is the dorsum sella, with the superolateral posterior clinoid processes on either side. The dorsum sella is continuous posteriorly with the clivus. The chiasmatic sulcus lies just anterior to the tuberculum sella and medial to optic canals. The planum sphenoidale, a part of the anterior cranial fossa, lies in front of the tuberculum sellae and chiasmatic sulcus. The medial processes along lesser wings of sphenoid bilaterally form the sella's anterior clinoid processes. The floor of the pituitary fossa has a well corticated, less than 1-mm-thick bony wall known as the lamina dura. The diaphragma sellae is a slightly inferior, convex, thin dual fold covering the superior aspect of sella and is perforated centrally by the pituitary stalk. The pituitary stalk passes through the cerebrospinal fluid (CSF) filled suprasellar cistern on its way to the hypothalamus. The suprasellar cistern also houses the optic chiasm and circle of Willis. Large sellar or suprasellar lesions, including pituitary adenomas and craniopharyngiomas, can produce optic chiasm compression.

Cavernous Sinus

The cavernous sinuses, dural venous sinuses lying on either side of the sella connected by intercavernous sinuses, are fed by multiple tributaries, including the superior ophthalmic veins

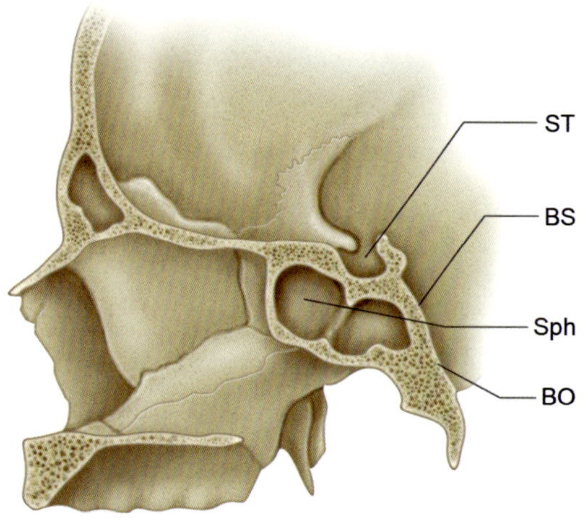

Fig. 3.4 Sagittal illustration through the central skull base demonstrates the bony anatomy of the sella trurcica (ST). The anterior wall of the sella is very thin and separates the sella from the sphenoid sinus (Sph). The clivus is formed by the basisphenoid (BS) superiorly and the basiocciput (BO) inferiorly.

in the orbits, sphenoparietal sinuses seen along the anterior aspect of middle cranial fossa, basal vein of Rosenthal seen in the perimesencephalic cisterns draining toward the vein of Galen, pterygoid venous plexus seen in the masticator space, and the basilar venous plexus near the petrous apex. They drain through the superior petrosal sinus into the sigmoid sinus and through the inferior petrosal sinus into the internal jugular vein. In a carotid-cavernous fistula, venous channels may be engorged with high pressure arterialized flow and appear enlarged on magnetic resonance imaging (MRI) and CT scan images.[9]

The cavernous sinus has five walls.[1,10] The medial wall of the cavernous sinus consists of an upper sellar component with a single-layered, thin, dural membrane separating it from the lateral margin of the pituitary gland, and a lower, thicker component adherent to the carotid sulcus. Tumor obliteration of the medial venous compartment of the cavernous sinus inferior to the cavernous ICA in a coronal MRI scan (called carotid sulcus venous compartment of cavernous sinus) has been shown to have a 95% positive predictive value (PPV) for cavernous sinus invasion by a pituitary adenoma.[11] Perimeter encasement of 67% or more of the cavernous segment of the ICA (100% PPV) and tumor spread beyond the border joining the lateral wall of the intracavernous and supracavernous ICAs (85% PPV), as seen on coronal MRI, both suggest cavernous sinus invasion. If the percentage of encasement of the perimeter of the intracavernous ICA is less than 25%, or if adenoma invasion does not cross beyond the adjoining medial wall of the intracavernous and supracavernous ICAs, cavernous sinus invasion can then be ruled out with a negative predictive value of 100%.

Forming the medial margin of the temporal lobe, the bilaminar lateral wall of the cavernous sinus consists of a thin outer meningeal layer and a thicker inner dural layer that extends from the region of superior orbital fissure and the anterior clinoid process anteriorly to the petrous apex posteriorly. The oculomotor nerve (cranial nerve III, or CN III), the trochlear nerve (CN IV), and the ophthalmic segment of the trigeminal nerve (CN V1) are contained within the lateral wall layers, and the only truly intracavernous nerve, namely, the abducens nerve (CN VI), lies within the cavernous sinus itself, along with the cavernous segment of ICA (**Fig. 3.5**). Inferiorly, the medial and lateral walls fuse along the lateral margin of the body of sphenoid bone. It is interesting to note that this fusion occurs just superior to the maxillary nerve (second division of the trigeminal nerve, CN V2) and that the CN V2 and mandibular nerve (third division of the trigeminal nerve, CN V3) are not part of the cavernous sinus, even though they are invested by the contiguous dura.[1,12]

The cavernous sinus becomes contiguous with the inferior petrosal sinus (which in turn drains through the petroclival fissure into internal jugular vein) posteriorly. The posterior wall of the cavernous sinus extends from the lateral margin of the dorsum sella to the superomedial aspect of Meckel's cave. Just posteroinferior to this is the petrous apex, over which the abducens nerve (CN VI) travels underneath the petrosphenoid ligament, goes through the Dorello's canal, enters the posterior wall of the cavernous sinus, and is seen within the substance of the cavernous sinus lateral to the cavernous ICA (**Fig. 3.6**). Petrous apicitis can lead to Gradenigo syndrome with CN VI palsy (resulting from involvement in Dorello's canal) and trigeminal distribution pain from spread of inflammation into the adjacent Meckel's cave, where the trigeminal ganglion resides.[13]

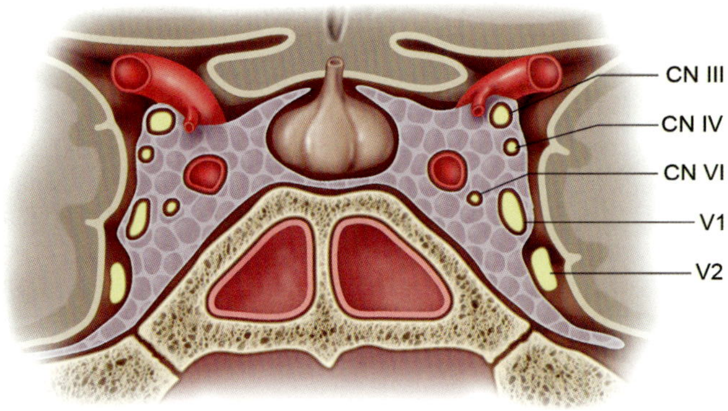

Fig. 3.5 Posterior view through the cavernous sinuses. The central location of the cavernous internal carotid artery is noted. Cranial nerve VI, the abducens, is the only nerve that is truly intracavernous. From superior to inferior, the oculomotor, trochlear, ophthalmic, and maxillary nerves are seen along the lateral margin of the cavernous sinus. The lateral wall is divided into two layers, an outer meningeal layer and an inner dural layer. The inner dural layer envelops the oculomotor, trochlear, and ophthalmic nerves.

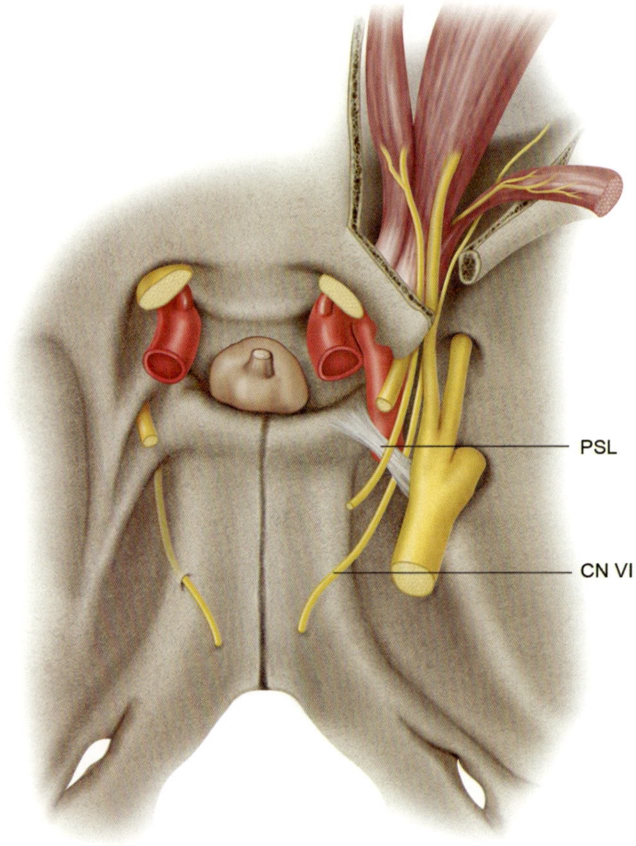

Fig. 3.6 The right cranial nerve (CN VI), the abducens nerve, enters the posterior wall of the cavernous sinus, beneath the petrosphenoid ligament, through Dorello's canal, and travels within the cavernous sinus, lateral to the cavernous internal carotid artery.

The rectangular anterior wall of the cavernous sinus extends from the optic strut under the anterior clinoid process toward the superior orbital fissure, and its inferior margin forms the superior end of foramen rotundum carrying CN V2. The cavernous sinus roof extends from the optic strut and superior orbital fissure anteriorly to the petrous apex and the edge of the tentorium posteriorly. It is contiguous with the diaphragma sellae medially and is separated laterally from the lateral wall of cavernous sinus by the anterior petroclinoid fold. The anterior petroclinoid fold is a cordlike thickening of the dura extending from the anterior clinoid process anteriorly to tentorial edge posteriorly. The posterior petroclinoid fold is a separate fold extending from the posterior clinoid process to the tentorial edge, whereas the interclinoid fold is a thin band of dura that extends from the anterior clinoid process to the posterior clinoid process. The anatomical importance of these three folds is that they form a landmark triangle at the cavernous sinus roof—the oculomotor triangle (**Fig. 3.7**). CN III pierces the oculomotor triangle from a posterosuperior aspect to pass through a short oculomotor cistern and enters within the bilaminar lateral wall of the cavernous sinus near the anterior clinoid process. CN IV enters the oculomotor triangle posterolaterally, just posterior to the oculomotor nerve.[14]

Internal Carotid Artery

The ICAs are important structures that are intimately related to the middle skull base, except for the proximal cervical and distal communicating segments. The widely used Bouthillier system divides the ICA into a seven-segment numerical scale along the superiorly oriented direction of blood flow according to a detailed understanding of the surrounding anatomy and the compartments through which it travels (**Fig. 3.8**),[15] including the following segments from its origin in the neck to its termination at the circle of Willis: cervical (C1), petrous (C2), lacerum (C3), cavernous (C4), clinoid (C5), ophthalmic (C6), and communicating (C7) segments. Cervical C1 segment of the ICA has no branches, enters the carotid canal at the skull base, and travels medially in the carotid canal as the petrous C2 segment, surrounded by bone at its most solid posteromedial and relatively thinner anterolateral and inferior walls, with the roof being covered by dura. The petrous segment of ICA branches are the small caroticotympanic arteries, which enter the middle ear and the occasionally present vidian artery that usually arises from the maxillary artery, which in turn is a branch of the external carotid artery. The petrous carotid artery ends medially partially surrounded by fibrocartilaginous tissue contiguous with the cartilage of the foramen lacerum, over which the ICA passes as the lacerum C3 segment. The foramen lacerum is not within a single bone; rather, it is actually a cartilage-filled gap separating the petrous apex from the basisphenoid medially and the basiocciput posteriorly. Meningeal branches of the ascending pharyngeal artery pass through the cartilage-filled foramen.[1] Then the ICA turns superiorly on its way to the cavernous sinus, passing under a fibrous band called the *petrolingual ligament* (which extends from the petrous apex to the lingula of the carotid sulcus of the sphenoid body), after which the cavernous C4 segment begins. The petroshenoid ligament or Gruber's ligament (which extends from the petrous apex to posterior clinoid process) is situated superior to the petrolingual ligament, and the abducens nerve (CN VI) lies just lateral and parallel

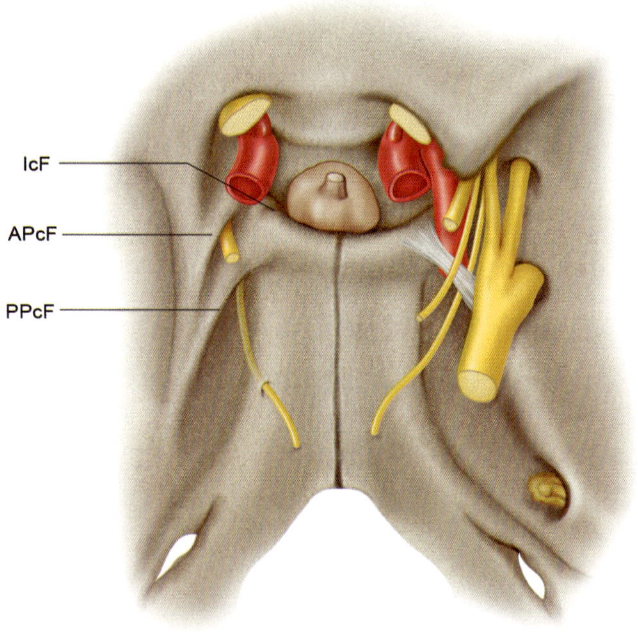

Fig. 3.7 Cranial nerve III, the oculomotor nerve, pierces the roof of the cavernous sinus on the left. Marginal thickening of the dura forms three distinct folds: the anterior petroclinoid fold (APcF), the posterior petroclinoid fold (PPcF), and the interclinoid (IcF) fold; these folds form the oculomotor triangle.

to the horizontal portion of the cavernous ICA underneath the petroshenoid ligament.[16–18]

The cavernous C4 segment travels superiorly and then turns anteriorly with a horizontal course along the cavernous sinus. This horizontal portion of cavernous ICA lies in a shallow sulcus along the lateral aspect of body of sphenoid, called the carotid sulcus. Dehiscence of the bone in this location allows the ICA to project into the sphenoid sinus, potentially posing a risk during endoscopic trans-sphenoidal surgery. The characteristically described three named branches of the cavernous ICA are the meningohypophyseal trunk, inferolateral trunk, and capsular artery. The meningohypophyseal trunk (dorsal mainstem artery) arises from the cavernous ICA at the center of the outer convexity of its posterior genu, where the initial ascending segment turns anteriorly to become the horizontal segment, and subdivides into three vessels: the tentorial artery (artery of Bernasconi and Cassinari), the dorsal meningeal artery, and the inferior hypophyseal artery. The inferolateral trunk (lateral mainstem artery or artery of the inferior cavernous sinus) arises from the horizontal portion of the cavernous ICA segment itself and supplies small arterial branches to the intracavernous cranial nerves and tentorium. This artery is clinically important because it is anastomosed with the external carotid artery branches through the foramen rotundum, ovale, and spinosum. McConnell's capsular artery arises from the most superior segment of the intracavernous ICA and supplies the inferior and peripheral aspect of the anterior lobe of the pituitary gland and the diaphragma sellae.

The ICA then turns vertically near the anterior margin of the cavernous sinus and continues medially to the anterior clinoid process, where it passes through two dural rings, the proximal dural ring (which forms the true roof of the cavernous sinus anteriorly), and the distal dural ring (which represents the anatomical border between the extradural and intradural ICA). This short vertical segment of ICA medial to the anterior clinoid process between the proximal and distal dural rings is called the clinoid C5 segment, and it has no named branches. Differentiation of an ICA aneurysm, which has a neck in the proximal intra-

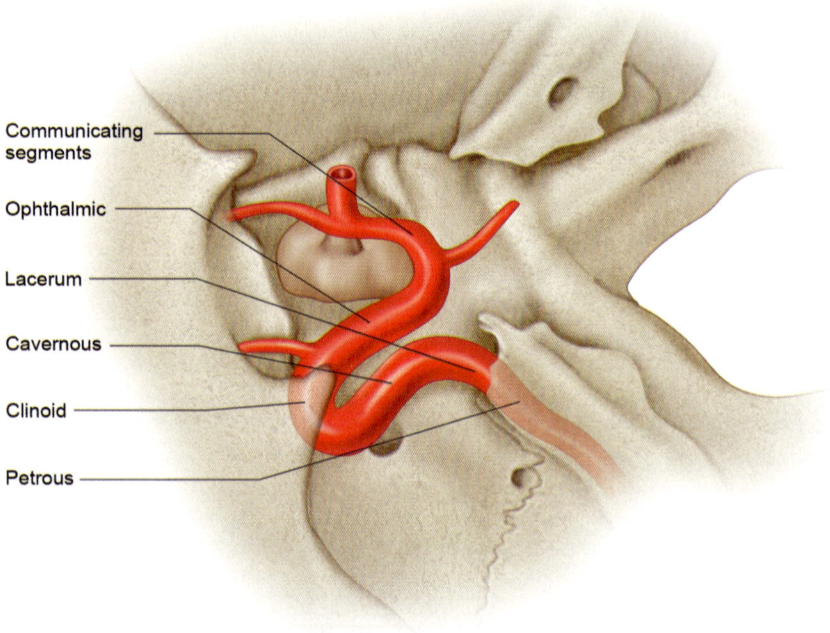

Fig. 3.8 The seven-segment classification system for the internal carotid artery. From proximal to distal, these include the (1) cervical (not shown), (2) petrous, (3) lacerum, (4) cavernous, (5) clinoid, (6) ophthalmic, and (7) communicating segments. All but the cervical segment are intimately related to the central skull base region.

dural segment that could produce a carotid–cavernous fistula if it bleeds, from one with a neck in the distal intradural segment, which can produce life-threatening subarachnoid hemorrhage, is extremely important. Although the dural rings are not seen at imaging, the location of the proximal dural ring can be assumed by the knowledge that (1) it forms the superomedial margin of the easily identifiable optic strut, a tiny bony process connected to the anterior clinoid process of the lesser wing of sphenoid; and (2) it separates the medial optic canal from the superior orbital fissure laterally.[19] The distal dural ring, lying superior to the proximal dural ring, forms the real line of demarcation between the extradural and intradural ICA and can be assumed to be at the junction of the CSF and cavernous sinus on high-resolution coronal 3D CT cisternography or 3D T2 MRI.[20]

After this, the ICA continues into the intradural subarachnoid space as the ophthalmic C6 segment, giving rise to the ophthalmic artery anteriorly and superior hypophyseal artery projecting posteroinferomedially into the sella. The terminal communicating C7 segment of the ICA begins just before the origin of its branch called the posterior communicating artery (PCOM) and ends by bifurcating into the anterior cerebral artery and middle cerebral artery. The anterior choroidal artery arises from the communicating segment immediately distal to the origin of the PCOM.

Structures Filling Posterior Aspect of the Sphere

Petrous Apex and Petroclival Junction

The petrous apex, the pyramidal obliquely oriented anteromedial extension of petrous temporal bone, must be considered a part of the 3D configuration of the middle skull base. Petrous apex pneumatization varies, being filled with bone marrow in 60%, pneumatized in 33%, and sclerotic in 7% (**Fig. 3.9**). A pneumatized petrous apex may communicate directly with the mastoid or middle ear cavity and provide direct pathways for disease spread. Pneumatization is asymmetric in 5 to 10%, and the T1 hyperintense marrow fat on the nonpneumatized side has the potential to mimic a lesion in MRI. Pneumatized petrous apices are more prone to apical petrositis and nonpneumatized marrow containing apices to disease processes like metastasis.[21–23] The clinically important Dorello's canal, petro-occipital fissure, and Meckel's cave are in close relation to the petrous apex. Dorello's canal is a small channel between two layers of dura overlying the superomedial aspect of the petrous apex, where it is fused to the posterolateral sphenoid body below the posterior clinoid process. This channel transmits the abducens nerve (CN VI) and is surrounded by the inferior petrosal sinus, which in turn is continuous with the cavernous sinus anteriorly and drains into inferior petrosal sinus. Petro-occipital (petroclival fissure) fissure is the oblique cartilaginous junction of inferomedial petrous temporal bone and inferolateral clivus. This cartilage-filled fissure appears lucent on CT scans, but it can be variably ossified and dense and is the classic site of origin for skull base chondrosarcoma.[24]

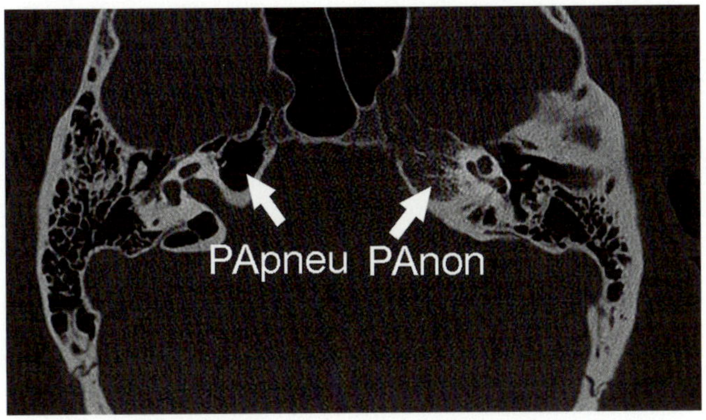

Fig. 3.9 Axial computed tomography image through the petrous apex demonstrates the variability in pneumatization of the petrous apex. The petrous apex on the right is well pneumatized and demonstrates air density (PApneu); the contralateral petrous apex is nonpneumatized and demonstrates bone trabecular bone density (PAnon).

Meckel's Cave

Meckel's cave is a localized dural outpouching over the petrosphenoid junction at the posteromedial aspect of middle cranial fossa. It houses the trigeminal (Gasserian) ganglion within its anteroinferior aspect and the caval segment of trigeminal nerve more posteriorly. Immediately posterior to Meckel's cave, the trigeminal nerve lies in close relation to a small depression in the superior aspect of the petrous apex, just lateral to petrosphenoid junction, called the trigeminal impression. The trigeminal nerve then travels into the posterior fossa as the cisternal segment and enters the pons at the root entry zone. Anteromedially, Meckel's cave is closely opposed to the posteroinferolateral aspect of the cavernous sinus and is just lateral to the ICA near the lacerum or proximal cavernous segment, where the artery begins to run anterosuperiorly into the cavernous sinus. The three major divisions of trigeminal nerve arise within the Meckel's cave. The ophthalmic division (V1) runs anteromedially to enter the lateral wall of cavernous sinus, whereas the maxillary division (V2) runs anteriorly underneath the cavernous sinus to enter into foramen rotundum, and the mandibular division (V3) extends inferolaterally along the foramen ovale into the masticator space.[25]

Extracranial Structures Lying Anterior/Inferior to Center of the Sphere

Orbital Apex and Pterygopalatine Fossa

The orbital apex is contiguous with the middle skull base through the optic canal in the lesser wing of the sphenoid, superior orbital fissure between the lesser and greater wings and the pterygopalatine fossa through the inferior orbital fissure. Orbital tumors like optic nerve sheath meningioma, inflammatory lesions like orbital apex pseudotumor, and infections like invasive fungal disease can extend into the middle skull base and vice versa. Orbital apex syndrome can produce vision loss, ophthalmoplegia, and multiple cranial neuropathies as a result of the connections with cavernous sinus and pterygopalatine fossa. Superior ophthalmic vein thrombosis, which usually arises from infections in the dangerous triangle of the face, can lead to cavernous sinus thrombosis. Despite classic assumptions that the absence of valves in the facial and superior ophthalmic veins is thought to facilitate infectious spread from the midface region to the cavernous spread, a recent cadaveric stereomicroscopic study has demonstrated valves in these veins. The consistent communications between the facial vein and cavernous sinus and the direction of blood flow are important in the spread of infection rather the than absence of valves.[26]

The optic canal is the pathway of optic nerve and ophthalmic artery and lies entirely within the lesser wing of sphenoid. The optic strut (inferior root of lesser wing), along with the anterior clinoid process of the lesser wing of sphenoid, which it is connected to, separates the optic canal from the superior orbital fissure laterally. The fatty bone marrow in the optic strut may have high T1 MRI signal and may be seen projecting inferomedially from the anterior clinoid process, separating the optic nerve from the oculomotor and other cranial nerves. The anterolateral aspect of body of the sphenoid bone forms the medial boundary of optic canal, and a thin bony bridge called the superior root of the lesser wing forms its roof.[27] Within the dural sheath in optic canal, the ophthalmic artery lies inferolateral to optic nerve. It later leaves the dura and crosses above the optic nerve from lateral to medial sides, giving rise to the central retinal artery as it winds around the nerve. The ciliary ganglion lies in the posterior orbit between the optic nerve and lateral rectus muscle at the lateral aspect of ophthalmic artery.

The superior orbital fissure (SOF) is an oblique gap between the lesser wing of sphenoid superomedially and the greater wing of sphenoid inferolaterally (**Fig. 3.10**). It connects the orbit and middle cranial fossa via the cavernous sinus. It is divided by the annulus of Zinn, a tough fibrous aponeurotic ring at the orbital apex, into a medial intraconal compartment (containing CN III, CN VI, and the nasociliary nerve) and a lateral extraconal compartment (containing CN IV, frontal, and lacrimal nerves, and the superior ophthalmic vein). The extraocular muscles arise from the annulus of Zinn, except the inferior oblique muscle, which originates at anteroinferior orbital rim. In addition to the medial SOF compartment, the annulus also surrounds the optic canal, and hence the optic nerve and ophthalmic artery become intraconal structures.

The intraconal medial SOF is wider, lies directly anterior to the cavernous sinus, and contains the oculomotor nerve (CN III), which immediately divides into the superior division (to supply superior rectus and levator palpebrae superioris muscles) and the inferior division (to supply the medial rectus, inferior rectus, and inferior oblique muscles). The medial compartment also contains the abducens nerve (CN VI to supply lateral rectus muscle) lying immediately lateral to the CN III superior division and the nasociliary nerve further superiorly. Note that the nasociliary nerve is one of the three branches of the sensory ophthalmic division of trigeminal nerve (CN V_1) branching within the distal cavernous sinus before entering the orbit.

The other two branches of the ophthalmic CN V_1, namely, the frontal and lacrimal nerves, lie within the smaller extraconal lateral compartment of SOF inferiorly and superolaterally respectively. The trochlear nerve (CN IV to supply the superior oblique muscle) enters the orbit at the extraconal lateral SOF compartment outside the annulus of Zinn and lies here above the frontal nerve and inferomedial to the lacrimal nerve. The

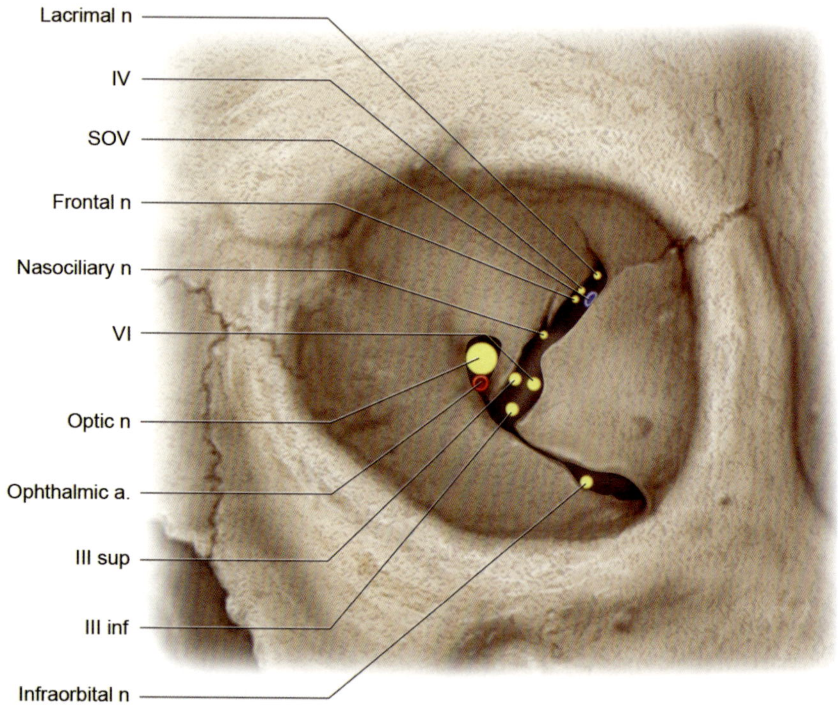

Fig. 3.10 Orbital apex. The superior, medial, inferior, and lateral rectus muscles converge posteriorly and attach to a dense fibrous ring, the annulus of Zinn. The ring circumscribes the optic canal and the inferomedial aspect of the superior orbital fissure. The optic canal contains the optic nerve and ophthalmic artery. The oculomotor nerve (CN III) enters the medial superior orbital fissure and divides into superior and inferior divisions. The nasociliary and abducens (CN VI) nerves also enter through the medial compartment. Laterally, the superior orbital fissure contains the trochlear nerve (CN IV), the lacrimal nerve, the frontal nerve, and the superior ophthalmic vein (SOV).

superior ophthalmic vein lies further lateral to the nerves in the lateral SOF compartment.

The inferior orbital fissure is an oblique gap situated between the floor and lateral wall of orbit (greater wing of sphenoid). It communicates with the pterygopalatine fossa and masticator space and contains the infraorbital nerve and zygomatic nerve (branches of the maxillary division of the trigeminal nerve CN V2), inferior ophthalmic vein division, or emissary veins between the inferior ophthalmic vein and the pterygoid plexus.[28,29]

The pterygopalatine fossa (PPF) is a fat-filled space between the maxillary sinus anteriorly and pterygoid process of sphenoid bone posteriorly. Medially, it is partially bound by a portion of the perpendicular plate of the palatine bone (**Fig. 3.11**). The PPF contains the small pterygopalatine ganglion at its medial aspect, the maxillary nerve (V2) entering via the foramen rotundum, and the distal internal maxillary artery entering via the pterygomaxillary fissure. It is difficult to differentiate the ganglion from nerves and vessels in the PPF, even with high-resolution CT/MRI. Although it is quite small, the PPF has important connections with the middle skull base, orbit, palate, and nasal cavity and can act as a junctional area for the spread of infiltrating or perineural tumor and infection.

Masticator Space

The pterygomaxillary fissure is the lateral opening of PPF into the nasopharyngeal masticator space (infratemporal fossa). The sphenopalatine foramen is its mucosa-covered medial opening into the superior meatus of the nose through a gap in its medial boundary formed by the palatine bone. Nasopharyngeal angiofibromas arise in this region. The PPF communicates superiorly with the SOF. The inferior orbital fissure is its anterior opening into the orbit, which transmits the infraorbital nerve (CN V2 continuation branch) and artery. The foramen rotundum is the pathway along which the intracranial maxillary nerve (CN V2) passes into the PPF after traveling in the dura underneath the lateral wall of the cavernous sinus. The canal can be easily identified in axial CT and MRI connecting the PPF to middle cranial fossa alongside the lateral wall of the cavernous sinus and in coronal imaging superior to an occasionally pneumatized lateral recess of the sphenoid sinus. The vidian canal is a channel that runs through the body of the sphenoid bone connecting the PPF to the foramen lacerum, which in turn is the anteroinferomedial cartilaginous floor of the horizontal petrous ICA canal situated between the sphenoid and temporal bones. In coronal sections, the vidian canal is seen inferomedial to the foramen rotundum with an occasionally pneumatized lateral recess of the sphenoid sinus between them. The pterygopalatine canal is the common inferior canal leading from the PPF and carrying the palatine nerves, and ultimately it divides into an anterior greater palatine foramen and posterior lesser palatine foramen at the hard palate.[30,31]

The masticator space, containing the mastication muscles, is intimately related to the middle skull base through (1) the foramina in the greater wing of sphenoid (e.g., foramen ovale transmitting mandibular division of trigeminal nerve, CN V3); (2) the lesser petrosal nerve, accessory meningeal branch of maxillary artery and emissary vein; and (3) the tiny foramen spinosum, just posterolateral to it (transmitting the middle meningeal artery and vein and meningeal branch of CN V3). These foramina are easily identified on CT images just anterolateral to the horizontal petrous carotid canal. As described already herein, the masticator space is connected with the PPF through the pterygomaxillary fissure. These connections allow perineural

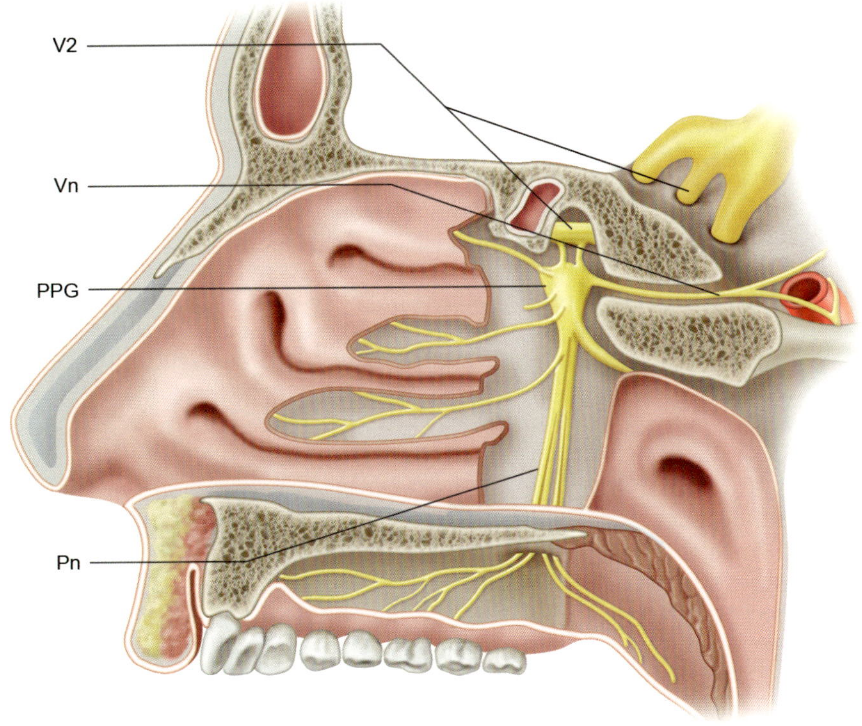

Fig. 3.11 Pterygopalatine fossa (PPF). The posterior aspect of the lateral nasal wall has been dissected, exposing the sphenopalatine foramen and pterygopalatine fossa. The pterygopalatine ganglion (PPG) has multiple neural connections. The maxillary nerve (V2) traverses the upper aspect of the PPF. The vidian nerve (VN) is seen passing from the ganglion into the vidian canal. The greater and lesser palatine nerves (Pn) descend into the palatine canal and into the submucosa of the palate.

tumor spread within the middle skull base. Aggressive masticator space lesions can also erode bone and extend intracranially. The superficial layer of the deep cervical fascia splits to enclose this space, which extends inferiorly to the attachment of medial pterygoid and masseter muscles onto the mandible and superomedially abuts the skull base, with the foramen ovale and foramen spinosum included in this space. Superolaterally, the masticator space extends along the outer surface of the skull as far as the temporalis muscle.[32]

Nasopharynx

The nasopharynx lies immediately inferior to the basisphenoid and clival region of the middle skull base and is an important area to evaluate for contiguous intracranial spread of tumor or aggressive infection (**Fig. 3.12**). It extends from the posterior nasal choana anterosuperiorly to the retropharyngeal and prevertebral space posteriorly and the parapharyngeal spaces lie laterally. Anteroinferiorly, the soft palate separates it from the oropharynx with the posterior side of the soft palate considered part of nasopharynx and its anteroinferior side part of oropharynx. The separation posterior to the soft palate is arbitrary, using an imaginary horizontal line along the hard palate or superior edge of the anterior arch of C1 or through the atlantoaxial articulation.[33,34]

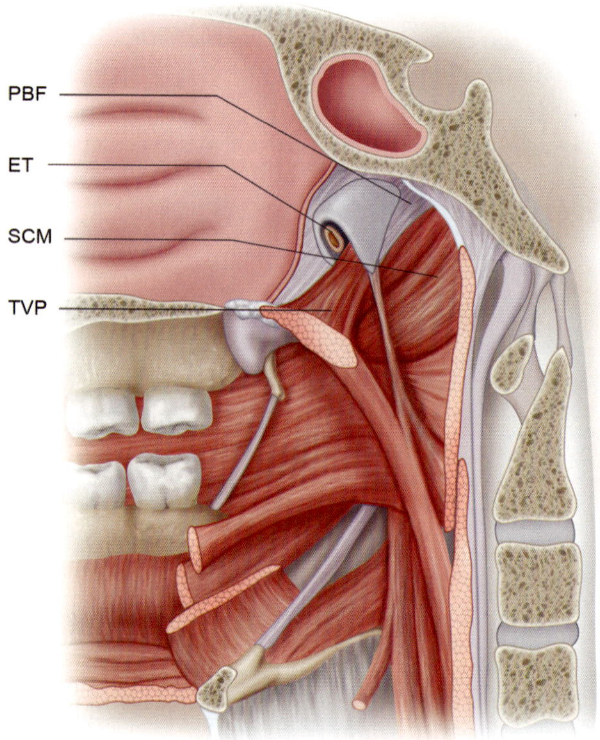

Fig. 3.12 Illustration of the submucosal nasopharynx. The superior constrictor muscle (SCM) attaches to the skull base via the pharyngobasilar fascia (PBF). The eustachian tube (ET) passes through a defect in the PBF referred to as the sinus of Morgagni. The tensor veli palatini (TVP) muscle is seen arising from the cartilaginous eustachian tube and extending inferiorly to the lateral margin of the soft palate.

The middle visceral or pharyngeal mucosal layer of the deep cervical fascia encloses the pharynx; hence, the oropharynx and nasopharynx are collectively called the visceral space or pharyngeal mucosal space (PMS). The nasopharyngeal superficial mucosa consists of epithelium of the PMS and can give rise to nasopharyngeal squamous cell carcinoma.[5] The submucosal space contains lymphoid tissue, accessory salivary glands, and cellular notochord remnants, which can give rise to benign and malignant lesions like lymphoma, salivary gland tumors, and chordoma. The nasopharyngeal tonsils are called adenoids; they lie at the midline roof of the nasopharynx and are usually prominent in children.

The pharyngeal tubercle of the occipital bone provides posterior attachment to the midline pharyngeal raphe and the paired superior constrictor muscles of the pharynx; however, the superior constrictor muscle of either side fans forward to attach to the lower portion of the medial pterygoid plate. This exposes a gap between the muscles and the skull base, which is filled by the pharyngobasilar fascia, a tough aponeurosis that surrounds the pharynx and attaches to the skull base. The pharyngobasilar fascia attaches to the medial pterygoid plate anteroinferiorly and extends superiorly to the skull base. It fills the gap between the muscles and skull base as it proceeds posteriorly, attaching to the body of sphenoid bone, petrous apex, foramen lacerum, and more posteriorly as it processes to the occipital pharyngeal tubercle and prevertebral muscles. Therefore, the foramen lacerum lies within the attachment of this fascia to the skull base, whereas the foramen ovale is seen lateral to this fascia. The eustachian tube and levator veli palatini muscle enter the nasopharynx through a posterolateral defect of the pharyngobasilar fascia called the sinus of Morgagni. Protection from tumor spread from the nasopharynx to the middle skull base and vice versa by the tough pharyngobasilar fascia is deficient at the sinus of Morgagni and at the foramen lacerum, even though fibrocartilage closes this foramen.[35]

The tensor veli palatini and levator veli palatini muscles reside in the nasopharynx. The torus tubarius is the prominent medial end of the cartilaginous eustachian tube, which together with the levator veli palatini muscle and the overlying mucosa forms a ridgelike protrusion into the nasopharynx.[33] The eustachian tube orifice is a mucosa-lined recess in front of the torus tubarius. The lateral pharyngeal recess or fossa of Rosenmüller is another mucosa-lined recess located posterosuperior to the torus tubarius. The fossa of Rosenmüller is an important site of origin of nasopharyngeal carcinoma and appears to be posterior to the eustachian tube orifice on axial images and superior on coronal images owing to the configuration of the torus tubarius.

The eustachian tube connects the middle ear to the nasopharynx (**Fig. 3.13**). The posterolateral bony portion begins along the anterior wall of the tympanic cavity and travels anteroinferomedially toward the nasopharynx and is seen just inferolateral to the prominent landmark of proximal petrous carotid canal in axial CT scan images. The bony portion of the tube continues as the cartilaginous portion at the sphenopetrosal groove, which is the gap between the posterior margin of the greater wing of sphenoid and the anterior margin of petrous temporal bone. The cartilaginous portion can be seen as a soft tissue density immediately posterior to the foramen ovale and foramen spinosum on axial CT scans and continues into the nasopharynx as described already. Mass lesions in the nasophar-

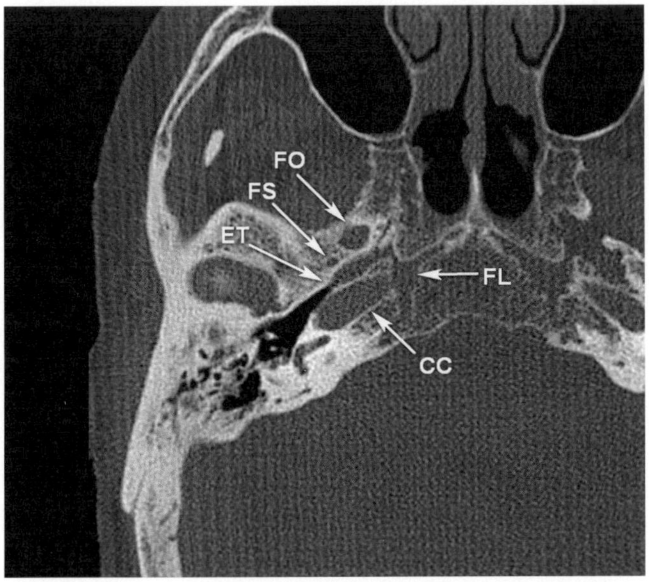

Fig. 3.13 Axial computed tomographic image through the skull base demonstrates the relationships between various foramina, fissures, and canals along the lateral margin of the central skull base region. The internal carotid artery passes obliquely through the carotid canal (CC) and exits the canal just above cartilage-filled gap, the foramen lacerum (FL). The eustachian tube (ET) consists of bony and cartilaginous segments and passes both medially and inferiorly from the middle ear to the nasopaharynx. Note the intimate relationship between the eustachian tube, the carotid canal and the foramen spinosum (FS).

ynx, especially those in the fossa of Rosenmüller, can compress the eustachian tube opening and lead to the development of middle ear and mastoid effusions. It is extremely important to evaluate for any nasopharyngeal mass lesion when unilateral middle ear or mastoid effusion is identified on a brain or paranasal sinus CT scan.

The retropharyngeal space (RPS) lies behind the pharynx, immediately posterior to the middle (visceral) layer of deep cervical fascia and anterior to deep (prevertebral) layer of deep cervical fascia. The nasopharyngeal RPS extends superiorly to the basiocciput and the thin horizontal alar fascia extending from the skull base to cervicothoracic region divides the space into an anterior true RPS and posterior danger space. Anywhere between the C6 and T4 level, the alar fascia fuses with the anterior middle (visceral) layer of the deep cervical fascia and terminates at the inferior extent of the true RPS; however, the posterior danger space continues inferiorly as a potential source of skull-base infection spread into the posterior mediastinum. The RPS harbors normal fat and retropharyngeal lymph nodes, especially laterally. The retropharyngeal lymph nodes (RPLNs) are divided into a lateral group that overlie the prevertebral fascia at the level of the upper cervical vertebral transverse processes and are more commonly involved by pathology especially from squamous cell carcinomas of the nasopharynx, oropharynx, hypopharynx, and nasal cavity and an inconsistent small medial group. It is important to note that only those nodes lying medial to the ICA and within 2 cm of the skull base are classified as RPLN on imaging-based classification. If a lymph node situated within 2 cm of the skull base lies anterior, lateral, or posterior to the carotid sheath, it is classified as a level II node. Nodes inferior to a level 2 cm below the skull base are not named RPLN.[36]

The prevertebral space (PVS), which lies immediately posterior to the RPS, is surrounded by the deep (prevertebral) layer of deep cervical fascia. In the suprahyoid neck, the PVS contains prevertebral muscles longus colli and capitis, vertebral body, cervical intervertebral disk, spinal canal, vertebral arteries, and the phrenic nerve. Specifically, at the nasopharyngeal level, the larger longus capitis and the smaller anterior rectus capitis muscles behind it reside in this location. Differentiation of PVS lesions from the anterior RPS and lateral carotid space lesions is sometimes challenging, especially if the lesions are large. Useful hints for imaging include the fact that a PVS abscess elevates the prevertebral muscles, whereas a RPS abscess does not. Likewise, bony erosion of adjacent anterior portion of vertebral body favors a PVS tumor like rhabdomyosarcoma, whereas erosion along the lateral aspect of a vertebra favors a carotid space tumor like neuroblastoma.[1,29]

References

1. Chapman PR, Bag AK, Tubbs RS, Gohlke P. Practical anatomy of the central skull base region. Semin Ultrasound CT MR 2013;34(5): 381–392
2. Borges A. Imaging of the central skull base. Neuroimaging Clin N Am 2009;19(3):441–468
3. Morani AC, Ramani NS, Wesolowski JR. Skull base, orbits, temporal bone, and cranial nerves: anatomy on MR imaging. Magn Reson Imaging Clin N Am 2011;19(3):439–456
4. Laine FJ, Nadel L, Braun IFCT. CT and MR imaging of the central skull base. Part 1: Techniques, embryologic development, and anatomy. Radiographics 1990;10(4):591–602
5. Laine FJ, Nadel L, Braun IFCT. CT and MR imaging of the central skull base. Part 2. Pathologic spectrum. Radiographics 1990;10(5): 797–821
6. Rhoton AL Jr. The sellar region. Neurosurgery 2002;51(4, Suppl) S335–S374
7. Unal B, Bademci G, Bilgili YK, Batay F, Avci E. Risky anatomic variations of sphenoid sinus for surgery. Surg Radiol Anat 2006;28(2): 195–201
8. Hamid O, El Fiky L, Hassan O, Kotb A, El Fiky S. Anatomic variations of the sphenoid sinus and their impact on trans-sphenoid pituitary surgery. Skull Base 2008;18(1):9–15
9. Vattoth S, Cherian J, Pandey T. Magnetic resonance angiographic demonstration of carotid-cavernous fistula using elliptical centric time resolved imaging of contrast kinetics (EC-TRICKS). Magn Reson Imaging 2007;25(8):1227–1231
10. Miyazaki Y, Yamamoto I, Shinozuka S, Sato O. Microsurgical anatomy of the cavernous sinus. Neurol Med Chir (Tokyo) 1994;34(3): 150–163
11. Cottier JP, Destrieux C, Brunereau L, et al. Cavernous sinus invasion by pituitary adenoma: MR imaging. Radiology 2000;215(2):463–469
12. Tubbs RS, Hill M, May WR, et al. Does the maxillary division of the trigeminal nerve traverse the cavernous sinus? An anatomical study and review of the literature. Surg Radiol Anat 2008;30(1):37–40
13. Hardjasudarma M, Edwards RL, Ganley JP, Aarstad RF. Magnetic resonance imaging features of Gradenigo's syndrome. Am J Otolaryngol 1995;16(4):247–250

14. Isolan GR, Krayenbühl N, de Oliveira E, Al-Mefty O. Microsurgical anatomy of the cavernous sinus: measurements of the triangles in and around it. Skull Base 2007;17(6):357–367
15. Bouthillier A, van Loveren HR, Keller JT. Segments of the internal carotid artery: a new classification. Neurosurgery 1996;38(3):425–433
16. Liu XD, Xu QW, Che XM, Mao RL. Anatomy of the petrosphenoidal and petrolingual ligaments at the petrous apex. Clin Anat 2009; 22(3):302–306
17. Chapman PR, Gaddamanugu S, Bag AK, Roth NT, Vattoth S. Vascular lesions of the central skull base region. Semin Ultrasound CT MR 2013;34(5):459–475
18. Tubbs RS, Hansasuta A, Loukas M, et al. Branches of the petrous and cavernous segments of the internal carotid artery. Clin Anat 2007;20(6):596–601
19. Hashimoto K, Nozaki K, Hashimoto N. Optic strut as a radiographic landmark in evaluating neck location of a paraclinoid aneurysm. Neurosurgery 2006;59(4):880–895, discussion 896–897
20. Watanabe Y, Nakazawa T, Yamada N, et al. Identification of the distal dural ring with use of fusion images with 3D-MR cisternography and MR angiography: application to paraclinoid aneurysms. AJNR Am J Neuroradiol 2009;30(4):845–850
21. Connor SE, Leung R, Natas S. Imaging of the petrous apex: a pictorial review. Br J Radiol 2008;81(965):427–435
22. Isaacson B, Kutz JW, Roland PS. Lesions of the petrous apex: diagnosis and management. Otolaryngol Clin North Am 2007;40(3): 479–519, viii
23. Razek AA, Huang BY. Lesions of the petrous apex: classification and findings at CT and MR imaging. Radiographics 2012;32(1):151–173
24. Balboni AL, Estenson TL, Reidenberg JS, Bergemann AD, Laitman JT. Assessing age-related ossification of the petro-occipital fissure: laying the foundation for understanding the clinicopathologies of the cranial base. Anat Rec A Discov Mol Cell Evol Biol 2005;282(1): 38–48
25. Woolfall P, Coulthard A. Pictorial review: Trigeminal nerve: anatomy and pathology. Br J Radiol 2001;74(881):458–467
26. Zhang J, Stringer MD. Ophthalmic and facial veins are not valveless. Clin Experiment Ophthalmol 2010;38(5):502–510
27. Daniels DL, Mark LP, Mafee MF, et al. Osseous anatomy of the orbital apex. AJNR Am J Neuroradiol 1995;16(9):1929–1935
28. Aviv RI, Casselman J. Orbital imaging: Part 1. Normal anatomy. Clin Radiol 2005;60(3):279–287
29. Vattoth S, Sullivan JC. Face and neck anatomy. In: Canon CL, ed. McGraw-Hill Specialty Board Review: Radiology. 1st ed. New York: McGraw-Hill; 2010:99–114
30. Daniels DL, Mark LP, Ulmer JL, et al. Osseous anatomy of the pterygopalatine fossa. AJNR Am J Neuroradiol 1998;19(8):1423–1432
31. Curtin HD, Williams R. Computed tomographic anatomy of the pterygopalatine fossa. Radiographics 1985;5(3):429–440
32. Harnsberger HR. Anterior skull base. In: Harnsberger HR, Osborn AG, Macdonald AJ, Ross JS AJ, eds. *Diagnostic and Surgical Imaging Anatomy: Brain, Head & Neck, Spine.* 1st ed. Philadelphia, PA, Amirsys; 2010:II26–II35
33. Siddiqui A, Connor SEJ. Imaging of the pharynx and larynx. Imaging 2007;19:83–103
34. Dubrulle F, Souillard R, Hermans R. Extension patterns of nasopharyngeal carcinoma. Eur Radiol 2007;17(10):2622–2630
35. Som PM, Curtin HD. Fascia and Spaces of the Neck. In: Som PM, Curtin HD, eds. *Head and Neck Imaging.* Vol 2. 3rd ed. St. Louis: Mosby; 2003:1805–1827
36. Som PM, Curtin HD, Mancuso AA. Imaging-based nodal classification for evaluation of neck metastatic adenopathy. AJR Am J Roentgenol 2000;174(3):837–844

4 Soft Tissue of the Scalp and Temporal Regions

Noriyuki Koga

Introduction

The scalp is the soft tissue covering the calvaria. It anatomically positioned in the cranial side of the line connecting the supraorbital border of the forehead, the frontal process of the zygomatic bone, the superior margin of the zygomatic arch, the external acoustic foramen, the mastoid process of the temporal bone, and the superior nuchal line of the occipital bone.[1] The major difference between the scalp and other skin in terms of appearance is that it has hair in almost all areas, excluding the forehead. In a cross-section, the scalp reveals a layered structure, usually divided into five layers, excluding the temporal region, as follows, from the outermost layer down: skin, subcutaneous fat (dense connective tissue), galea aponeurotica (aponeurotic layer), loose connective tissue; and pericranium (**Fig. 4.1**). Among these layers, the skin, subcutaneous tissue, and galea aponeurotica layer are closely connected, making it difficult to bluntly separate each layer. Therefore, these layers from the skin to galea aponeurotica are lumped together and also called the superficial fascial layer, whereas loose connective tissue is also called the deep fascial layer.[2]

Scalp (Skin) and Subcutaneous Fat Layer

The structure of the scalp is fundamentally similar to the skin in other regions; however, the dermis is thick compared with that in other parts of the body and is rich in blood vessels. Furthermore, it has an abundance of hair.

Subcutaneous tissue comprises an abundance of hair follicles and sweat glands. Moreover, there are many fibrous septa, similar to that of the palms of the hands and soles of the feet, closely connecting the skin and the galea aponeurotica layer. Therefore, subcutaneous fat is separated into small fat lobes by these fibrous septa. In this layer are many perforating arteries and veins heading to the skin from the main vascular network of the scalp inside the galea aponeurotica, along with the small sensory nerves transmitting cutaneous sensation.

Galea Aponeurotica

The galea aponeurotica is the intermediate aponeurosis of the occipitofrontalis muscle and is connected to the frontalis muscle at the front as well as to the occipitalis muscle at the rear (**Fig. 4.2**). The frontalis muscle originates from the galea aponeurotica and attaches to the dermis of the eyebrow after intersecting with the orbicularis oculi muscle and procerus muscle near the supraorbital border. Generally, frontalis muscles run obliquely downward superolaterally to inferomedially; therefore, there is a V-shaped area in the center of the forehead between the bilateral frontails muscles and the galea aponeurotica that extends to the front in this V-shaped part of the forehead. The occipitalis muscle originates from the highest nuchal line of the occipital bone, runs upward, and attaches to the galea aponeurotica. These frontalis and occipitalis muscles are both innervated by the facial nerve; the temporal branch innervates the frontalis muscle, and the occipitalis muscle is innervated by the posterior auricular nerve. It is the role of the frontalis muscle to lift the eyebrows, thereby forming horizontal wrinkles on the forehead. The occipitalis muscle has a role of pulling the galea aponeurotica and placing tension on the scalp; however, it is degenerative and weak, only having the effect of supporting the frontalis muscle. In the temporal region, the galea aponeurotica transitions to the superficial temporal fascia, which is a part of the superficial musculoaponeurotic system (SMAS).[3,4] The superficial temporal fascia contains the temporoparietal muscle and superior auricular muscle in the same plane. Major blood vessels of the scalp run in the galea aponeurotica layer and give off multiple branches toward the skin and subcutaneous fat layer. Therefore, massive bleeding is commonly observed when separating the galea aponeurotica and subcutaneous fat layer.

Loose Connective Tissue

This layer is also known as the subgaleal fascia and subaponeurotic plane (**Fig. 4.3**). It is found between the galea aponeurotica or pericranium, providing mobility to the scalp. It is approximately 1 to 3 mm thick and is grossly observed as a semitransparent, foamy layer. Chayen et al reported that this loose connective tissue layer is a three-layer structure comprising two loose areolar tissue layers and a dense fascial layer between two loose areolar tissue layers, an outer layer (loose areolar tissue), a dense fascial layer, and a deep layer (loose areolar tissue).[5] Although blood vessels are not grossly observed in this layer, it is macroscopically observed as layers having blood vessels. The blood circulation of this layer is supplied via two strains wherein the first is the perpendicular blood flow from the vascular plexus inside the galea aponeurotica layer using perforating vessels; the second is the blood flow by the blood vessel system directly flowing in from the main blood vessel of the scalp to the loose connective tissue layer, such as a superficial temporal artery, supraorbital artery, and supratrochlear artery. Using these blood circulations, it is used as a flap when very thin soft tissue flaps are required during auricular reconstruction and such procedures.[6]

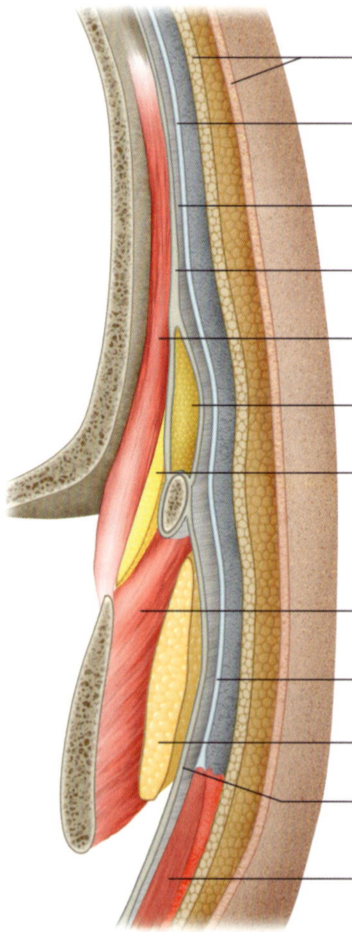

Fig. 4.1 The layers of the scalp. The scalp is divided into five layers from the surface down: skin (S), subcutaneous fat (dense connective tissue) (C), galea aponeurotica (A), loose connective tissue (L), and pericranium (P).

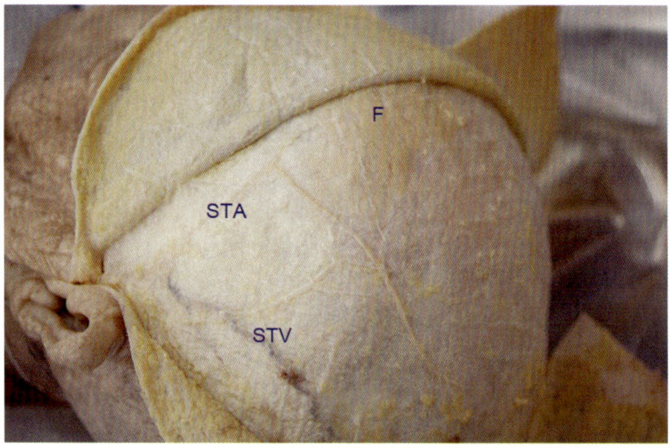

Fig. 4.2 Galea aponeurotica (cadaver dissection picture of the left superior view.) Left frontalis muscle, galea aponeurotica, and superficial temporal fascia are exposed. F, frontalis muscle; STA, superficial temporal artery; STV, superficial temporal vein.

Pericranium

This soft tissue layer is positioned in the deepest subcutaneous tissue. The pericranium of the head is continuous with the temporal fascia in the temporal region and is not observed underneath the temporalis muscle of the temporal fossa.

Blood Circulation Morphology of the Scalp

Regarding the arterial blood supply to the scalp, the supraorbital artery and supratrochlear artery, branching from the

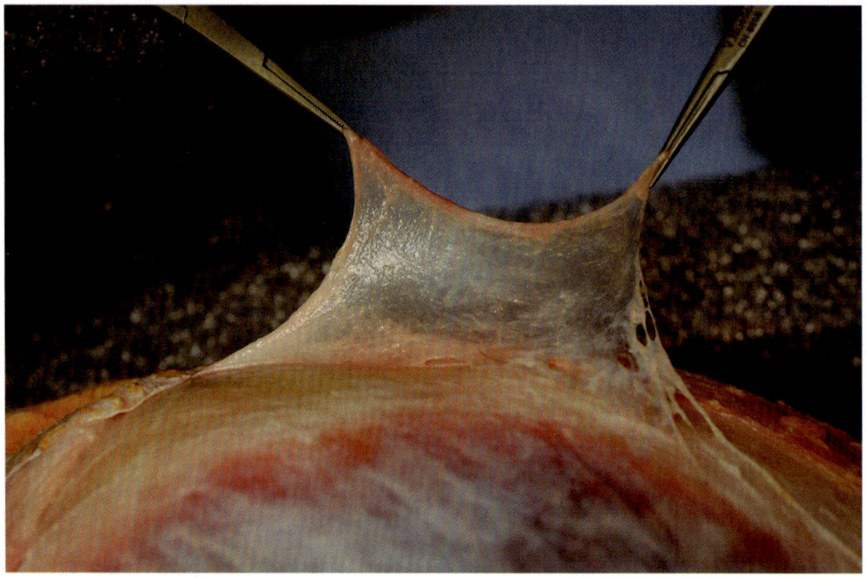

Fig. 4.3 Loose connective tissue layer (cadaver dissection picture).

Table 4.1 Blood circulation morphology of the scalp

Artery	Origin	Distribution
Supraorbital artery	Ophthalmic artery (a branch of the internal carotid artery)	Anterior part of the scalp
Supratrochlear artery	Ophthalmic artery (a branch of the internal carotid artery)	Anterior part of the scalp
Superficial temporal artery	External carotid artery	Lateral part of the scalp
Posterior auricular artery	External carotid artery	Posterior part of the scalp
Occipital artery	External carotid artery	Posterior part of the scalp

ophthalmic artery, supply blood flow to the anterior scalp; the superficial temporal artery, posterior auricular artery, and occipital artery, branching from the external carotid artery, supply blood flow to the lateral and posterior sides of the scalp, respectively (**Table 4.1**). These arteries are connected to each other in the parietal region, forming a dense vascular network. These blood vessels form the vascular plexus in the galea aponeurotica layer, thereby branching blood vessels vertically toward the superficial layer (that is, the subcutaneous fat layer) or deep layer (loose connective tissue layer and the pericranium). These main arteries of the scalp form the vascular plexus also in the loose connective tissue, and this vascular network connects with the perforator vessels from the network in the galea aponeurotica.

The veins mainly run parallel with the arteries, flowing into the internal jugular vein via veins with the same names as the arteries, that is, the supratrochlear vein, supraorbital vein, superficial temporal vein, posterior auricular vein, and occipital vein. The supratrochlear and supraorbital veins flow into the internal jugular vein via the facial vein; however, some flow inside the orbit toward the intracranial cavernous sinus. Moreover, the superficial temporal vein is connected to the superior sagittal sinus in the cranial cavity via the emissary vein passing through the parietal foramen. This vein causes sustained bleeding from the parietal bone during subperiosteal dissection in the parietal region.

Surgical Annotation

Scalp Flap

This skin flap is the first considered in cases requiring various reconstructions of the soft tissue defect in the head. Although known as a skin flap, it is actually raised underneath the galea aponeurotica. Although it is often fundamentally used as a random pattern flap, it may also be used as an axial pattern flap, including the main arteries distributing the scalp, such as the superficial temporal artery.

Frontal Musculopericranial Flap

The frontal musculopericranial flap is useful in the reconstruction of the anterior cranial base required after injury or tumor excision because it provides good blood circulation in addition to being strong but thin and flexible (**Fig. 4.4**). A periosteal flap in the frontal region is sometimes used for repairing anterior skull-base defects. When creating a large periosteal flap such as covering the entire anterior skull base, the blood circulation in the peripheral region of the flap often becomes unstable; then, in cases of large defects, the frontalis muscle flap should be raised with the periosteum.

Characteristics of the Layered Structures of Soft Tissue in the Temporal Region

The layered structures of the soft tissues in the temporal region is greatly different from the layered structures of other parts of the scalp. The following are the two main differences: (1) the temporalis muscle is in the deepest layer, and (2) the pericranium is not present underneath the temporalis muscle, and the pericranium of other parts of the head is continuous with the deep temporal fascia. From these differences, the layered structure of the temporal region is basically as follows, from the surface down: skin, subcutaneous tissue, superficial temporal fascia, subgaleal fascia (also called innominate fascia or loose areolar tissue layer), deep temporal fascia (divided into two layers inferiorly: the superficial layer and the deep layer), temporalis muscle, and subperiosteum (tissues below the pericranium).

The superficial temporal fascia is continuous with the galea aponeurotica layer in other parts of the head upward, in addition to being continuous with the SMAS in the face and continuous with the platysma in the neck.[3,4] The superficial temporal fascia layer anatomically has the superior auricular muscle, temporoparietal muscle, and so forth, which are mimetic muscles in relation to the auricle; however, these muscles are difficult to appreciate during surgery and to recognize as the fascia of the superficial layer.

The subgaleal fascial layer consists of a loose connective tissue covering the entire calvarial region, as well as the temporal region, and it has a role of supporting the mobility of the scalp. Blood circulation of this layer is rich in the temporal region as a result of the abundant axial blood supply from the superficial

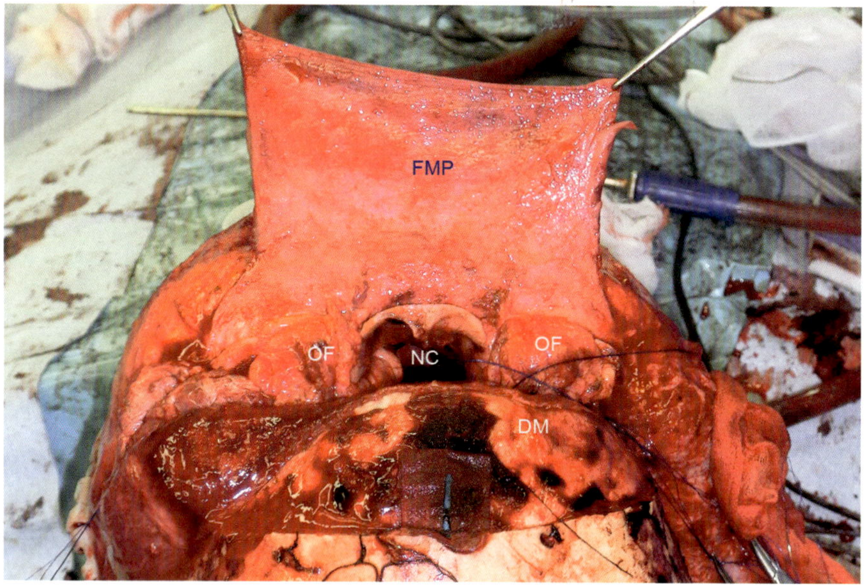

Fig. 4.4 Frontalis muscle-pericranial flap. A case of anterior skull base tumor. The anterior skull base reconstruction was performed by using the frontal musclopericranial flap. After frontal craniotomy and supraorbital bar osteotomy, the frontalis muscle-pericranial flaps were raised and transplanted to the anterior skull base tissue defect. FMP, frontalis muscle-pericranial flap; DM, dura mater; OF, orbital fat; NC, nasal cavity.

temporal artery. Thin fat tissue is observed between the subgaleal fascia layer and the deep temporal fascia. Regarding the structure of the layers around the suprazygomatic arch region, Moss et al reported a fibrous partition called the inferior temporal septum, which is located along a line connecting the external acoustic meatus and temporal ligamentous adhesion (near the forefront edge of the temporal line and the lateral margin of the orbit) and connecting to the deep temporal fascia and superficial temporal fascia. In addition to reporting that there is a triangular fibrofatty compartment on the caudal side, they found that the temporal branch of the facial nerve runs directly underneath the superficial temporal fascia in this fat tissue in the temporal region above the zygomatic arch.[7]

The deep temporal fascia is a fascia covering the temporalis muscle, which may be seen as a thick white-colored fascial layer. This layer is a single layer, the upper two-thirds, and it is continuous with the pericranium above the temporal line upward. It splits into two lobes: the superficial layer and deep layer downward above the zygomatic arch. Then these two layers of the deep temporal fascia are attached so as to cover the superficial and deep surfaces of the zygomatic arch (**Fig. 4.5**). The superficial temporal fat pad can be found in the space surrounded by these two layers of the deep temporal fascia and zygomatic arch. Opinions differ regarding the continuation of the temporal fascia to the pericranium. Casanova et al mentioned that the pericranium of the head transitions to a membrane of a thin connective tissue known as the innominate fascia, which is the layer between the layer underneath the galea aponeurotica and the temporal fascia.[8]

Beneath the deep temporal fascia, the deep temporal fat pad can be found, and this fat tissue is continuous with the buccal fat pad passing under the zygomatic arch. The aforementioned superficial temporal fat pad is bound fat tissue and does not continue to the deep temporal fat pad.[9]

The temporalis muscle can be found in the substratum of the deep temporal fascia. The temporalis muscle is a masticatory muscle; it arises from the infratemporal fossa and inserts into the coronoid process of the mandible (**Fig. 4.6**). The temporal fossa does not have periosteum as seen at the external skull base; therefore, the pericranium is not present on the underside of the temporalis muscle, this area being composed of thin, coarse connective tissue.

Blood Circulation Morphology of the Temporal Region

The superficial temporal artery, middle temporal artery, and deep temporal artery are mainly involved in blood circulation of the temporal region (**Table 4.2**). The superficial temporal artery is one of two terminal branches of the external carotid artery, which passes inside the parotid gland after the maxillary artery is separated below the neck of mandible, appearing from the deep part to the subcutaneous fat layer at the inferior border at the posterior end of the zygomatic arch and running toward the vertex perpendicularly in front of the auricle. The superficial temporal artery is distributed widely from the skin to the subgaleal layer. The middle temporal artery is a branch of the superficial temporal artery, which turns to the deeper layer and pierces the deep temporal fascia just after arising at the superior margin of the zygomatic arch, enters the deeper layer, and is

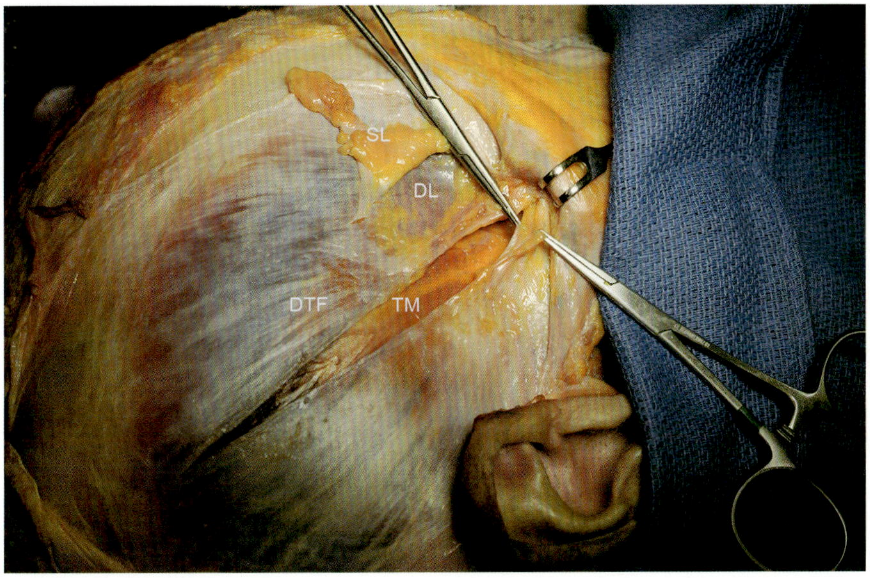

Fig. 4.5 Deep temporal fascia (cadaver dissection; right temporal region). Deep temporal fascia is cut, and the temporalis muscle is exposed. Each superficial and deep layer of the deep temporal fascia is held by Kocher forceps. The fat tissue between the superficial and deep layer of the deep temporal fascia is the superficial fat pad. DL, deep layer of the deep temporal fascia; DTF, deep temporal fascia; SL, superficial layer of the deep temporal fascia and superficial temporal fat pad; TM, temporalis muscle.

distributed mainly in the deep temporal fascia. Moreover, some branches of the middle temporal artery travel to the temporalis muscle and are distributed in the posterior region of the muscle. Usually, two branches arise from the maxillary artery and lead to the temporalis muscle. These are the posterior deep temporal artery and anterior deep temporal artery. These deep temporal arteries run on the surface of the superior head of the lateral pterygoid muscle after arising from the maxillary artery and enter the temporalis muscle on its deep surface, with the posterior deep temporal artery supplying the intermediate part of the temporalis muscle; the anterior deep temporal artery supplies the anterior part of the temporalis muscle. Three kinds of anastomoses between these arteries have been observed. Nakajima et al provide a detailed report.[10] These anastomoses include the following: (1) a connection between the vascular plexus of the superficial temporal artery branching from the skin to the superficial temporal fascia and the subgaleal vascular plexus via perforators, (2) a connection between the terminal branch of the middle temporal artery branching in the temporal fascia and vascular plexus inside the temporalis muscle, and (3) a connection near the temporal line between the vascular plexus of the lower layer of the galea aponeurotica and the vascular plexus inside the temporalis muscle over the temporal fascia. When forming the soft tissue flap of the temporal region,

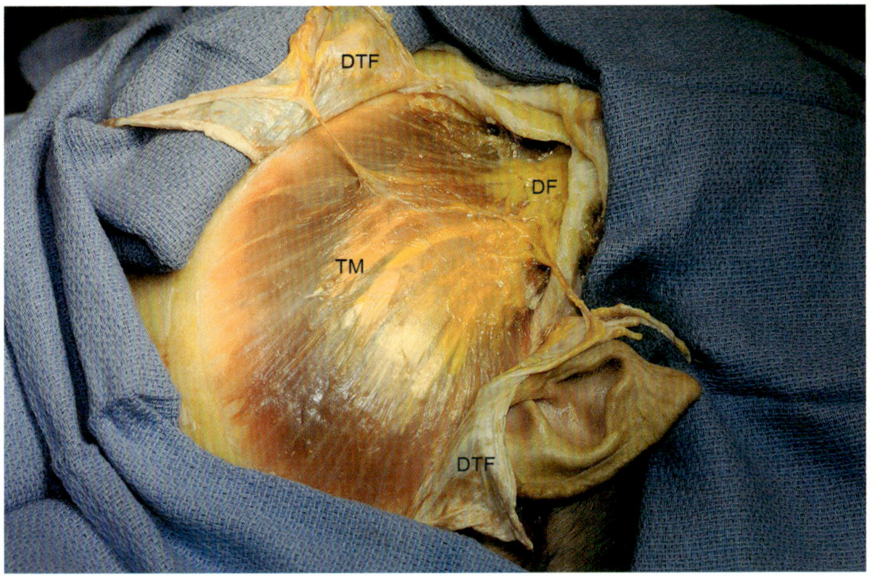

Fig. 4.6 Temporalis muscle (cadaver dissection; right temporal region). Deep temporal fascia was cut in the middle part and opened. The zygomatic arch was removed and the stump of the zygomatic bone can be seen. Deep temporal fat pad, which continues to the buccal fat pad, lies on the temporalis muscle. DF, deep temporal fat pad; DTF, deep temporal fascia; TM, temporal muscle.

Table 4.2 Blood circulation morphology of the temporal region

Artery	Origin	Distribution
Superficial temporal artery	One of the terminal branches of the external carotid artery	Skin to subgaleal layer
Middle temporal artery	A branch of the superficial temporal artery	Deep temporal fascia and posterior region of the temporalis muscle
Anterior deep temporal artery Posterior deep temporal artery	Branches of the maxillary artery	Anterior part of the temporalis muscle (anterior deep temporal artery) Intermediate part of the temporalis muscle (posterior deep temporal artery)

sufficient consideration is required regarding its blood circulation and the respective anastomoses.

Surgical Annotation

Superficial Temporal Fascial Flap (Temporoparietal Fascial Flap)

The superficial temporal fascial flap is a thin muscle flap with superficial temporal arteries as a vascular pedicle. These are used for vascularization when reconstructing the face, auricle, and dura mater and for the reconstructing the limbs as a free flap.[11,12]

Deep Temporal Fascial Flap

This fascial flap involves the middle temporal arteries as a vascular pedicle. It can be used not only as a single fascial flap but also as a bilobed flap or combined flap together with the superficial temporal fascial flap with the superficial temporal artery as a vascular pedicle.[13]

Temporalis Muscle-Pericranial Flap

This thin, flexible pericranial flap uses the temporalis muscle as the pedicle (**Fig. 4.7**). The vascular pedicle of this flap is the deep temporal arteries supplying the temporalis muscle. When creating the flap, the parietal pericranium and the loose connecting tissue layers are raised along with the temporalis muscle so as not to detach the temporalis muscle and the deep temporal fascia in an area that is about 2 cm wide from the temporal crest down because there is a vascular plexus connecting the temporalis muscle and subgaleal fascial layer. Therefore, blood flow from the deep temporal arteries can reach the pericranium in the midparietal region via this vascular network.[14] Creating the bilateral pericranial flaps becomes possible by dividing the pericranium at the midparietal region, which is used for reconstructing the anterior cranial base and middle cranial base of the skull.

Temporalis Muscle Flap

The temporalis muscle flap is usually used as a pedicle flap for dynamic reconstruction of the eyelids and the lip for facial palsy.[15,16]

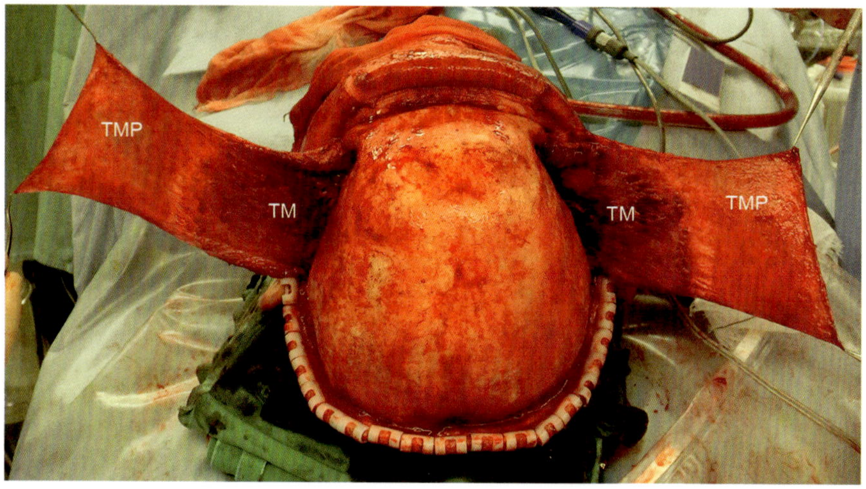

Fig. 4.7 Temporalis muscle-pericranial flap. Bilateral temporalis muscle-pericranial flap are raised after bicoronal skin incision. Bilateral pericranial flaps were raised with the temporalis muscles, and the deep temporal arteries, which supply the temporalis muscle, provide the blood circulation of this flap. TM, temporalis muscle; TMP, temporalis muscle-pericranial flap.

References

1. Tolhurst DE, Carstens MH, Greco RJ, Hurwitz DJ. The surgical anatomy of the scalp. Plast Reconstr Surg 1991;87(4):603–614
2. Tremolada C, Candiani P, Signorini M, Vigano M, Donati L. The surgical anatomy of the subcutaneous fascial system of the scalp. Ann Plast Surg 1994;32(1):8–14
3. Mitz V, Peyronie M. The superficial musculo-aponeurotic system (SMAS) in the parotid and cheek area. Plast Reconstr Surg 1976; 58(1):80–88
4. Stuzin JM, Baker TJ, Gordon HL. The relationship of the superficial and deep facial fascias: relevance to rhytidectomy and aging. Plast Reconstr Surg 1992;89(3):441–451
5. Chayen D, Nathan H. Anatomical observations on the subgaleotic fascia of the scalp. Acta Anat (Basel) 1974;87(3):427–432
6. Carstens MH, Greco RJ, Hurwitz DJ, Tolhurst DE. Clinical applications of the subgaleal fascia. Plast Reconstr Surg 1991;87(4):615–626
7. Moss CJ, Mendelson BC, Taylor GI. Surgical anatomy of the ligamentous attachments in the temple and periorbital regions. Plast Reconstr Surg 2000;105(4):1475–1498
8. Casanova R, Cavalcante D, Grotting JC, Vasconez LO, Psillakis JM. Anatomic basis for vascularized outer-table calvarial bone flaps. Plast Reconstr Surg 1986;78(3):300–308
9. Stuzin JM, Wagstrom L, Kawamoto HK, Baker TJ, Wolfe SA. The anatomy and clinical applications of the buccal fat pad. Plast Reconstr Surg 1990;85(1):29–37
10. Nakajima H, Imanishi N, Minabe T. The arterial anatomy of the temporal region and the vascular basis of various temporal flaps. Br J Plast Surg 1995;48(7):439–450
11. Brent B, Upton J, Acland RD, et al. Experience with the temporoparietal fascial free flap. Plast Reconstr Surg 1985;76(2):177–188
12. Tegtmeier RE, Gooding RA. The use of a fascial flap in ear reconstruction. Plast Reconstr Surg 1977;60(3):406–411
13. Hirase Y, Kojima T, Bang HH. Double-layered free temporal fascia flap as a two-layered tendon-gliding surface. Plast Reconstr Surg 1991;88(4):707–712
14. Kiyokawa K, Tai Y, Inoue Y, et al. Efficacy of temporal musculopericranial flap for reconstruction of the anterior base of the skull. Scand J Plast Reconstr Surg Hand Surg 2000;34(1):43–53
15. Gillies SH, Millard DR. The Principles and Art of Plastic Surgery. London: Butterworths; 1957
16. Frey M, Giovanoli P, Tzou CHJ, Kropf N, Friedl S. Dynamic reconstruction of eye closure by muscle transposition or functional muscle transplantation in facial palsy. Plast Reconstr Surg 2004; 114(4):865–875

5 Arterial Supply of the Facial Skin

Nobuaki Imanishi

Introduction

Arterial supply of the facial skin is chiefly provided by the facial and superficial temporal arteries and also by branches of the maxillary and ophthalmic arteries, which accompany the cutaneous branches of the trigeminal nerve. Branches from the source arteries run within the subcutaneous soft tissue and reach the dermis and then form the subdermal plexus. In this chapter, the detailed arterial vascularity of each region of the face on the basis of angiograms I have performed is described. Because the arterial supply of the face is substantial, necrosis of most local flaps here rarely occurs; however, knowledge of the arterial anatomy of the face is important when various local flaps of the face are elevated.

Arteries of the Facial Skin

The superficial temporal, facial, and ophthalmic arteries are three major source arteries of the facial skin. The superficial temporal artery gives off the transverse facial and zygomatico-orbital arteries and divides into the frontal and parietal branches. The facial artery gives off the submental, inferior labial, superior labial, and lateral nasal arteries and then becomes the angular artery. The ophthalmic artery gives off the supratrochlear, supraorbital, dorsal nasal, and medial and lateral palpebral arteries. The branches from the source arteries form an intimate vascular network in the face (**Fig. 5.1**). In addition, the infraorbital, zygomaticofacial, and mental arteries, which are derived from the maxillary artery, accompany cutaneous branches of the trigeminal nerve. The skin territories supplied by the zygomaticofacial and mental arteries are small and play only a supplemental role in the blood supply of the face.

Vasculature of Each Region of the Face

Forehead

Blood supply to the forehead is provided by the supratrochlear and supraorbital arteries and the frontal branch of the superficial temporal artery (**Fig. 5.2**). An intimate vascular plexus is formed by the arteries and their branches. The supratrochlear artery is dominant in the median forehead. The main trunk of the artery penetrates the orbital septum above the medial palpebral ligament and then ascends between the corrugator supercilii and orbicularis oculi muscles after sending vessels to the loose areolar tissue under the corrugator supercilii muscle.[1,2] It penetrates the frontalis muscle about 1 cm above the eyebrow and runs approximately a few centimeters just above the muscle to reach the subdermal plane (**Fig. 5.3**). During its course, small vessels branch off toward the dermis and frontalis muscle. The supratrochlear artery does not travel far into the frontalis muscle. The forehead flap originally included the frontalis muscle, but from the point of view of arterial anatomy, it is not essential to include the muscle itself. Therefore, the forehead flap is not a musculocutaneous flap but rather a fasciocutaneous flap.

Upper Eyelid

Blood supply of the upper eyelid is provided by four arterial arcades—the marginal, peripheral, superficial orbital, and deep orbital arcades—and by ascending and descending branches from these arcades[3] (**Fig. 5.4, Fig. 5.5**). Among these arcades, the marginal one along the margin of the upper eyelid and the peripheral one along the upper margin of the tarsus are formed by vascular anastomoses of medial and lateral palpebral arteries from the ophthalmic artery.

The marginal arcade runs along the front lower edge of the tarsus, giving off branches that ascend on the anterior and posterior surfaces of the orbicularis oculi muscle and tarsus. Among these ascending branches, the arteries on the anterior surface of the orbicularis oculi muscle and on the posterior surface of the tarsus pass under the lower margin of the muscle and tarsus. From the ascending branches, additional small vessels reach the skin, orbicularis oculi muscles, and tarsus. The margin of the eyelid is also supplied by small direct vessels from the marginal arcade.

The peripheral arcade runs along the attachment of Müller's muscle to the tarsus, giving off branches that descend on the anterior and posterior surfaces of the tarsus. These descending branches communicate with the ascending branches from the marginal arcade.

The superficial and deep orbital arcades run on the anterior and posterior surfaces of the orbicularis oculi muscle along the superior margin of the orbit. The main blood supply of the ar-

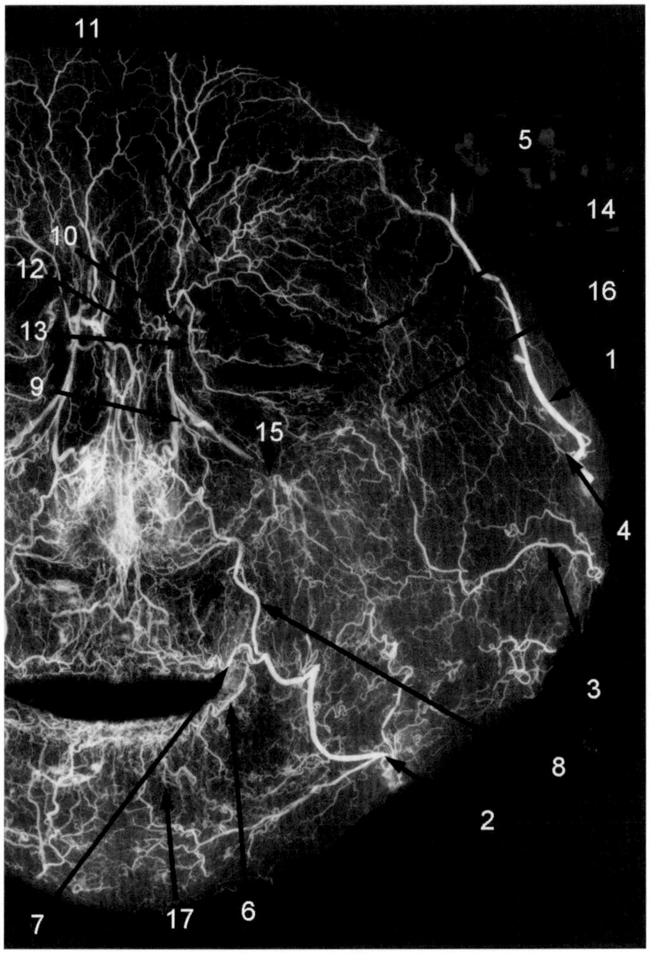

Fig. 5.1 Angiogram of the face. (1) Superficial temporal artery. (2) Facial artery. (3) Transverse facial artery. (4) Zygomatico-orbital artery. (5) Frontal branch. (6) Inferior labial artery. (7) Superior labial artery. (8) Lateral nasal artery. (9) Angular artery. (10) Supratrochlear artery. (11) Supraorbital artery. (12) Dorsal nasal artery. (13) Medial palpebral artery. (14) Lateral palpebral artery. (15) Infraorbital artery. (16) Zygomaticofacial artery. (17) Mental artery.

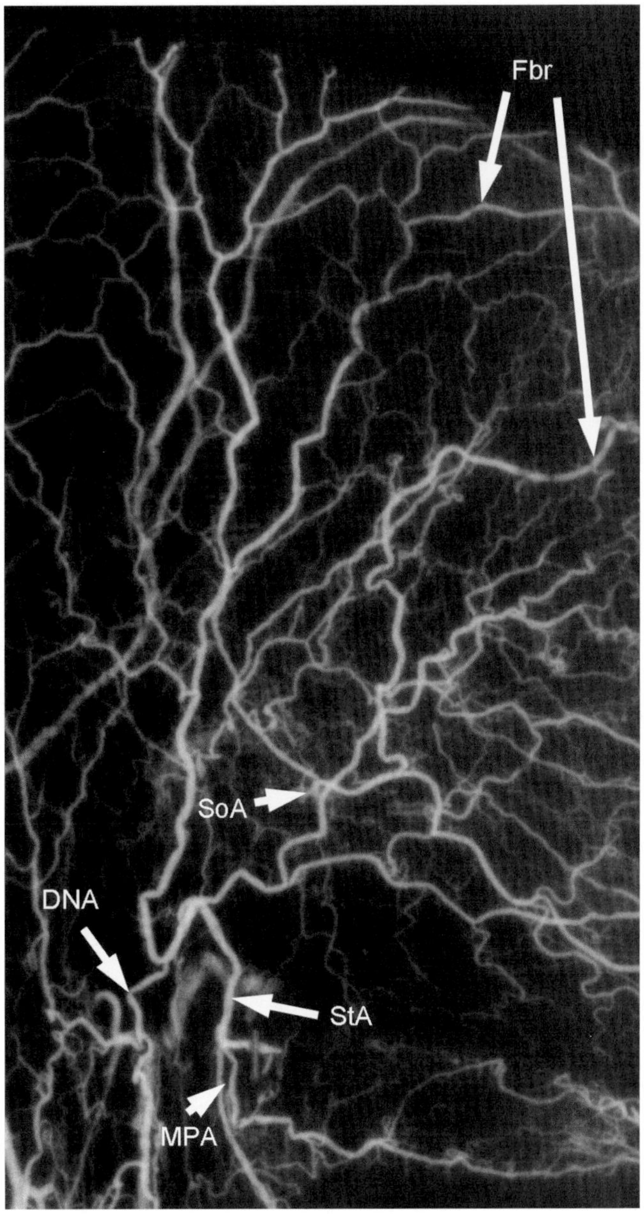

Fig. 5.2 Angiogram of the left forehead. Enlarged image of **Fig. 5.1**. DNA, dorsal palpebral artery; Fbr, frontal branch of the superficial temporal artery; MPA, medial palpebral artery; SoA, supraorbital artery; StA, supratrochlear artery.

cades is provided by the supratrochlear artery. The supraorbital and medial palpebral arteries on the medial side of the orbit and the zygomatico-orbital, transverse facial, and superficial temporal arteries on the lateral side participate in forming the superficial and deep orbital arcades. Descending vessels from the superficial orbital arcade on the anterior surface of the orbicularis oculi muscle and from the deep orbital arcade on the posterior of the muscle anastomose with the ascending branches of the marginal arcade.

Because the blood supply to the skin depends basically on the superficial orbital and marginal arcades and their connecting vessels, it is necessary for a local flap on the upper eyelid to be elevated just above the orbicularis oculi muscle, thereby preserving those vessels. There are no major arteries within the orbicularis oculi muscle, and blood supply of the muscle is provided by small branches from the ascending and descending vessels on the anterior and posterior surfaces of the muscle. In the case of a musculocutaneous flap, such as a V–Y advancement

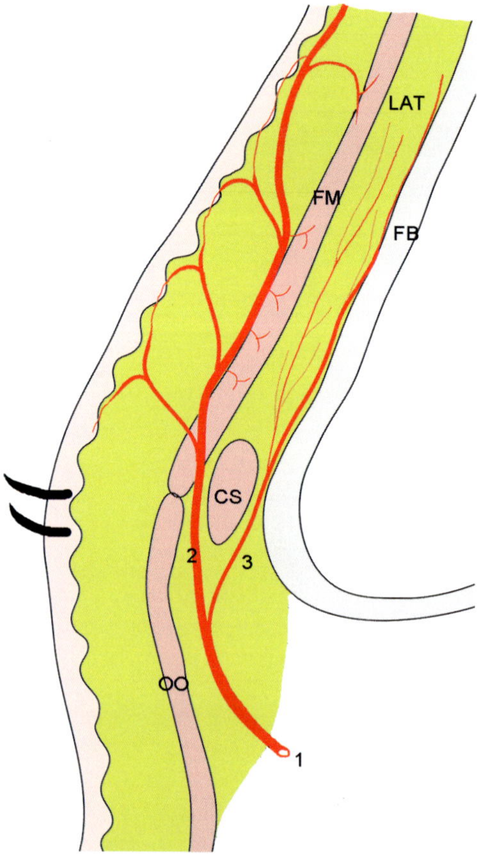

Fig. 5.3 Schematic sagittal section showing the course of the supratrochlear artery. (1) Supratrochlear artery. (2) Main trunk ascending between the corrugator supercilii and orbicularis oculi muscles. (3) Branch to the loose areolar tissue. CS, corrugator supercilii muscle; FB, frontal bone; FM, frontalis muscle; LAT, loose areolar tissue; OO, orbicularis oculi muscle.

flap, its blood supply depends on the deep orbital and marginal arcades and their connecting vessels. Accordingly, surgical operations must not extend behind the orbicularis oculi muscle.

Nose and Upper Lip

The facial artery gives off the superior labial artery about at the angle of mouth and becomes the angular artery toward the medial canthus.[4] In 12% of our cases, the peripheral portion of the facial artery can certainly be recognized as the angular artery with a slight decrease in its diameter.[5] In 88%, the facial artery ends at the alar base, and the terminal portion of the facial artery toward the alar base is called the lateral nasal artery (**Fig. 5.6**). In these cases, a thin vessel or a vascular plexus connects the lateral nasal artery with vessels from the supratrochlear artery near the medial canthus.

The lateral nasal artery divides into two vessels surrounding the alar base. One is called the inferior alar branch, and it runs toward the columella along the lower margin of the nostril, supplying blood to the alar base and nostril floor. A few branches travel toward the upper lip from the inferior alar branch. The other vessel is called the superior alar branch, which ascends along the lateral side of the alar, giving off branches to the lateral portion of the alar, nasal tip, and dorsum of the nose.

The superior labial artery runs between the labial mucosa and orbicularis oris muscle at the level of the upper margin of the red lip. The superior labial artery does not always consist of one vessel; in 35% of cases, it consists of two vessels. This artery runs medially, giving off ascending branches at both sides of the labial mucosa and skin, and then it anastomoses with the contralateral artery of the same name.

The ascending vessels toward the cutaneous side penetrate the orbicularis oris muscle at the level of the upper margin of the red lip and give off branches to the red lip, skin, and orbicu-

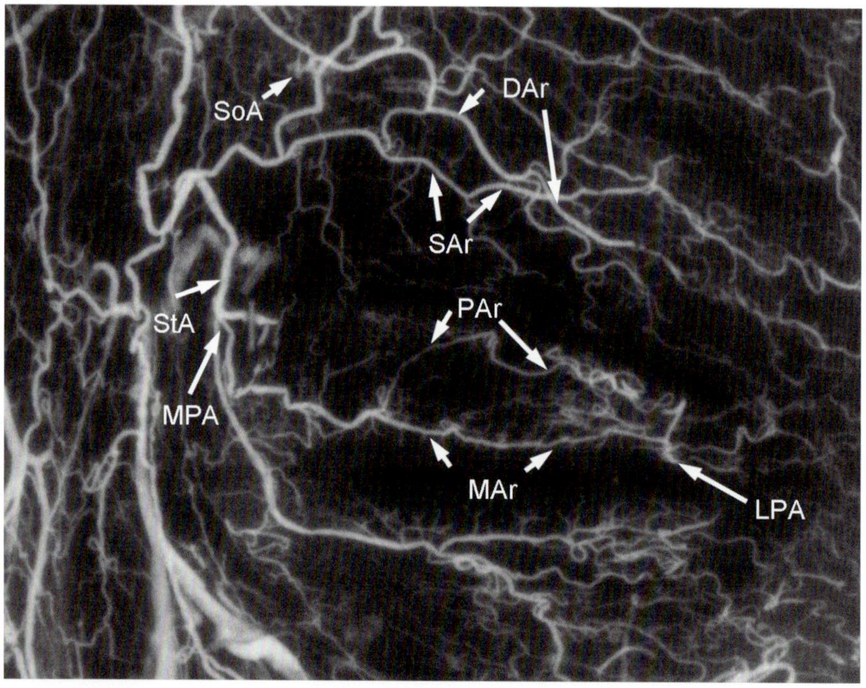

Fig. 5.4 Angiogram of the left eyelid; enlarged image of **Fig. 5.1**. DAR, deep orbital arcade; LPA, lateral palpebral artery; MAr. marginal arcade; MPA, medial palpebral artery; PAr. peripheral arcade. SAr, superficial orbital arcade; SoA, supraorbital artery; StA. supratrochlear artery.

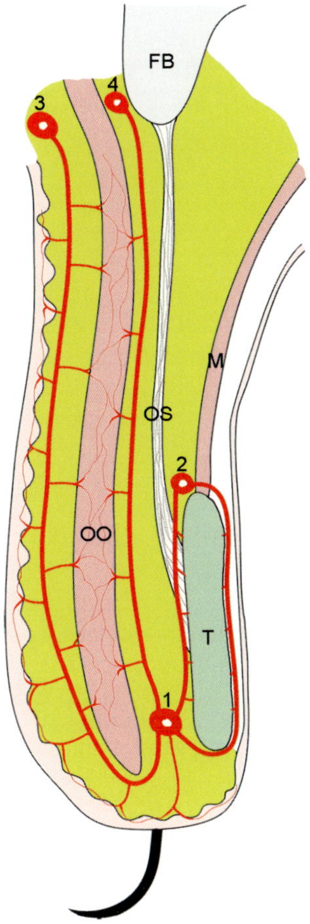

Fig. 5.5 Schematic sagittal section through the upper eyelid (1) marginal arcade. (2) peripheral arcade. (3) Superficial orbital arcade. (4) Deep orbital arcade. FB, frontal bone; M, Müller's muscle; OO, orbicularis oculi; OS, orbital septum; T, tarsus.

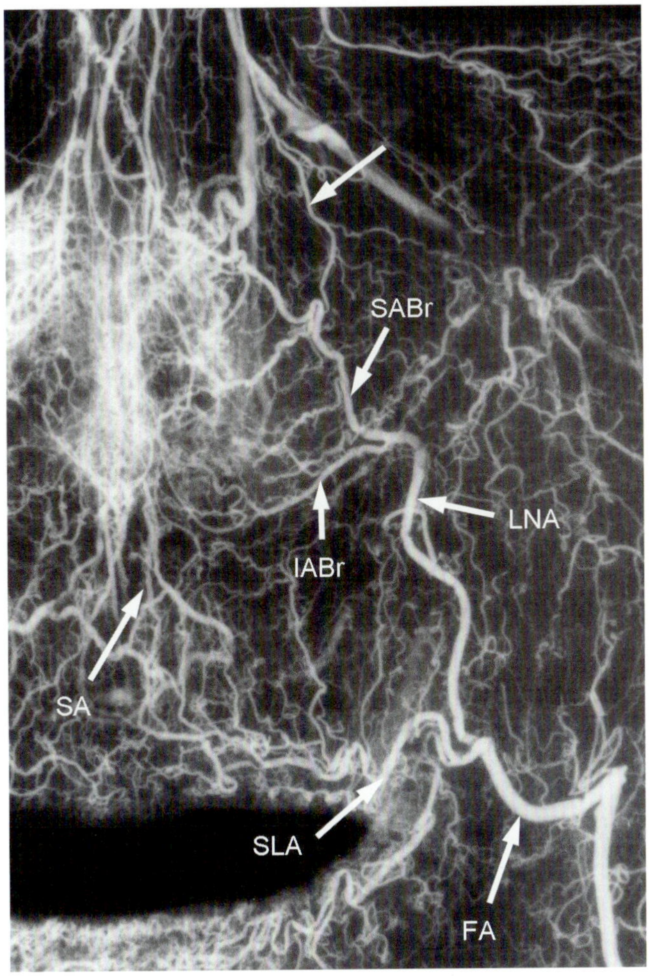

Fig. 5.6 Angiogram of the left upper lip and nose. Enlarged image of **Fig. 5.1**. FA. facial artery; IABr, inferior alar branch; LNA, lateral nasal artery; SA, septal artery; SABr, superior alar branch; SLA, superior labial artery. Artery: a thin vessel toward the medial canthus.

laris oris muscle (**Fig. 5.7**). A few vessels at the philtrum among the ascending vessels are sometimes large and are called the septal arteries. The ascending vessels at the mucosal side give off braches to both the orbicularis oris muscle and labial mucosa. At the base of the columella, the ascending vessels from both sides of the superior labial artery and the terminal portion of the inferior alar branch from the lateral nasal artery anastomose with each other and form a vascular network. At the columella base are two kinds of vessels from the vascular network that ascend toward the nasal tip. One is an artery that ascends within the columella and reaches vascular network at the nasal tip. The other is an artery that enters into the nasal septum and ascends along the anterior margin of the nasal septal cartilage. This artery also reaches the nasal tip vascular network through a small opening among the alar and lateral nasal cartilages. This artery gives off branches in both anterior and posterior directions. The anterior branches reach the medial crus of the alar cartilage and columella between the medial crura. The posterior branches reach the nasal septal cartilage. The vasculature of the skin of the upper lip and muscle is similar to that of the upper eyelid (**Fig. 5.3**).

Cheek

From the point of view of arterial anatomy, the cheek is roughly a region surrounded by the facial and superficial temporal arteries. Therefore, the blood supply of the cheek is chiefly provided by branches of the facial artery, transverse facial artery, and zygomatico-orbital artery (**Fig. 5.8**). A complementary relationship can be seen among these arteries. For example, when the zygomatico-orbital artery is small, the transverse facial artery is enlarged (**Fig. 5.1**). In addition, there are infraorbital and zygomaticofacial arteries. The zygomaticofacial artery plays the role of a supplementary blood supply.

A subdermal plexus is vessels in both the dermis and subdermal plane.[6] The subdermal plexus is not always random, but its vascular pattern shows some axiality.[7] In the nasolabial fold and its neighboring area, small branches from the facial or lateral nasal arteries ascend vertically.[8] The skin territory of each branch is also small (**Fig. 5.9**). Accordingly, a V-Y advancement flap on the nasolabial fold is suitable based on the vasculature by the small vertical vessels; however, branches of the transverse facial and zygomatico-orbital arteries and the proximal

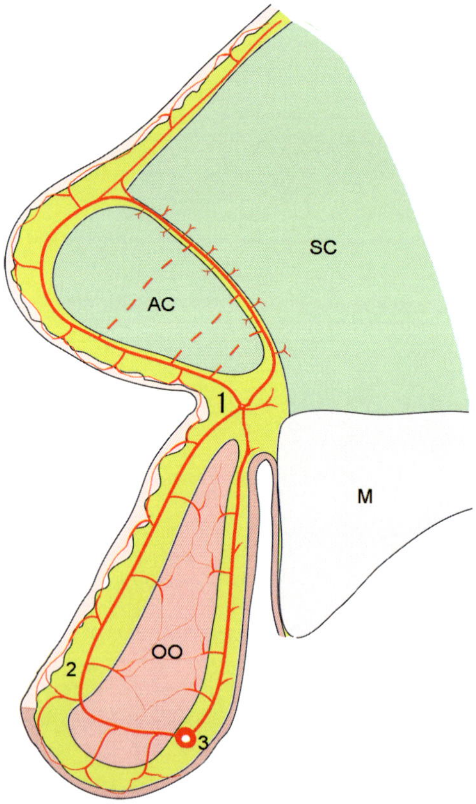

Fig. 5.7 Schematic sagittal section through the upper lip and nose. (1) Terminal portion of the inferior alar branch. (2) Septal nasal artery. (3) Superior labial artery. AC, medial crus of alar cartilage; M. maxilla; OO. orbicularis oris muscle; SC, septal cartilage.

portion of the facial artery are comparatively large, and vascular continuity by these branches is apparent. In this region, the subdermal plexus runs axially. In the infraorbital region, the infraorbital artery radiates just after passing through the infraorbital foramen, but the skin territory supplied by each branch is small.

Lower Lip

The blood supply of the lower lip is provided by the facial and submental arteries. There are two kinds of branches from the facial artery. One is the inferior labial artery, and the other is a branch that travels horizontally at a level between the lower lip and mentum.[9] In addition, ascending branches from the submental artery take part in this blood supply (**Fig. 5.10**).

The inferior labial artery is derived from the facial artery at the lower margin of the mandible in 67% of cases and at the corner of the mouth in 25%. It is sometimes derived from the superior labial artery in 8%. The inferior labial artery runs between the orbicularis oris and buccinator muscles and then reaches the lower lip. It passes transversely between the orbicularis oris muscle and labial mucosa at the level of the boundary of the red and white parts of the lips giving off descending branches at both sides of the skin and labial mucosa (**Fig. 5.11**). The descending branches of the cutaneous side cross over the upper margin of the orbicularis oris muscle or penetrate the muscle and descend, giving off small vessels to the skin and muscle. The descending branches of the mucosal side also give off small vessels to the muscle and mucosa.

The horizontal branch at the level between the lower lip and mentum is derived from the facial artery and arises at the lower

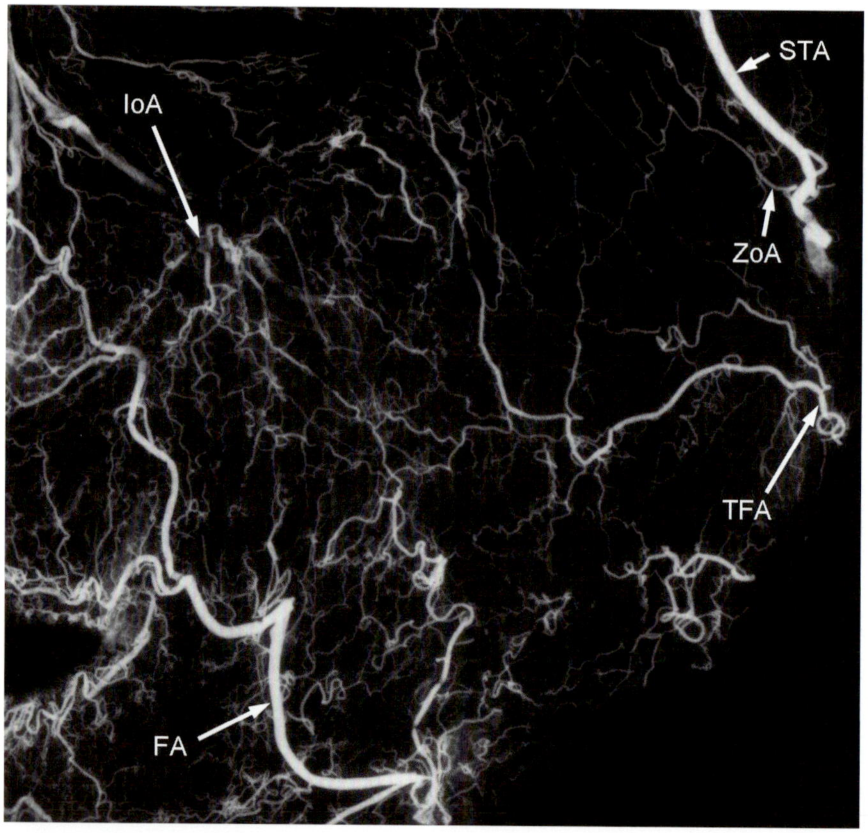

Fig. 5.8 Angiogram of the left cheek. Enlarged image of **Fig. 5.1**. FA, facial artery; IoA, infraorbital artery; STA, superficial temporal artery; TFA, transverse facial artery; ZoA, zygomatico-orbital artery.

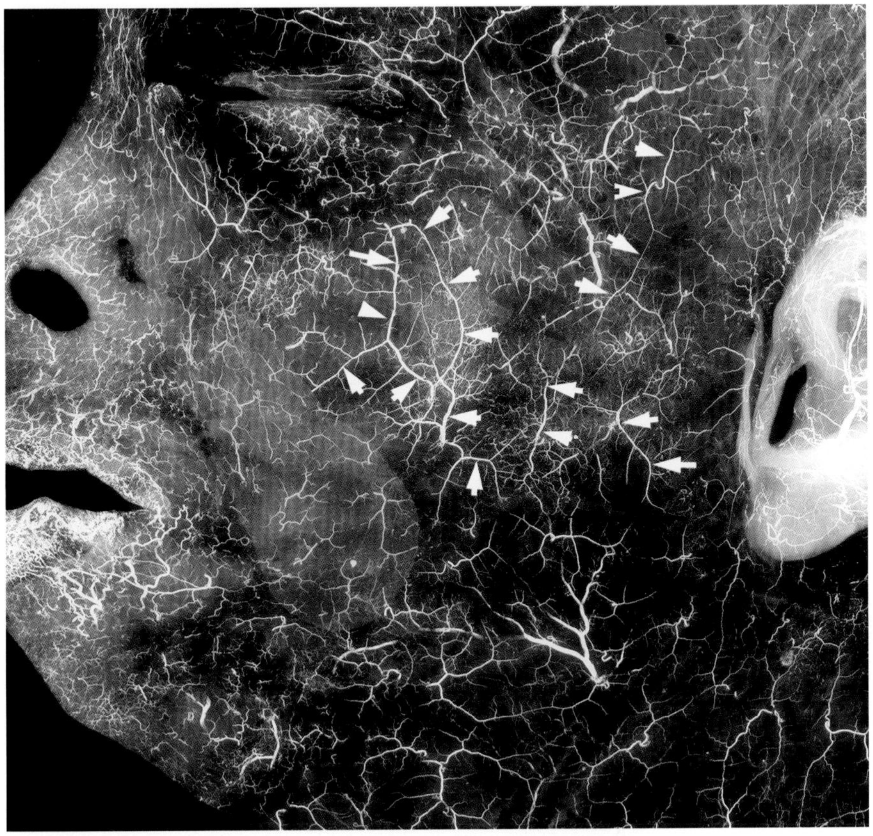

Fig. 5.9 Subdermal plexus of the cheek Angiogram shows the subdermal plexus of the cheek region. There are comparatively small vessels from the facial or lateral nasal arteries in the green area. Each small artery that enters the subdermal plane has a small skin territory. In other cheek regions, vessels that enter the subdermal plane are comparatively large, and their vascular continuity (*arrows*) is good.

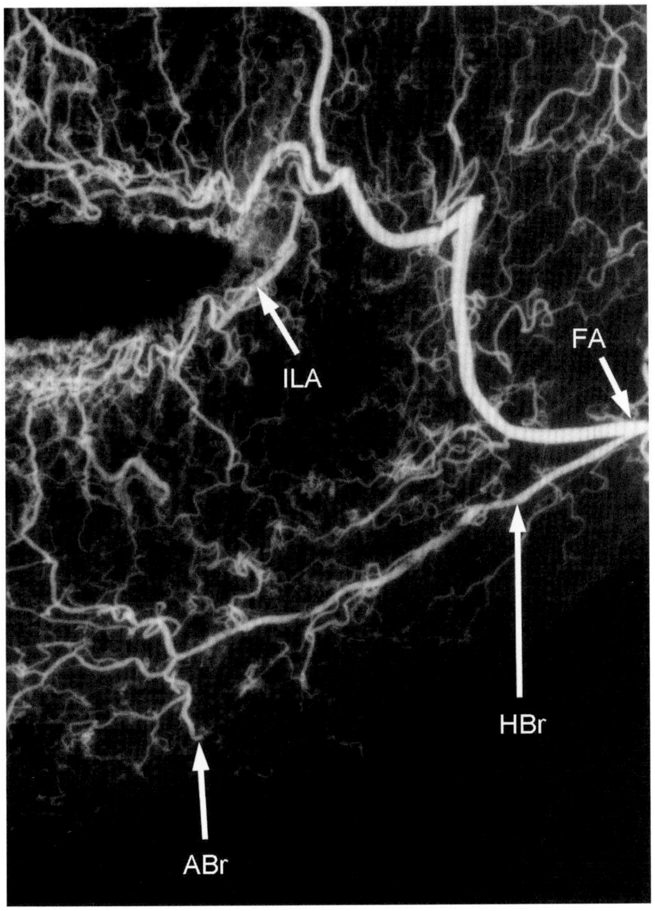

Fig. 5.10 Angiogram of the left lower lip. Enlarged image of **Fig. 5.1**. ABr, ascending branch from the submental artery; FA, facial artery; Hbr, horizontal branch at the level between the lower lip and mentum; ILA, inferior labial artery.

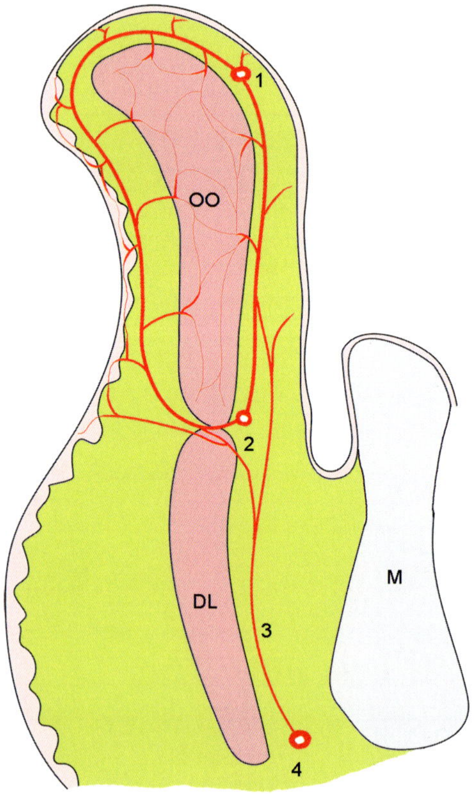

Fig. 5.11 Schematic sagittal section through the lower lip. (1) Inferior labial artery. (2) Horizontal branch at the level between the lower lip and mentum. (3) Ascending branch from the submental artery. (4) Submental artery. DL, depressor labii inferioris muscle; M, mandible; OO, orbicularis oris muscle.

margin of the mandible. The artery runs on the mucosal side between the orbicularis oris and depressor labii inferioris muscles. In 50% of cases, it anastomoses with the artery of the same name on the contralateral side without decreasing its diameter. In 33% of cases, its diameter decreases gradually, and it is not identified in the middle of the lower lip. In 17% of cases, its pathway changes from a horizontal direction to a vertical direction and it anastomoses with branches of the inferior labial artery. The artery is larger than the inferior labial artery in 50% of cases. The artery gives off ascending branches on both sides of the skin and labial mucosa behind the inferior margin of the orbicularis oris muscle. The ascending branches anastomose with the descending branches of the inferior labial artery. Ascending arteries from the mentum to the lower lip arise from the submental artery. At the beginning of their pathways, they run behind the depressor labii inferioris muscle. They bifurcate when they ascend near the orbicularis oris muscle. The bifurcating branches anastomose with the ascending branches from the horizontal branch of the facial artery. Blood supply of the lower lip and mentum is provided by not only the three dominant vessels, as mentioned, but also by direct branches from the facial artery and mental artery. Blood supply by the mental artery is only supplemental.

References

1. Nakajima H, Imanishi N. Nasal reconstruction by the median forehead flap. In: Ogawa Y, ed. *Facial Reconstruction by Various Local Flaps: Recent Advancement*. 1st ed. Tokyo: Kokuseidou Co.; 2000:93 (in Japanese)
2. Kishi K, Imanishi N, Shimizu Y, Shimizu R, Okabe K, Nakajima H. Alternative 1-step nasal reconstruction technique. Arch Facial Plast Surg 2012;14(2):116–121
3. Kawai K, Imanishi N, Nakajima H, Aiso S, Kakibuchi M, Hosokawa K. Arterial anatomical features of the upper palpebra. Plast Reconstr Surg 2004;113(2):479–484
4. Barry KB. Face and scalp. In: Standring S, ed. Gray's Anatomy, 40th ed. Edinburgh: Churchill Livingstone/Elsevier; 2008:467.
5. Nakajima H, Imanishi N, Aiso S. Facial artery in the upper lip and nose: anatomy and a clinical application. Plast Reconstr Surg 2002; 109(3):855–863
6. Imanishi N, Nakajima H, Minabe T, Aiso S. Angiographic study of the subdermal plexus: a preliminary report. Scand J Plast Reconstr Surg Hand Surg 2000;34(2):113–116
7. Chang H. Arterial anatomy of subdermal plexus of the face. Keio J Med 2001;50(1):31–34
8. Imanishi N. Arterial anatomy of the nasolabial flap. Jpn J Plast Surg 2014;57(3):223–230 (in Japanese)
9. Kawai K, Imanishi N, Nakajima H, Aiso S, Kakibuchi M, Hosokawa K. Arterial anatomy of the lower lip. Scand J Plast Reconstr Surg Hand Surg 2004;38(3):135–139

6 Arteries of the Face and Neck

Yelda Atamaz Pinar, Figen Govsa, and Servet Celik

Introduction

Safe and effective reconstructive surgical procedures rely on a clear knowledge of facial and neck arterial anatomy. Cadaveric angiographic and dissection studies have demonstrated that the external and internal carotids are the main arterial sources for the head and neck regions.

The skin and soft tissue of the face receive their arterial supply from the branches of the facial, maxillary, and superficial temporal arteries, all of which are branches of the external carotid. The exception is a masklike area that includes the central forehead, the eyelids, and the upper part of the nose and is supplied via the internal carotid artery system via the ophthalmic arteries. The ophthalmic artery gives off branches to the face, including the lacrimal, supraorbital, supratrochlear, dorsal nasal, and external nasal arteries.

Because there are communications between the external and internal carotid artery systems around the eye, external nose, and forehead through several anastomoses, knowledge of the arterial territories is important in flap anatomy. Most flaps are based on vascularization of the arteries, and anatomical variations must be considered when individual flaps are planned for patients. To elevate an arterial flap safely, routine use of a Doppler probe preoperatively and intraoperatively is recommended.

The primary arterial territories of the head and the neck have been defined by mapping their three-dimensional territories in the skin, the deep soft tissues, and the bones.[1–3] The external carotid artery supplies the exterior of the head, the face, and much of the neck. The internal carotid artery supplies the central face, which contains the eyes, the upper two-thirds of the nose, and the central forehead[4] (**Fig. 6.1, Fig. 6.2, Fig. 6.3**).

There is a rich anastomotic network between the branches of the internal carotid and ophthalmic artery systems (supraorbital or supratrochlear vessels) (**Fig. 6.4a**) and the angular artery and superficial temporal artery via the transverse facial artery to the facial artery (**Fig. 6.4b**). There are also multiple anastomoses between the facial and maxillary artery territories via the infraorbital and mental arteries (**Fig. 6.4c**).[3,5]

Reconstruction methods for facial defects include skin grafts, local flaps, pedicled flaps, and microvascular tissue transfers[6]; however, remote tissues do not provide ideal tissue contour, thickness, texture, or shape for the facial structures; hence, they often require multiple revisions and result in donor-site morbidity.[1,7] Muscles and other tissues have a vital role because they provide anastomotic networks for preventing vascular compromise.

The many changes undergone by embryonic arteries, such as regression or reappearance, can result in variations of the origin points, the courses, and the anastomotic features of the vessels. Arterial variations can be explained by the persistence of channels that normally disappear or by the disappearance of normally persisting vessels. These anatomical variations arising from embryologic development can be significant.[8,9] Doppler ultrasound helps to define arterial features and provides information about backflow and the potential for reverse flow in the artery.[7,10]

External Carotid Artery

The cervical part of the common carotid is usually divided into the external and the internal carotid arteries at the level of the upper border of the thyroid cartilage. The carotid bifurcation is located 13.2 ± 5.6 mm below the tip of the greater horn of the hyoid bone. The external carotid artery is covered by skin, superficial fascia, platysma, deep fascia, and the anterior margin of the sternocleidomastoid muscle. It begins by taking a slightly curved course and then passes upward and forward.[11] After branching on its anterior (superior thyroid, lingual, facial arteries) and posterior (ascending pharyngeal, occipital, posterior auricular arteries) sides, the artery inclines backward to the space behind the neck of the mandible, where it is divided into its terminal branches, the superficial temporal and maxillary arteries (**Fig. 6.1, Fig. 6.2**).

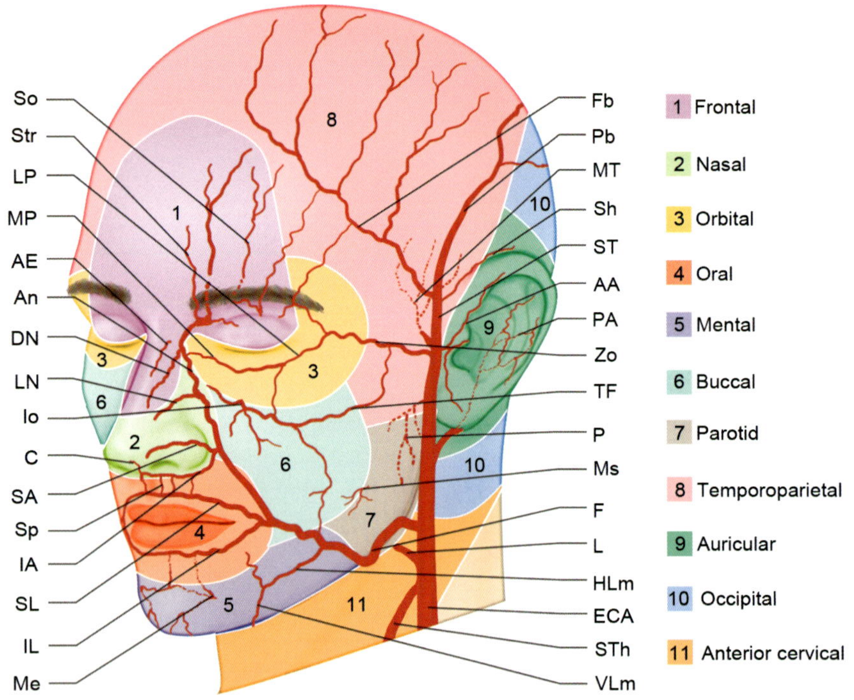

Fig. 6.1 The superficial arteries of the head and neck regions in anterolateral oblique view. Regions: Arterial territories include (1) frontal: Str, So, MP (O territory); (2) nasal: DN, AE, An (F-O territory); (3) orbital: MP, LP, Io (O-Max-Zo territory); (4) oral: SL, IL (F territory); (5) mental: Me, IL (Max-F territory); (6) buccal: Io, TF (Mx-ST territory); (7) parotid: TF, Ms (ST territory); (8) temporoparietal: Fb, Pb, MT (ST territory); (9) auricular: AA, PA (ST-ECA territory); (10) occipital: O (ECA territory); (11) anterior cervical: STh (ECA territory). AA, anterior auricular artery, AE: anterior ethmoidal artery; An, angular artery; C, columellar artery; DN, dorsal nasal artery; ECA, external carotid artery; F, facial artery; Fb, frontal branch of the superficial temporal artery; HLm, horizontal labiomental artery; IA, inferior alar artery; IL, inferior labial artery; Io, infraorbital artery; MP, medial palpebral artery; Ms, masseteric artery; Me, mental artery; Mx, maxillary artery; MT, middle temporal artery; L, lingual artery; LN, lateral nasal artery; LP, lateral palpebral artery; P, parotid branch; PA, posterior auricular artery; Pb, parietal branch of the superficial temporal artery; SA, superior alar artery; Sh, suprahelical artery; SL, superior labial artery; So, supraorbital artery; Sp, septal artery; ST, superficial temporal artery; STh, superior thyroid artery; Str, supratrochlear artery; TF, transverse facial artery; VLm, vertical labiomental artery; Zo, zygomatico-orbital artery.

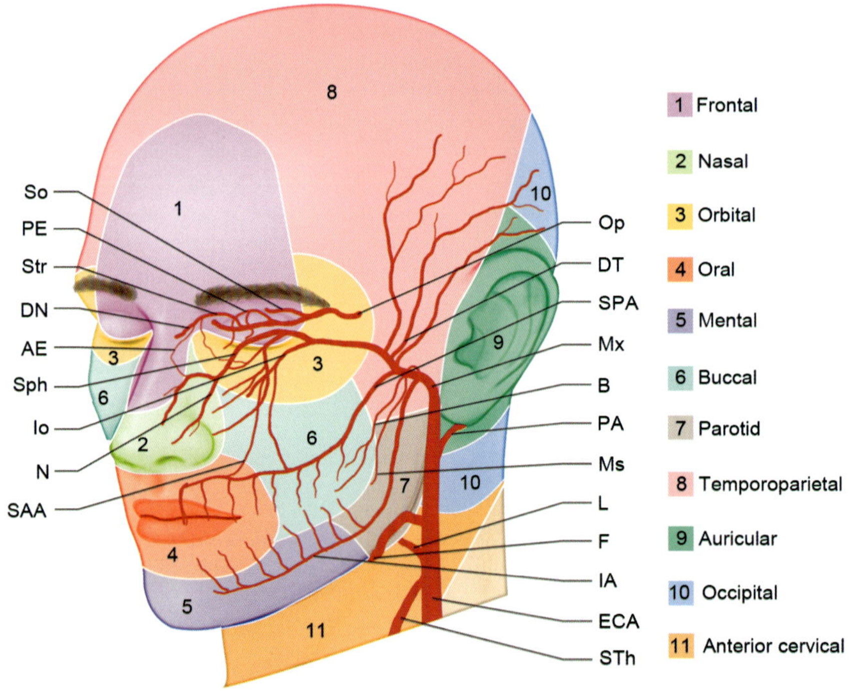

Fig. 6.2 The deep arteries of the head and neck regions in anterolateral oblique view. Regions: arterial territories: (1) frontal: Str, So, MP (O territory); (2) nasal: DN, AE, An (F-O territory); (3) orbital: MP, LP, Io (O-Max-Zo territory); (4) oral: SL, IL (F territory); (5) mental: Me, IL (Max-F territory); (6) buccal: Io, TF (Mx-ST territory); (7) parotid: TF, Ms (ST territory); (8) temporoparietal: Fb, Pb, MT (ST territory); (9) auricular: AA, PA (ST-ECA territory); (10) occipital: O (ECA territory); (11) anterior cervical: STh (ECA territory). AE, anterior ethmoidal artery; B, buccal artery; DN, dorsal nasal artery; DT, deep temporal artery; ECA, external carotid artery; F, facial artery; IA, inferior alveolar artery; Io, infraorbital artery; L, lingual artery; Ms, masseteric artery; Mx, maxillary artery; N, nasopalatine artery; PA, posterior auricular artery; PE, posterior ethmoidal artery; Op, ophthalmic artery; SAA, superior alveolar artery; SPA, superior posterior alveolar artery; Sph, sphenopalatine artery; So, supraorbital artery; Str, supratrochlear artery; STh, superior thyroid artery.

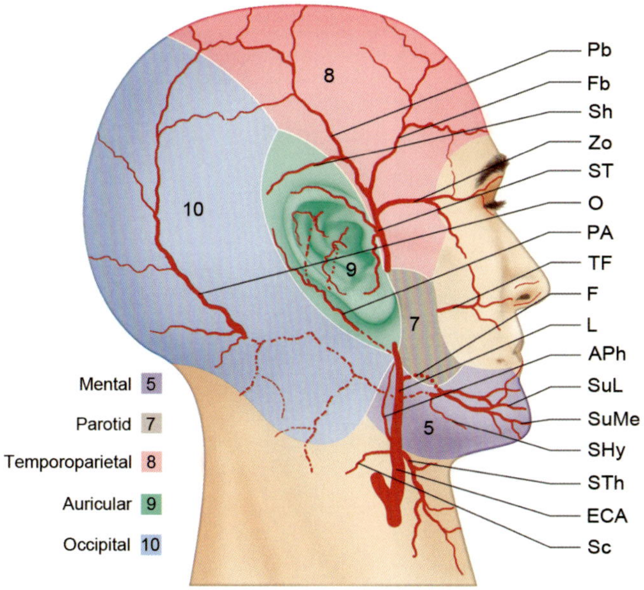

Fig. 6.3 Branches of the external carotid artery, posterolateral view. Regions: Arterial territories (5) mental: Me (Mx), Shy, SuL (L), SuMe (F) territory; (7) parotid: TF, Ms (ST territory); (8) temporoparietal: Fb, Pb, MT (ST territory); (9) auricular: AA, PA (ST-ECA territory); (10) occipital: O (ECA territory). APh, ascendening pharyngeal artery; ECA: external carotid artery; F, facial artery; Fb, frontal branch of the superficial temporal artery; L, lingual artery; PA, posterior auricular artery; Pb, parietal branch of the superficial temporal artery; O, occipital artery; Sc, sternocleidomastoid branch; SHy, suprahyoid artery; Sh, suprahelical artery; ST, superficial temporal artery; STh, superior thyroid artery; SuL, sublingual artery; SuMe, submental artery; TF, transverse facial artery; Zo, zygomatico-orbital artery.

Surgical Annotation

The superior thyroid, lingual, and facial arteries originate as separate branches in 50 to 80%; a lingulofacial trunk exists in 18 to 31%, a thyrolingual trunk in 1 to 18%, and a thyrolingulofacial trunk in about 2.5% (**Fig. 6.5**).[8,9,11,12] The carotid bifurcation is commonly located at the superior border of the thyroid cartilage. The distance from the origin of the superior thyroid artery to the carotid bifurcation is 3.3 ± 4.3 mm, from the origin of the superior thyroid artery to that of the lingual artery is 10.5 ± 5.2 mm, and from the origin of the superior thyroid artery to that of the facial artery is 18.2 ± 8.8 mm.[8,9,12]

Superior Thyroid Artery

The superior thyroid artery typically arises from the anterior surface of the external carotid just below the level of the greater cornu of the hyoid bone, although there are variations (**Fig. 6.6**).[8,9,11,12] The superior thyroid artery usually has a sharp downward angle at its origin. From its origin under the anterior border of the sternocleidomastoid muscle, it runs upward and forward for a short distance in the carotid triangle; it then arches downward beneath the infrahyoid muscles (**Fig.6.5a**). It distributes twigs to the adjacent muscles and numerous branches to the thyroid gland, anastomosing with its fellow on the opposite side and with the inferior thyroid arteries.

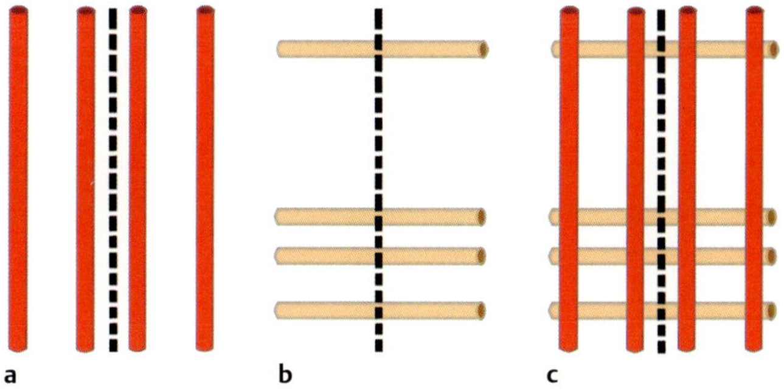

Fig. 6.4 Schematic representation of the arterial anastomoses in three patterns. **(a)** Intercarotid anastomoses (angular and dorsal arteries). **(b)** Transfacial anastomoses (radix, lateral nasal, marginal, and subnasal arteries). **(c)** Polygonal system (intercarotid and transfacial). Red: intercarotid; orange: transfacial interconnected arteries.

Surgical Annotation

The origin of the superior thyroid artery can be identified 13 ± 4.5 mm below the tip of the greater horn of the hyoid. The distance from its origin to the thyroid cartilage's upper edge is 7.1 ± 6.4 mm and to the horizontal plane passing through the upper edge of the thyroid gland is 26.1 ± 12.1 mm.[8,9,12]

Lingual Artery

The lingual artery arises from the external carotid artery between the origin of the superior thyroid and facial arteries. It first runs obliquely upward and medially to the greater cornu of the hyoid bone (**Fig. 6.5**). It then curves downward and forward and passes beneath the digastric and stylohyoid muscles. It runs horizontally forward, beneath the hyoglossus muscle, finally ascending as the deep lingual artery.

Surgical Annotation

The branching patterns can vary. These anatomical variations arise from embryological development and can be significant in clinical cases (**Fig. 6.5, Fig. 6.6**). The anatomical characteristics and variations of the external carotid, superior thyroid, lingual, and facial arteries, such as their branching patterns, lengths, and outer diameters, are crucial for safe implementation of intra-arterial catheterization for administering anticancer drugs to the head and the neck, surgical excision of benign and malignant tumors, and microsurgical arterial implantations.[8,9,12]

The distance from the origin of the lingual artery to the carotid bifurcation is 12 ± 5.9 mm, to the origin of the facial artery is 5.3 ± 5.2 mm, and to the thyroid cartilage's upper edge is 15.6 ± 7.7 mm.

Occipital Artery

The occipital artery arises from the external carotid (89–95%) or as a common trunk with the posterior auricular artery from the external carotid artery (5–10%). From the mandibular angle, the origin of the occipital artery is on average 13.4 mm (5–22 mm) above in 29% cases, 17.6 mm (4–32 mm) below in 57%, and

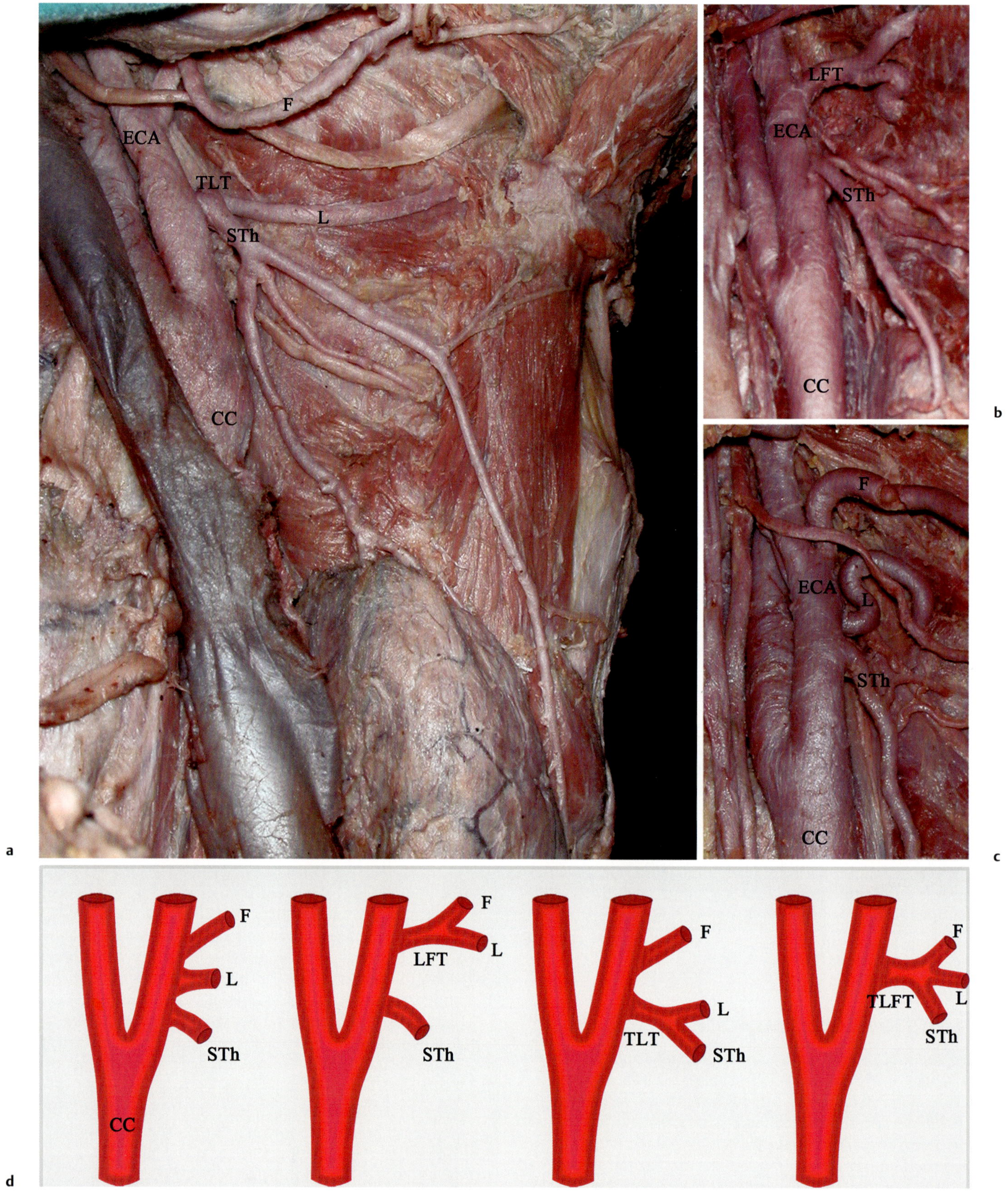

Fig. 6.5 The anterior branches of the external carotid artery. **(a)** Case of thyrolingual trunk, **(b)** case of lingulofacial trunk, **(c)** case of separate branches, and **(d)** the branching types of the anterior branches of the external carotid artery. CC, common carotid artery; ECA, external carotid artery; F, facial artery; L, lingual artery; LFT, lingulofacial trunk; TLFT, thyrolingulofacial trunk; TLT, thyrolingual trunk; STh, superior thyroid artery.

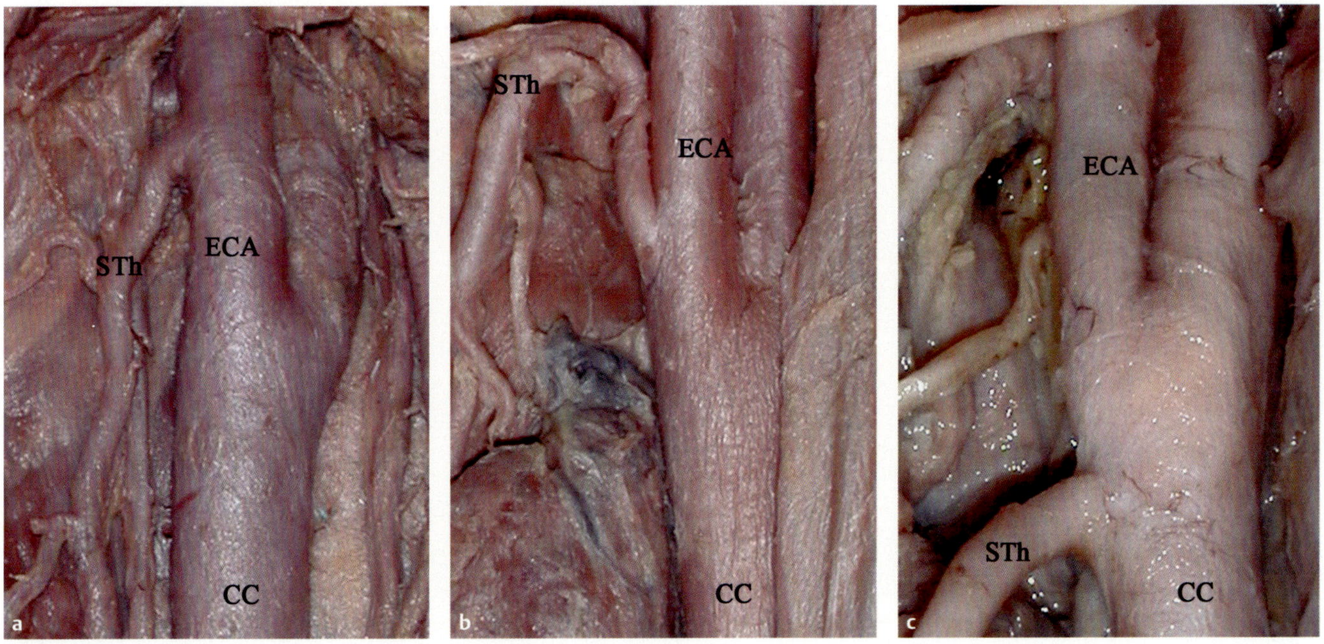

Fig. 6.6 Origin of the superior thyroid artery. **(a)** From the external carotid artery, **(b)** from the carotid bifurcation, **(c)** from the common carotid artery. CC, common carotid artery; ECA, external carotid artery; STh, superior thyroid artery.

at the same level in 14%. From the external carotid artery, the artery emerges from the posterior side in 88%, from the lateral side in 8%, and from the medial side in 4%. It takes a tortuous course superiorly and posteriorly toward the base of the scalp, traveling beneath the splenius capitis and the sternocleidomastoid muscles.[11,13,14] The mean length of the artery is 9 cm (3.4–12.5 cm). It is divided into descending, horizontal, and vertical branches (**Fig. 6.3**). The horizontal branch runs along the nuchal ridge, connecting across the midline to branches of the contralateral occipital artery. The vertical branch runs superiorly along the posterior skull and anastomoses with the posterior auricular, superficial temporal, and supraorbital arteries (**Fig. 6.7c,d**). The descending branch is divided over the trapezius, and it supplies the trapezius, splenius, and sternocleidomastoid muscles. The descending branch anastomoses with the deep cervical and the ascending branch of the transverse cervical arteries.[2,15]

The sternocleidomastoid artery generally arises from the occipital artery, but sometimes it springs directly as a separate branch from the external carotid artery (**Fig. 6.3**). The distance from the origin of the sternocleidomastoid branch to the external carotid artery is 14.4 mm. It passes downward and backward over the hypoglossal nerve and supplies the sternocleidomastoid muscle and the integument.[11]

Surgical Annotation

The occipital artery is the main artery of the suboccipital region. The vascular network of the cervico-occipital flap consists of the cutaneous and musculocutaneous perforators of the descending branch of the occipital artery anastomosing with the cervical arteries and the cutaneous branches of spinal arteries in the region around the nape of the neck. The cervico-occipital flap is used to reconstruct defects after resection of the mandible or the floor of the mouth and the tongue or to close pharyngoesophageal and tracheal fistulae. As the content of the cervico-occipital flap is richly vascularized and as the two-headed sternocleidomastiod muscle has minimal donor-site morbidity, it is preferred as a myocutaneous flap for stable and durable reconstruction. The upper third of the sternocleidomastoid muscle is supplied by branches of the occipital artery. The middle third receives a branch from the superior thyroid artery (42%), the external carotid artery (23%), or both (27%). The lower third is supplied by a branch arising from the suprascapular artery.[2,15] In the suboccipital region, the mean distance between the point at which the occipital artery pierces the sternocleidomastoid muscle and the inion is 4.8 cm (3.9–6.5 cm). The mean distance between the piercing point of the artery in the muscle and the lower part the mastoid process is 5.1 cm (3.9–5.9 cm). Classically, the occipital artery enters the sternocleidomastoid muscle 1.5 to 2 cm below the anterior margin. The point where the occipital artery enters the sternocleidomastoid and then comes out to the surface up to 4 cm under the process is determined as the reference point. Studies suggest that the greater occipital nerve crosses the occipital artery lateral to the inion. Occipital artery biopsy should be performed between 4 to 5 cm lateral and 1 to 3 cm proximal to the inion to avoid injury to this artery in vasculitis cases.[2,4,15]

Posterior Auricular Artery

The posterior auricular artery arises from the external carotid artery, above the digastric and stylohyoid muscles, opposite the apex of the styloid process.[7,16,17] It has a mean distance of 0.29 cm anterior to the mastoid tip, just deep to the lobule and in the posterior auricular sulcus. It ascends, under cover of the parotid gland, on the styloid process of the temporal bone and, immedi-

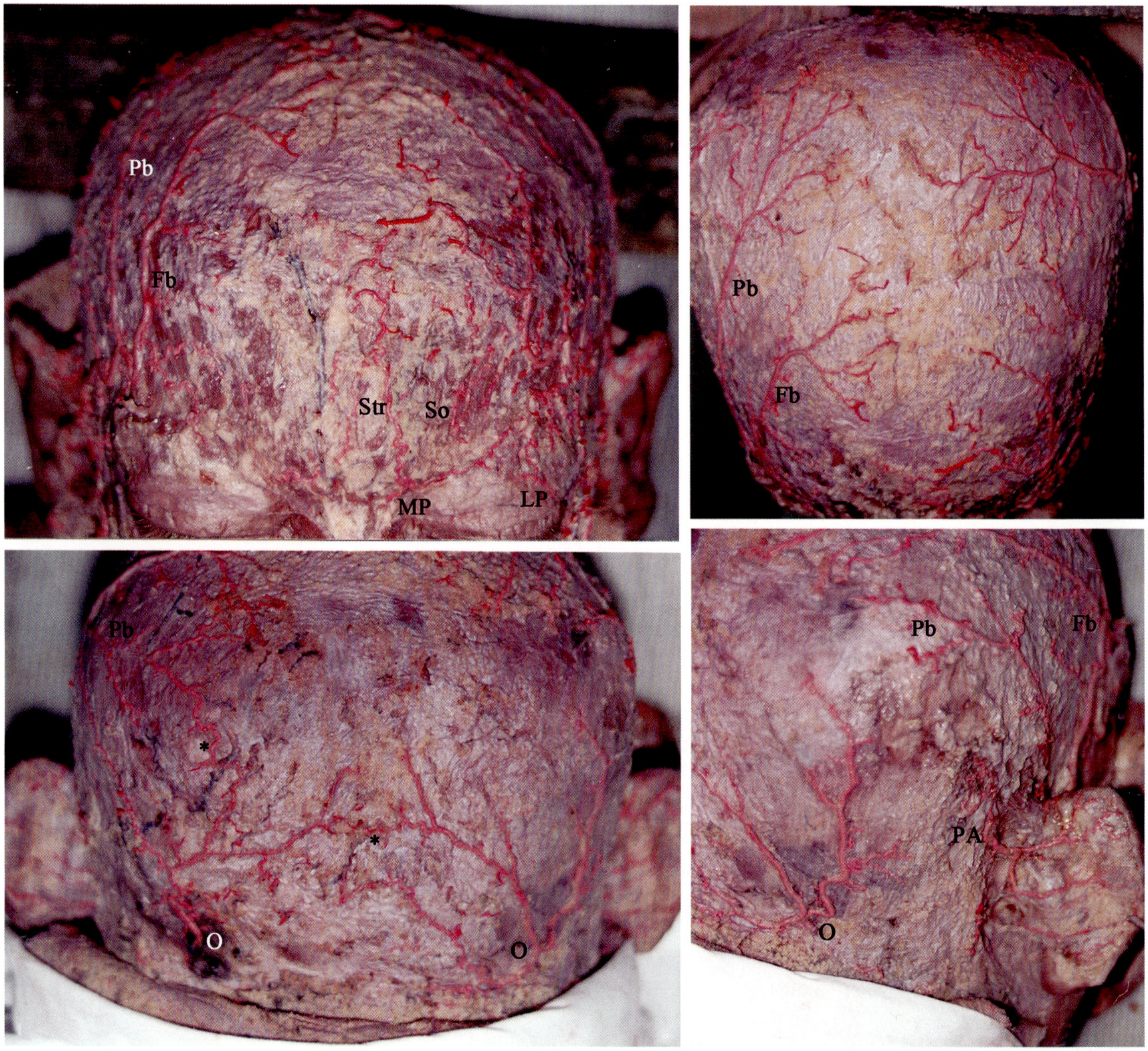

Fig. 6.7 Blood supply of the (**a, b**) forehead, (**c**) occipital, and (**d**) retroauricular regions. Red latex is injected into the common carotid arteries before dissection. Fb, frontal branch of the superficial temporal artery; LP, lateral palpebral artery; MP, medial palpebral artery; O, occipital artery; PA, posterior auricular artery; Pb, parietal branch of the superficial temporal artery; So, supraorbital artery; Str, supratrochlear artery; *, anastomoses.

ately above this point, divides into its auricular and occipital branches (**Fig.6.1, Fig. 6.2, Fig. 6.3, Fig. 6.7c,d**). The occipital branch passes backward, over the sternocleidomastoid muscle, to the scalp above and behind the ear. It anastomoses with the occipital artery (**Fig. 6.7c,d**).

Surgical Annotation

The arterial network in the upper ear is formed from the posterior auricular artery. The mean length of this artery before it penetrates the temporoparietal fascia measured from the mastoid tip is 75.6 mm. The posterior auricular artery gives off a retroauricular branch to the posterior surface of the auricle and an occipital branch to the postauricular skin, which travels in the postauricular sulcus. The mean distances from the mastoid tip is 8.4 mm to the occipital branch and 6.8 mm to the auricular branch. The arterial network of the triangular fossa and scaphoid fossa is provided by branches of the superficial temporal and posterior auricular arteries.

Facial Artery (External Maxillary Artery)

The facial artery arises at the level of the greater horn of the hyoid bone a little above the lingual artery's origin from the external carotid. It can arise from various trunks from the external carotid (**Fig. 6.5**). Hence, the level of the origin is situated

19.6 ± 8.7 (10–35 mm) away from the bifurcation of the common carotid artery. The distance from the origin of the facial artery to a horizontal plane passing over the top side of the thyroid cartilage is 15.4 ± 8.4 mm. It ascends under cover of the posterior belly of the digastric and stylohyoid muscles and grooves the submandibular gland by making a loop. It curves upward over the body of the mandible at the anteroinferior angle of the masseter muscle. It then passes forward and upward across the cheek to the labial commissure. The distances from the facial artery are 13.5 mm (8–23 mm) to the labial commissure and 45 mm (28–60 mm) to the midline. It then ascends along the side of the nose and ends at the medial commissure of the eye as the angular artery (**Fig. 6.1, Fig. 6.8**).

The course of the artery can vary.[6,18–20] Branches to the face include the ascending palatine, inferior labial, tonsillar, superior labial, glandular, lateral nasal, submental, angular, and muscular arteries. The facial artery and its branches mainly supply the mental region, the lips, the inferior part of the parotidomasseteric region, and the buccal, orbital, infraorbital, and nasal regions (**Fig. 6.1, Fig. 6.3**).[3–5,7,11]

Submental Artery

The submental artery is usually the largest of the cervical branches (**Fig. 6.3**). The distances of the origin of the submental artery are 27.5 mm (19–41 mm) to that of the facial artery and 23.8 mm (1.5–39 mm) to the mandibular angle.[2,21] The artery is deep to the anterior belly of the digastric muscle in 70–80%. It passes superficial to the mylohyoid nerve, 16.8 mm (9–34 mm) from its origin. A visible anastomosis between the two submental arteries is noted in 92%.[20] It anastomoses with the sublingual artery and with the mylohyoid branch of the inferior alveolar artery; at the symphysis menti, it turns upward over the border of the mandible and then is divided into superficial and deep branches. The superficial branch passes between the integument and depressor labii inferioris and anastomoses with the inferior labial artery; the deep branch runs between the muscle and the bone, supplies the lip, and anastomoses with the inferior labial and mental arteries.[20]

Surgical Annotation

The axial myocutaneous platysma flap using the upper part of the mylohyoid muscle is supplied by the submental artery.[2,21] Dissection of the pedicle back to the origin of the facial artery and vein to extend the arc of rotation of the flap is recommended. The diameter of the submental artery is suitable for safe microvascular transfer (1.7–2.2 mm).[5,21] The length of the submental artery is 58.9 mm (35–108 mm); its length from the origin to the anterior belly of the digastric muscle is 31.5 mm (26–38 mm).[21]

The facial artery crosses the inferior border of the mandible obliquely to enter the face at the anteroinferior angle of the masseter muscle. The distance between the mandibular angle and the point where the facial artery crosses the lower border of the mandible is 26.6 mm (15.5–38 mm).[21] It is extremely tortuous. It gives off small muscular branches to the masseter and the depressor anguli oris muscles (**Fig. 6.8a**).

Inferior Labial Artery

The inferior labial artery arises near the angle of the mouth; it passes upward and forward beneath the depressor anguli muscle or penetrates the orbicularis oris muscle (**Fig.6.1, Fig. 6.8a**). The distance from the origin of the inferior labial artery from the labial commissure is 19.3 ± 10 mm (4–35 mm). It follows a tortuous course along the edge of the lower lip between the muscle and the mucous membrane. The length of the inferior labial artery is 34.5 ± 20.8 mm (29–67 mm).[18,20,21] It supplies the labial glands, the mucous membrane, and the muscles of

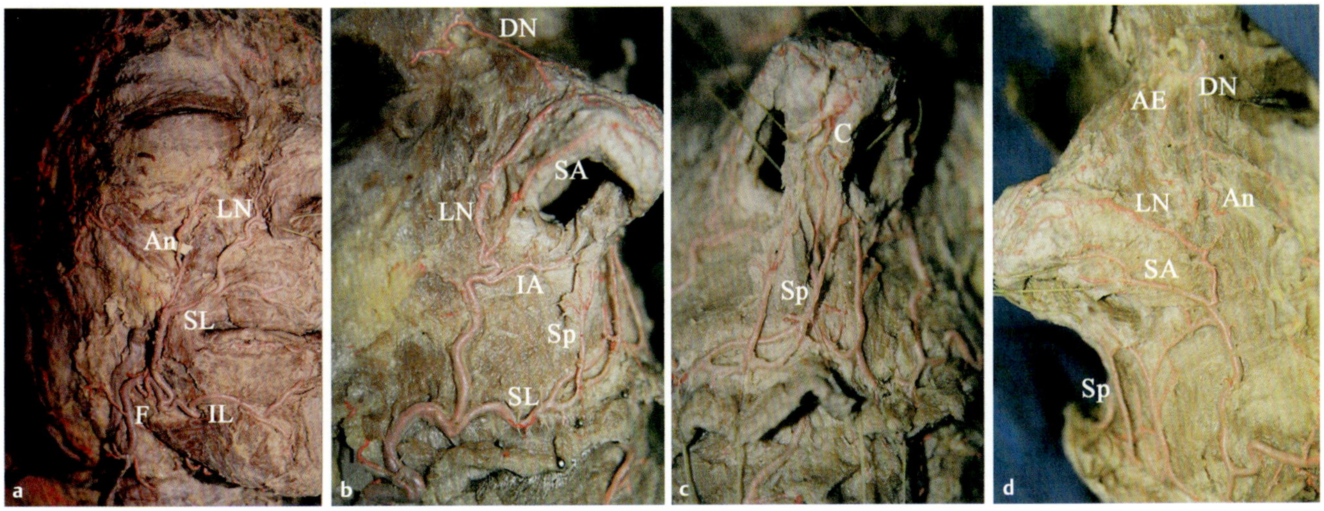

Fig. 6.8 Course of the facial artery and its branches. Red latex is injected into the common carotid arteries before dissection. **(a)** A doubled facial artery, **(b)** nasal-type facial artery. The anastomoses between alar branches and branches of the superior labial artery, and **(c)** septal branch are continued as the columellar artery. **(d)** Angular type facial artery. The anastomoses between the superficial ascending artery and inferior alar branch. AE, anterior ethmoidal artery; An, angular artery; C, columellar artery; DN, dorsal nasal artery; F, facial artery; IA, inferior alar artery; IL, inferior labial artery; LN, lateral nasal artery; SA, superior alar artery; SL, superior labial artery; Sp, septal artery.

the lower lip. It anastomoses with the artery on the opposite side and with the mental branch of the inferior alveolar artery.

Surgical Annotation

The origins of the inferior labial artery vary between the labial commissure and the lower margin of the mandible. The inferior labial artery can arise from the facial artery above the labial commissure (8%), below the labial commissure (22%), and at the labial commissure (60%).[10,18,20] The inferior labial and labiomental arteries come off at the level of the inferior border of the buccinator muscle and run anteriorly, passing deep to the depressor anguli oris. Different arterial distributions exist in the lower lip such as end-to-end anastomosis between the bilateral inferior labial arteries and the inferior labial arteries anastomose with the submental artery. The vertical and horizontal labiomental arteries are situated between the lower lip and the submental region (transfacial anastomosis). The distances from the labial commissure are 29.1 ± 24.2 mm (7–71 mm) to the origin of the horizontal labiomental arteries and 28 ± 12.1 mm (10–52 mm) to the origin of the vertical labiomental arteries. The lengths of the horizontal labiomental arteries are 26.8 ± 10.7 mm (16–49 mm) and the vertical labiomental arteries are 13 ± 4 mm (1–17 mm).[10,18,20,21] The labiomental arteries, which form anastomoses between the facial, inferior labial, and submental arteries, vary in their course in the labiomental region (**Fig. 6.1**).[10,18,20,21] To elevate a labiomental arterial flap safely, routine use of a Doppler probe preoperatively and intraoperatively is recommended.[7,10]

Superior Labial Artery

The facial artery passes deep to the risorius and zygomaticus major muscles but superficial to the buccinator muscle. It gives off one of its major branches, the superior labial artery. Near the labial commissure, it gives off three to five branches to the anterior part of the buccinator and zygomaticus major muscles (**Fig. 6.8**).[20]

The arterial supply to the lips is based on the superior and inferior labial arteries at the level of the labial commissure, where it terminates in the form of a perilabial arterial network (**Fig. 6.4b**, transfacial anastomosis). The arterial supply to the upper lip arises mainly from the superior labial artery and from the subseptal and subalar arteries. The arterial supply to the lower lip arises from the inferior labial artery and the branches of the mental artery.[11,18]

Surgical Annotation

The superior labial artery is larger and more tortuous than the inferior labial artery. It originates as follows: at the level of the labial commissure in 5% of cases, superior to the commissure in 25%, and inferior to the commissure in 70%. It can be identified usually 8 ± 4.4 mm (1–18 mm) lateral to the medial labial commissure. Its length is 4.8 ± 12.2 mm (29–67 mm). In 84.8%, the artery travels exclusively between the orbicularis oris muscle and the oral mucosa; in 15.2%, it travels partially invested by the orbicularis oris. It supplies the upper lip and gives off two or three vessels that ascend to the nose: a septal branch ramifies on the nasal septum, and an alar branch supplies the ala of the nose (**Fig. 6.1, Fig. 6.8**).[10,18,20,21] A relatively large branch that courses along the inferior margin of the nostril on its ascent toward the columellar base is called the inferior alar branch, and the artery running to the nasal tip over the ala nasi is called the superior alar branch. The inferior alar branch supplies the alar base, the nostril floor, and the upper lip; the superior alar branch participates in the vascular plexus of the nasal dorsum and the tip. The length of the superior alar branch is 14.6 ± 5.9 mm (7–26 mm), and that of the septal branch is 15.6 ± 6.2 mm (10–27 mm).[10,18,20]

The superior labial artery runs between the mucosa and orbicularis oris at approximately the border between the white and the red parts of the lips and anastomoses with the opposite artery in the middle of the lip.[6,7] The distances from the superior labial artery at midlip are 6.9 ± 2.5 mm (0.7–11 mm) to the inferior border of the red upper lip, 5.4 ± 1.8 mm (3–9 mm) to its anterior border, and 3.2 ± 0.7 mm to its posterior border.[10,18,20]

These branches are named as two groups: those running between the skin and the muscle are called superficial ascending branches, and those running through the muscle or between the muscle and the mucosa are called deep ascending branches. At the columellar base, there are anastomoses among the superficial ascending and inferior alar arterial branches. Ramifications of the deep ascending and inferior alar branches pass to the nasal septum and ascend along the anterior margin of the septal cartilage. Columellar branches are the continuation of the superficial ascending branches and become part of the vascular plexus of the nasal tip (**Fig. 6.8b–d**). The columellar artery is observed as a single branch in 48.9% and a double pattern in 38.7%.[20]

Lateral Nasal Artery

The lateral nasal artery arises from the facial artery at the nasolabial sulcus level. It runs 2 to 3 mm superior to the alar groove, extends between the nose and the cheek, and gives off the superior and inferior alar arteries to supply the nose (**Fig. 6.1, Fig. 6.8**). The lateral nasal artery anastomoses with its fellow, with the septal and alar branches, with the dorsal nasal branch of the ophthalmic, and with the infraorbital branch of the maxillary arteries (**Fig. 6.1**). The facial artery continues as the angular artery and proceeds to the medial palpebral commissure.[6,7]

Surgical Annotation

Small distal branches of the lateral nasal artery form several anastomoses with contralateral have branches and with the columellar arteries.[5,6,18] Some studies demonstrated the existence of an anastomotic system, situated in the superior musculoaponeurotic system plane, connecting the external and the internal carotid artery systems and the transfacial nasal vascular blood supply, which gives rise to the subdermal plexus. This network explains why many different pedicles can be safely used for local flaps in nasal reconstruction (**Fig. 6.4c,** polygonal system anastomosis). Furthermore, after skin tumor resections, the presence of these anastomotic vessels enables a large vessel ligation to be performed without skin necrosis; however, the presence of so many anastomotic vessels in the nasal area can be easily injured during injections, and creates a risk of embolism or microembolism, especially with rhinoplasties using fillers (**Fig. 6.4a,** intercarotid anastomosis).

Angular Artery

The angular artery is the terminal part of the facial artery; it ascends to the medial angle of the orbit and is accompanied by the angular vein. It is easily found on a vertical line about 6 to 8 mm medial to the medial canthus and 5 mm anterior to the lacrimal sac. In 60% of specimens, the terminal branch is formed by the lateral nasal artery, and in 22% it is formed by the angular artery. It anastomoses with the infraorbital artery on the cheek after supplying the lacrimal sac and the orbicularis oculi. The angular artery ends by anastomosing with the dorsal nasal branch of the ophthalmic artery (**Fig. 6.1, Fig. 6.8c**).[11] Its branches are a communicating branch with the dorsal nasal artery (96%), a communicating branch with the supratrochlear artery (67%), the infratrochlear artery, and the paracentral artery. The paracentral artery originates from the angular artery as the main continuation into the forehead (71%) or from the communicating branch with the supratrochlear artery (30%).[7,11,20,22]

Surgical Annotation

Difficult oronasal mucosal defects, including defects of the palate, alveolus, nasal septum, antrum, upper lip and lower lip, floor of the mouth, and soft palate, can be reconstructed using an axial musculomucosal flap based on the facial artery and its branches. Their diameters are suitable for microvascular anastomosis.[6,7,11,20] Most of these flaps are based on local axial vascularization via the labial arteries, but anatomical variations can lead to problems; its branching pattern shows great variability (**Fig. 6.8a, Fig. 6.9**). The distribution patterns of the artery are categorized into six types, A–F (**Fig. 6.9**).[6,7,11,20] In type A (47–78%) the artery bifurcates into the superior labial and lateral nasal arteries (the latter gives off the inferior and superior alar and ends as the angular artery). Type B (38–60%) is similar to type A except the lateral nasal terminates as the superior alar (the angular artery is absent). In type C (8–12%), the facial artery terminates as the superior labial artery. In type D (3.8%), the angular artery arises directly from the facial arterial trunk rather than as the termination of the lateral nasal, with the facial artery ending as the superior alar. In type E (1.4–3%), the facial artery terminates as a rudimentary twig without providing significant branches. Type F presents a doubled facial artery.[23] On the basis of anatomical studies, the degree of vascular territory lost as a result of vessel damage during the myocutaneous flap procedure can be estimated. For example, ligation of the superior labial artery in a patient with type A, B, or C would not result in ischemic injury to the nose, as the blood supply is provided by a separate lateral nasal artery. In contrast, ligation of the superior labial artery in a patient with type D or E distribution is more likely to result in loss of the vascular supply to the lateral nose.[7,10]

The facial musculomucosal flap is an axial flap based on the superior labial artery in an anterograde fashion or the angular artery in a retrograde fashion.[3,7,10] The nasolabial flap can be based on the angular artery either inferiorly or superiorly in an anterograde or retrograde fashion, respectively. Doppler ultrasound helps to locate the facial vessels and provides information about backflow and the potential for inverted flow in the facial artery.[7,10]

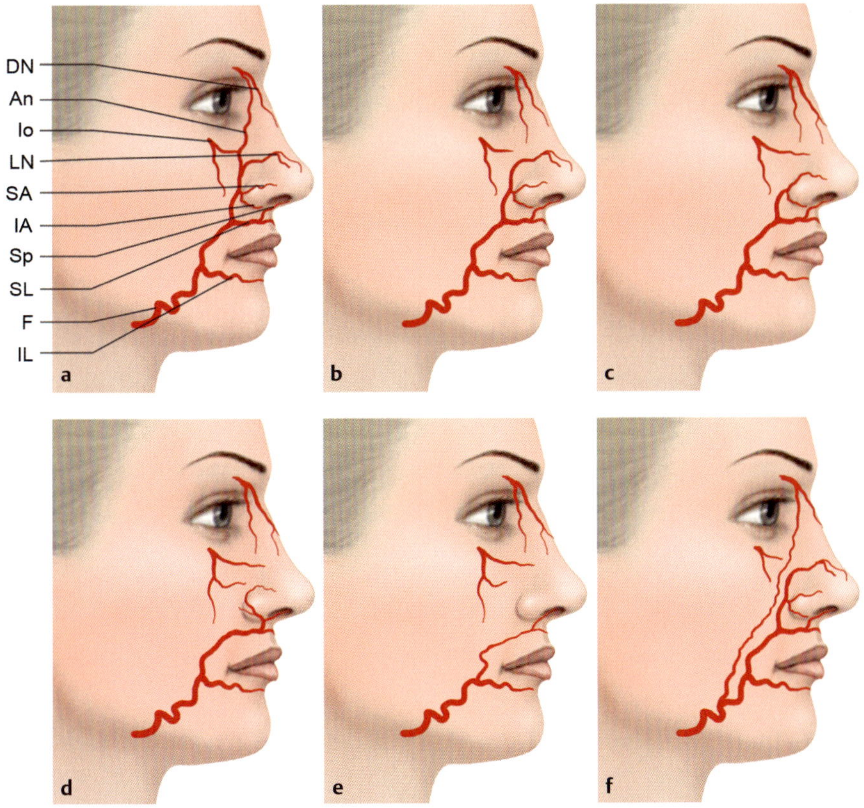

Fig. 6.9 Schematic drawing of the types of facial artery. **(a)** Angular, **(b)** nasal, **(c)** alar, **(d)** labial, **(e)** hypoplastic, **(f)** double type. An, angular artery; DN, dorsal nasal artery; F, facial artery; IA, inferior alar artery; IL, inferior labial artery; Io, infraorbital artery; LN, lateral nasal artery; SA, superior alar artery; SL, superior labial artery; Sp, septal artery.

Maxillary Artery

The maxillary artery, the larger of the two terminal branches of the external carotid artery, arises behind the neck of the mandible (**Fig. 6.2**). It runs in the infratemporal fossa superficial to the lateral pterygoid muscle and is easily found about 6.64 ± 6.33 mm from the infratemporal crest. It supplies the deep structures of the face and can be divided into mandibular, pterygoid, and pterygopalatine parts.[11] Its total length is 57.38 ± 7.1 mm.

Its first, or mandibular, part lies deep behind the mandibular ramus. From this part, the inferior alveolar artery arises. The distance between the origin of the maxillary artery and the inferior alveolar artery is 10.8 ± 6 mm.[11] It descends with the inferior alveolar nerve to the mandibular foramen on the medial surface of the ramus of the mandible. As it enters the foramen, it runs along the mandibular canal. The mental artery is the terminal branch of the inferior alveolar artery that passes with the nerve through the mental foramen to supply the chin and the lower lip. The mental branch anastomoses with the submental and inferior labial arteries.

The second, or pterygoid, part runs obliquely forward and upward under the cover of the ramus of the mandible. It runs either superficially or deep to the lateral pterygoid to the pterygopalatine fossa. Branches of this second part are the deep temporal, the masseteric, the pterygoid, and the buccinator arteries.[7,20,21] The deep temporal branches (i.e., three branches) ascend anteriorly and posteriorly between the temporalis muscle and the pericranium; they supply the muscle (**Fig. 6.2**). These arteries anastomose with the middle temporal artery; the anterior communicates with the lacrimal artery via small branches perforating the zygomatic bone (polygonal anastomosis). The masseteric artery passes laterally through the mandibular notch to the deep surface of the masseter muscle.[11] It supplies the muscle and anastomoses with the masseteric branches of the facial arteries and with the transverse facial arteries (**Fig. 6.2**). The buccinator artery runs obliquely forward, between the pterygoid and the insertion of the temporal muscles, to the outer surface of the buccinator muscle. It anastomoses with branches of the facial and with the infraorbital arteries (**Fig. 6.2**).

The third, or pterygopalatine, part lies in the pterygopalatine fossa near the pterygopalatine ganglion. The branches of this third part are the posterior superior alveolar artery; the artery of the pterygoid canal; and the infraorbital, pharyngeal, descending palatine, and sphenopalatine arteries (**Fig. 6.2**). The infraorbital artery appears, from its direction, to be a continuation of the trunk of the maxillary artery.[11,24] It runs along the infraorbital groove and canal with the infraorbital nerve. The infraorbital artery reaches the face through the infraorbital foramen and supplies the lower eyelid, the cheek, and the lateral nose (**Fig. 6.1, Fig. 6.2**). On the face, some branches pass upward to the medial angle of the orbit and the lacrimal sac. It anastomoses with the angular branch of the facial artery (**Fig. 6.2**); some run toward the nose, anastomosing with the dorsal nasal branch of the ophthalmic artery (**Fig. 6.4a**), and others descend between the levator labii superioris and the levator anguli oris and anastomose with the facial, transverse facial, and buccinator arteries (**Fig. 6.4c**).

Surgical Annotation

The location of the masseteric artery is easily determined in relation to three points in the anterioposterior plane between the mandibular condyle and the coronoid process: (1) the anterosuperior aspect of the condylar neck, (2) the most inferior aspect of the articular tubercle, and (3) the inferior aspect of the sigmoid notch. The mean distance of the masseteric artery to the most anterosuperior aspect of the condylar neck is reported as 10.3 mm; to the most inferior aspect of the articular tubercle, 11.4 mm; and to the most inferior aspect of the sigmoid notch, 3 mm.[25]

The temporalis muscle flap has been widely used for surgery of the skull base and the reconstruction of oral cavity and oropharyngeal defect. The vascular network of the temporalis muscle flap comes from three main pedicles: the anterior deep artery, the posterior deep artery (both collateral branches of the maxillary artery), and the middle temporal artery (a collateral branch of the superficial temporal artery).[25] The distance between a temporalis muscle flap and a temporalis muscle split on its superficial artery is 57 mm. The flap allows the midline to be crossed easily, thus broadening its indication. The gain obtained is greater than that obtained with a flap split on the deep temporal pedicles, and it can easily cross the midline; this is an important point.

Superficial Temporal Artery

The superficial temporal artery arises from the external carotid artery deep to the parotid gland. It ascends behind the condyle of the mandible.[25–27] The important branches of the superficial temporal artery are the transverse facial, anterior auricular, middle temporal, frontal and parietal arteries (**Fig. 6.1, Fig. 6.3**). Just before it reaches the zygomatic arch, the superficial temporal artery gives off the transverse facial artery.

The transverse facial artery arises from the superficial temporal artery in the parotid gland after branching off the maxillary artery. Its number ranges from one to three (mean, 1.34). It runs parallel about a finger's breadth inferior to the zygomatic arch (**Figs. 7.3, Fig. 6.10**). It passes transversely across the side of the face, between the parotid duct and the lower border of the zygomatic arch, and is divided into superior and inferior trunks after coursing 1 to 11 mm within the gland. The superior trunk is usually larger than the inferior trunk. The superior trunk is located below the level of the glandular border, 5.0 to 26.1 mm from the zygomatic arch (mean, 14.0 mm). Most perforators (76.8%) arise from the superior trunk, which can be useful when the structures are visible during surgery. The transverse facial artery is crossed by the temporal and zygomatic branches of the facial nerve. It anastomoses with the facial, masseteric, buccinator, and infraorbital arteries (**Fig. 6.10**, transfacial anastomosis).

The middle temporal artery arises immediately above the zygomatic arch and perforates the temporal fascia. It gives branches to the temporalis muscle and anastomoses with the deep temporal branches of the maxillary artery.

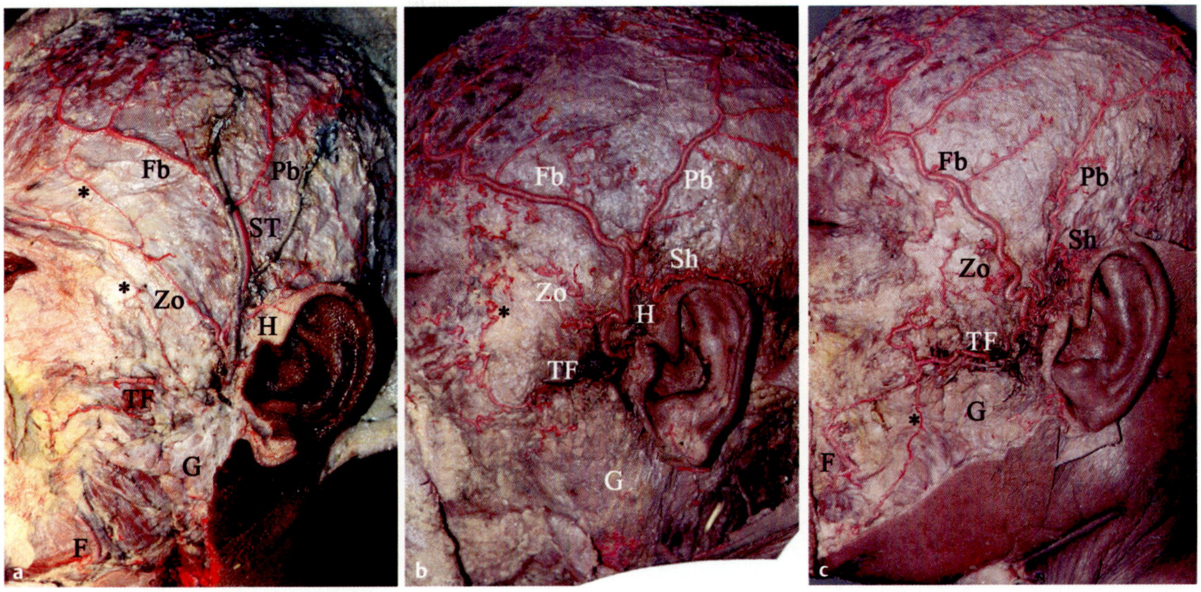

Fig. 6.10 Course of the superficial temporal artery and its branches. Red latex is injected into the common carotid arteries before dissection. **(a, b)** Bifurcation of the artery above the zygomatic arch, the anastomoses between the zygomatico-orbital artery and transverse facial artery; **(c)** bifurcation of the artery over the zygomatic arch; the frontal branch is larger than the parietal branch. F, Facial artery; Fb, frontal branch; G, parotid gland; H, helicial artery; Pb, parietal branch; Sh, suprahelical artery; ST, superficial temporal artery; TF, transverse facial artery; Zo, zygomatico-orbital artery; *, interfacial anastomosis.

The anterior auricular arteries run to the helix and the tragus. They reach the helix by passing under the superficial temporal vein at the level of the arch. The arteries are distributed to the anterior portion of the auricle, the lobule, and part of the external meatus, and they anastomose with the posterior auricular artery. The helical artery arises from the parietal branch of the superficial temporal artery where it bifurcates over the arch (**Fig. 6.10a, b**).

Surgical Annotation

An arterial anastomosis formed in the shape of an arcade has clinical importance in providing a longer flap for reconstruction. For instance, the anastomosis between the superficial temporal and the posterior auricular arteries is used as the Ishio flap when postauricular skin is pedicled on the superficial temporal vessels to reconstruct the nose.[1,10]

The zygomatico-orbital artery is present in 78 to 92%, and it originates from the superficial temporal artery and sometimes from its frontal branch. It courses anteriorly parallel to the upper border of the zygomatic arch between two layers of the temporal fascia to the lateral orbital region.[19,26] In the lateral face, it supplies the parotid gland and duct, facial nerve, facial muscles, and skin of the lateral canthus.[19,26] It anastomoses with the lacrimal and palpebral branches of the ophthalmic artery (**Fig. 6.1, Fig. 6.3, Fig. 6.10**).

Entering the temporal fossa, about 2 cm above the zygomatic arch, the superficial temporal artery is divided into frontal and parietal branches. In various studies, the bifurcation point of the artery has been observed above the zygomatic arch in 61 to 88% of cases, directly over the arch in 3.8 to 26%, and below the arch in 7 to 11.5%.[11,26–28]

The parietal branch (posterior) extending posteriorly curves upward and backward on the side of the head as the continuation of the superficial temporal artery. The parietal branch has anastomotic connections with the ipsilateral and contralateral arteries with the epicranial aponeurosis (**Fig. 6.7, Fig. 6.10**). The sub-branches coursing toward the front anastomose with the frontal branch in the temporoparietal region. Those going backward anastomose with the posterior auricular artery and occipital artery in the back of the head. Its perforating branches pass the deep fascia.

The frontal branch (anterior) runs tortuously upward and forward to the forehead, parallel to the upper corner of the orbicularis oculi muscle. Its perforating branches pass the deep fascia and the frontalis muscle. The frontal branch supplies the muscles, the integument, and the pericranium in this region. It anastomoses with the opposite frontal branch on the galea, with the supraorbital and supratrochlear arteries on the forehead, and with the zygomatico-orbital artery around the orbit and the forehead (**Fig. 6.7, Fig. 6.10**).

Surgical Annotation

Temporoparietal, parieto-occipital, galeopericranial, or forehead flaps are prepared on the superficial temporal artery and its branches. Face and neck reconstructions performed by using the superficial temporal artery with flaps have some advantages.

First, an end-to-end microanastomosis technique is practical. Dissecting the artery distally makes it possible to turn it over cranially or caudally to facilitate anastomosis. The diameters of the superficial temporal artery and its branches make them suitable for microvascular anastomoses.[5,17,25,26] The diameter of the superficial temporal artery is 2.03 to 2.14 mm, that of the frontal branch is 1.61 to 2.1 mm, and that of the parietal branch is 1.44 to 2.1 mm.[5,17,25,26] An atrophic frontal branch is present in 2%, either the parietal branch or the frontal branch is atrophic in 4%, an atrophic superficial temporal artery is present in 2%, and double parietal branches are present in 4%.[5,17,25,26] Second, even if the superficial temporal artery has been ruptured during previous procedures, the zygomatico-orbital artery may be available and is easily identified using Doppler or ultrasonography and can readily be accessed by following the superficial temporal artery.[19] Third, the preserved superficial temporal artery can be used another time.

The distance between the superficial temporal artery and the tragus is important for designing preauricular flaps. A rotation of the flap is successfully performed to include the parietal branch according to the anterior hairline and the course of this branch.[25,26] Some landmarks are chosen on the head: the middle point to the bony lateral canthus (A), the tragus (B), the superior attachment of the ear to the head (C), and a point 2 cm directly above this attachment (D). These points are joined to the bony lateral canthus by straight lines: AB, AC, and AD. The DF line, which takes Juri's original flap as a base, begins at the point 2 cm above the ear and is directed anterosuperiorly 45 degrees above the AD line to the anterior hair line. The F point is over the anterior hairline. Whether the parietal branch has passed the DF line is checked. According to Juri's design, the DF line builds the base of the parieto-occipital flap, and the parietal branch has to be located in the flap.[27] Line A–B is 80 ± 5 mm (65–87 mm), line A–C 81.8 ± 5.3 mm (66.2–88 mm), line A–D 83.6 ± 4.7 mm (72–90 mm), and line D–F 11 ± 7.7 mm.

Knowing the location of the transverse frontal artery can be of value for designing a galeal frontalis flap. If it is low, then a hairline incision would be adequate for the transverse forehead flap. If it is higher in the forehead, a superior incision in the hairline would be needed to capture the veins, which are more superior or posterior to the arteries, and in order to avoid venous congestion in this flap. The level at which the transverse frontal artery enters the forehead is often easily palpable, and the frontal branch of the superficial temporal artery is often easily seen weaving tortuously in the temporal area and the lateral forehead. The frontal branch of the superficial temporal artery and the transverse frontal artery are always anterior to the frontalis muscle.[16,23,27] At this point, the transverse frontal artery or the frontal branch of the superficial temporal artery often bends. The anastomosis of the oblique branch of the supraorbital artery is clinically significant; therefore, the distinction between the transverse frontal artery and the frontal branch of the superficial temporal artery is important. This arcade is crucial for planning flaps.

On the basis of anatomical studies, the retroauricular free flap pedicled on the superficial temporal vessels has advantages over the retroauricular free flap pedicled on the posterior auricular artery because the superficial temporal vessels are more reliable in course and caliber when the posterior auricular artery and its comitantes are compared.[16,23,27]

Ophthalmic Artery

The ophthalmic artery provides blood supply to the eyes, the upper two-thirds of the nose, and the anterior part of the forehead. Its branches include the lacrimal, ethmoid, supraorbital, supratrochlear, and external nasal arteries (**Fig. 6.2**). It arises from the internal carotid artery and enters the orbital cavity through the optic foramen. It then passes to the medial wall of the orbit, and then forward beneath the lower border of the obliquus superior muscle, and divides into branches.

The supraorbital artery exits the orbit with the supraorbital nerve through the supraorbital foramen, or notch, to supply the skin and the muscles of the forehead and scalp (**Fig. 6.1, Fig. 6.2, Fig. 6.7a,b**). Its terminal branches anastomose to the opposite side via the supratrochlear and the frontal branch of the superficial temporal arteries. The supratrochlear artery supplies the medial forehead and scalp as well as the root of the nose. The dorsal nasal artery anastomoses with the lateral nasal and infraorbital arteries. It provides blood supply to the medial eyelids and dorsal nasal skin. The external nasal branch, a branch of the anterior ethmoidal artery, supplies the skin of the nasal dorsum and tip.

Surgical Annotation

There is significant communication between the external and internal carotid artery systems around the eye through several anastomoses. These anastomoses run between the collateral branches of the internal carotid—the ophthalmic, supraorbital, supratrochlear, dorsal nasal, and lacrimal arteries (**Fig. 6.4c**, intercarotid anastomosis)—and the collateral and terminal branches of the external carotid—the facial artery (angular artery), superficial temporal, transverse facial and middle temporal arteries, and the frontal and parietal branches (**Fig. 6.4c**, transfacial anastomosis).

The supraorbital and supratrochlear vessels are described as an "intricate system of anastomosing vessels" between the angular, the supratrochlear, and the superficial temporal arteries.[13,29] Inadvertent intra-arterial injection of soft tissue augmentation around the eye can lead to occlusion of the central retinal vessels and potentially to blindness.[7,19] To avoid this complication, fillers should be injected in small volumes via blunt cannulas, implementing a careful retrograde injection technique (**Fig. 6.4c**, polygonal anastomosis).[10,30]

Lateral Palpebral Artery

The lateral palpebral arteries arise from the lacrimal artery and distribute to the eyelids and conjunctiva. They run medially in the upper and lower lids respectively and anastomose with the medial palpebral arteries, forming an arterial circle. The medial palpebral arteries leave the orbit to encircle the eyelids near their free margins, forming a superior and an inferior arch, which lie between the orbicularis oculi and the tarsus (**Fig. 6.1, Fig. 6.11**). The lacrimal artery gives off one or two zygomatic branches, one of which passes through the zygomaticotemporal foramen to reach the temporal fossa and anastomoses with the deep temporal arteries. Another branch appears on the cheek through the zygomaticofacial foramen and anastomoses with the transverse facial artery.[10,11,30]

Medial Palpebral Artery

The medial palpebral arteries are usually divided into branches for the upper and lower lids as the superior and inferior medial palpebrals.[10,30] The superior branch passes under the medial palpebral ligament to enter the upper eyelid. The inferior branch courses downwards behind the medial palpebral ligament to enter the lower lid (**Fig. 6.11b,c**).

The main blood supplies to the upper and lower lids are provided by arterial arcades. The superior palpebral arcade is situated at the lateral angle of the orbit with the zygomatico-orbital artery and the upper two lateral palpebral branches from the lacrimal artery.[11,24] The inferior palpebral arcade is at the lateral angle of the orbit, with the lower of the two lateral palpebral branches from the lacrimal, transverse facial artery, and at the medial part of the lid, with a branch from the angular artery (**Fig. 6.11c**).

The blood supply to the upper eyelid is composed of three arcades: marginal, supratarsal, and preseptal, which communicate by an anastomotic network of vertical branches. These small vertical branches run under the orbicularis oculi muscle in the submuscular fibroelastic layer.[30] The preseptal arcade is supplied by the branches of the ophthalmic artery (supraorbital, supratrochlear, and medial palpebral arteries). The marginal arcade is supplied by an anastomotic network connecting the supratarsal (60%) and preseptal (20%) arcades. Small vertical branches arising out of these arcades provide a richer and more complex anastomotic network.[24]

Surgical Annotation

The color match, contour, thickness, and mobility of the skin flap must be similar to the normal upper eyelid. Upper eyelid flaps, whether they have a medial or lateral pedicle or are bipedicled or with island flaps, are centered on the supratarsal arcade or the preseptal arcade.

Hematomas can arise because of injury to a perforating branch of the marginal arcade. The marginal arcade is easily found on the tarsus just 3 mm from the lid margin. Unexpected bleeding may be due to variants of an artery communicating between the peripheral and marginal arcades.[30] If artery variants are anticipated, bleeding can be prevented during blepharoplasty by more careful dissection of the eyelid around 4.5 mm from the lateral canthus.

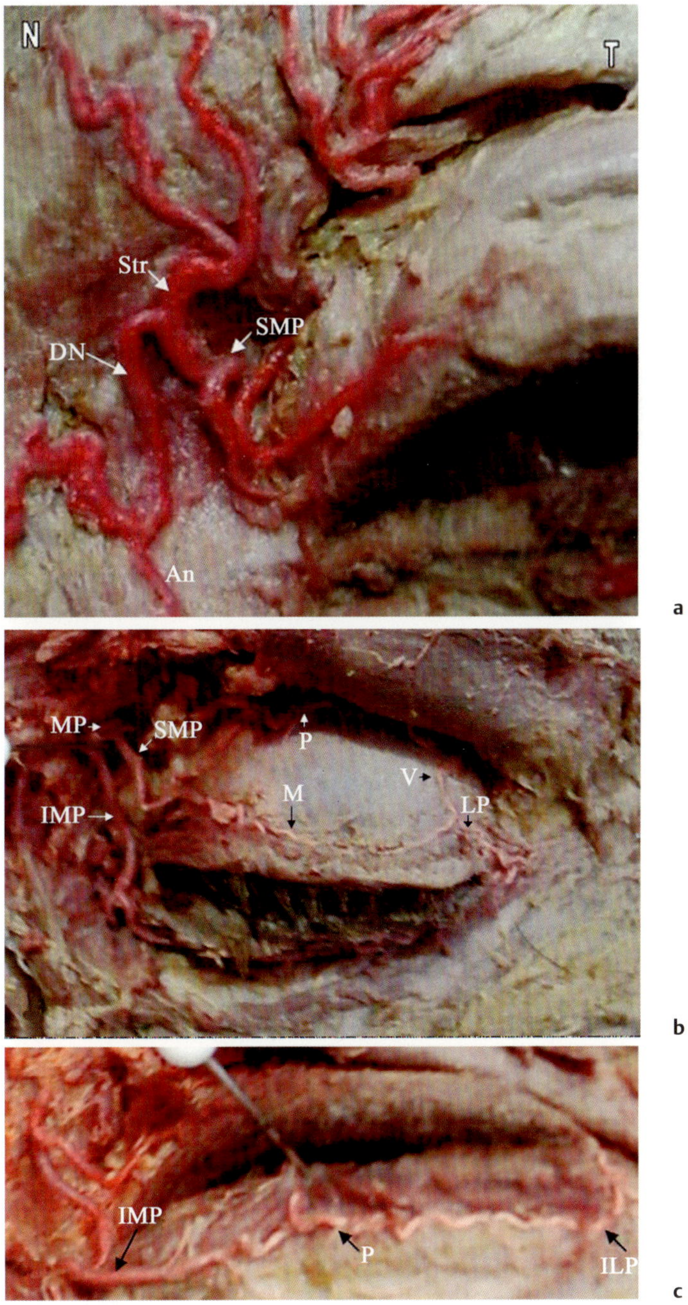

Fig. 6.11 Arteries of the **(a)** medial canthus, **(b)** upper eyelid, and **(c)** lower eyelid. Red latex is injected into the common carotid arteries before dissection. An, angular artery; DN, dorsal nasal artery; ILP, inferior lateral palpebral artery; IMP, inferior medial palpebral artery; LP, lateral palpebral artery; M, marginal arcade; MP, medial palpebral artery; P, peripheral arcade; SMP, superior medial palpebral artery; Str, supratrochlear artery; V, variant artery; N, nasal side, T, temporal side.

Ethmoidal Artery

The two ethmoidal arteries are posterior and the anterior. The posterior ethmoidal artery passes through the posterior ethmoidal canal. Its branches descend into the nasal cavity through apertures in the cribriform plate, anastomosing with the branches of the sphenopalatine artery. The anterior ethmoidal artery accompanies the nasociliary nerve through the anterior ethmoidal canal. It then descends into the nasal cavity, running along the groove on the inner surface of the nasal bone. Its terminal branch appears on the dorsum of the nose between the nasal bone and the lateral cartilage (**Fig. 6.1, Fig. 6.2**).

The frontal artery, one of the terminal branches of the ophthalmic artery, leaves the orbit at its medial angle with the supratrochlear nerve and, by ascending on the forehead, supplies the integument, the muscles, and the pericranium by anastomosing with the supraorbital artery and with the artery of the opposite side.

Supratrochlear Artery

The supratrochlear artery is relatively constant around the medial canthal vertical line and appears from the superomedial orbit (**Fig. 6.11a, Fig. 6.12**). The supratrochlear artery exits the orbit in a position 1.7 to 2.2 cm lateral to the midline. The course continues vertically in the forehead 1.5 to 2.0 cm lateral to the midline and goes across a transverse unnamed vessel to anastomose with the contralateral artery (**Fig. 6.1, Fig. 6.8d, Fig. 6.11a**).[11,29] The branches visible in the dissection are the medial communicating branch in 60%, lateral communicating branch in 23%, superior palpebral artery in 26%, periosteal branches in 7%, and cutaneous branches. Numerous additional muscular branches are present as oblique branches in 19%, medial and lateral vertical branches in 53%, and a single vertical branch in 47% (**Fig. 6.11a**).

Surgical Annotation

The supratrochlear artery travels under the orbicularis oculi muscle and over the corrugator muscle and then becomes superficial. The cutaneous branch is easily found at a position 11.8 to 3.6 mm superior to the supraorbital rim and 13.5 to 3.4 mm lateral to the midline (**Fig. 6.12**).[29] The supratrochlear artery enters a subcutaneous plane at average distances of 35 mm superior from the supraorbital rim and 56 mm from the supraorbital artery.[5,14] The superior one-third of the cutaneous branch travels under the dermis and over the fat layer.[29] The inferior two-thirds portion travels under the fat layer and over the frontalis muscle and gradually becomes superficial. The muscular branch travels through the frontalis muscle, but the cutaneous branch travels subcutaneously. The cutaneous branch anastomoses with the muscular branch or the supraorbital artery and the supratrochlear artery of the opposite side (**Fig. 6.12**).[5,29]

The artery can possibly have a periosteal course from the middle third of the forehead superiorly, which has clinical importance in flap planning. The paramedian forehead flap is supplied by the supratrochlear artery.[1,13] The common practice of removing fat from the superior third of the paramedian forehead flap could be quite risky if not done under direct vision because a variation has been reported in which the supratrochlear artery dives to a periosteal level in the middle third of the forehead and continues superiorly at the periosteal level. To avoid any possible risk of tip or distal partial necrosis or epidermolysis, the distal third flap should not be defatted at the first stage. The blood supply to the medial forehead is primarily from the supratrochlear and supraorbital arteries, ignoring the important contribution from the angular artery (dorsal nasal, central and paracentral arteries).[13,29]

Supraorbital Artery

The supraorbital artery appears over the supraorbital rim on a vertical line corresponding to the medial limbus of the cornea. It runs from medial to lateral over the supraorbital rim as it exits the orbit (**Fig. 6.1, Fig. 6.12**). The supraorbital artery passes through the supraorbital foramen and then divides into superficial and deep branches.[5,28] Five branches of the supraorbital artery are seen: the lateral rim (91%), oblique (91%), vertical (100%), medial, and brow (5%) branches. The medial, oblique, and lateral rim branches are always deep (periosteal or submus-

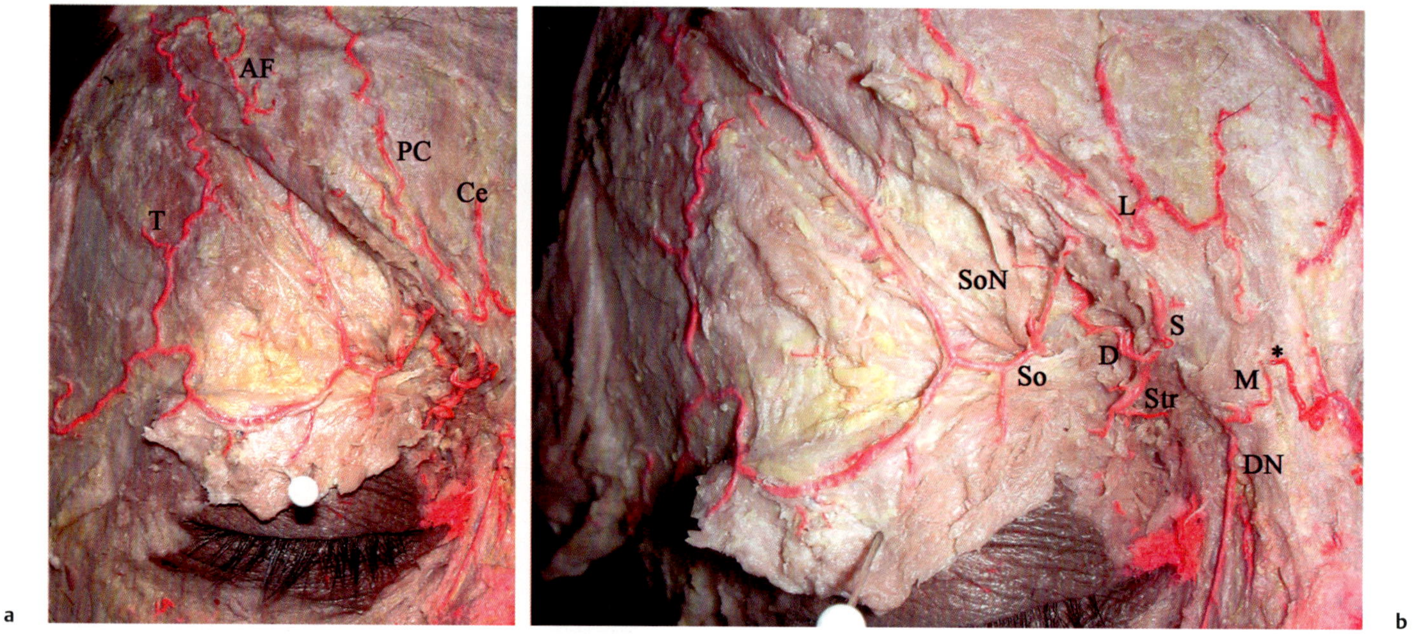

Fig. 6.12 Distribution of the neuroarterial structures on the orbitofrontal region (**a, b,** closer). Red latex is injected into the common carotid arteries before dissection. Photograph showing anastomosis of superficial temporal and supraorbital arteries; anastomosis of superficial temporal and supratrochlear arteries. AF, ascending frontal artery; Ce, central artery; D, deep (muscular) branch of the supratrochlear artery; DN, dorsal nasal artery; L, lateral communicating branch supratrochlear artery; M, medial communicating branch supratrochlear artery; PC, paracentral artery; S, superficial (cutaneous) branch of the supratrochlear artery; So, supraorbital artery; SoN, supraorbital nerve; Str, supratrochlear artery; T, transverse frontal artery; *, transfacial anastomosis.

cular). Often more than one vertical branch is present, or it subbranches soon after its origin.[7,13,29] The oblique branch runs on the periosteum toward either the frontal branch of the superficial temporal artery or the transverse frontal artery at the lateral orbital rim. The supraorbital artery is accompanied by the supraorbital nerve and the supraorbital vein. It supplies the integument, the muscles, and the pericranium of the forehead, anastomosing with the frontal branch of the superficial temporal and the artery on the opposite side.[16,28]

Surgical Annotation

The superficial arterial branches of the face cannot be recommended as the basis for any planned flap. The consistent presence of deep branches of the supraorbital artery makes them suitable for planning supraorbital artery–based flaps.[7,13] Potentially, a vascularized frontal bone flap could be developed using these deep branches. This flap could be useful for orbital roof or medial wall reconstruction.

Dorsal Nasal Artery

The dorsal nasal artery, the other terminal branch of the ophthalmic artery, emerges from the orbit above the medial palpebral ligament. It then gives off a twig to the upper part of the lacrimal sac. The artery is divided into two terminal branches, one of which crosses the root of the nose and anastomoses with the angular artery; the other runs along the dorsum of the nose, supplies its outer surface, and anastomoses with the artery on the opposite side and with the lateral nasal artery.[29,31]

Surgical Annotation

The dorsal nasal artery can be identified usually 5 to 7 mm above the medial canthal horizontal line. It gives off a superior central artery 3 to 5 mm after its origin.[32] It has many anastomoses with the angular artery, supratrochlear artery, alar branch of the facial artery, and superior labial artery (**Fig. 6.9, Fig. 6.12**). Two constant paramedian longitudinal branches from the dorsal nasal artery communicate freely across the midline.[1,28]

The central artery originates from the dorsal nasal artery. It supplies the glabella and inferior and middle transverse thirds of the central forehead. The central artery also has lateral anastomoses with the supratrochlear artery.

With an extensive surgical defect, such as eyelid trauma, periorbital cancer excision, cicatricial secondary healing, congenital anomalies, or nerve paralysis, a flap can be considered for eyelid reconstruction. Among the periorbital options, the goal of the reconstruction is to obtain functional and esthetic results.[31,33]

The branches of the ophthalmic artery (e.g., the dorsal nasal and supratrochlear arteries and the terminal branch of the angular artery) are responsible for the nutrition of the inner canthus region.[22,30] Dorsal nasal and angular artery flaps are repaired with a midline forehead flap, a paramedian forehead flap, a single-stage midline forehead flap, an interpolated melolabial flap, or a local nasal flap.[10,31–33]

Dual perfusion at the midline is consistent in the regions of the skin and soft tissue of the nasal dorsum, the forehead, and the lips. The vessels of the face form a series of plexuses, such as the deep facial, subcutaneous, and subdermal plexus. The deep facial plexus provides deep circulation to the anterior face lying deep behind or passing through the mimetic muscles.[6] This plexus communicates with the subdermal plexus via a dense population of small musculocutaneous penetrating branches of the facial, infraorbital, and supratrochlear arteries. The fasciocutaneous perforators of the transverse facial, submental, and posterior auricular arteries reach the subdermal plexus by passing through the deep facial planes and subcutaneous layers (**Fig. 6.4c**).[10]

References

1. Banks ND, Hui-Chou HG, Tripathi S, et al. An anatomical study of external carotid artery vascular territories in face and midface flaps for transplantation. Plast Reconstr Surg 2009;123(6):1677–1687
2. Behan FC, Rozen WM, Wilson J, Kapila S, Sizeland A, Findlay MW. The cervico-submental keystone island flap for locoregional head and neck reconstruction. J Plast Reconstr Aesthet Surg 2013;66(1):23–28
3. Houseman ND, Taylor GI, Pan WR. The angiosomes of the head and neck: anatomic study and clinical applications. Plast Reconstr Surg 2000;105(7):2287–2313
4. Marur T, Tuna Y, Demirci S. Facial anatomy. Clin Dermatol 2014;32(1):14–23
5. Pomahac B, Pribaz J. Facial composite tissue allograft. J Craniofac Surg 2012;23(1):265–267
6. Saban Y, Andretto Amodeo C, Bouaziz D, Polselli R. Nasal arterial vasculature: medical and surgical applications. Arch Facial Plast Surg 2012;14(6):429–436
7. Whetzel TP, Mathes SJ. Arterial anatomy of the face: an analysis of vascular territories and perforating cutaneous vessels. Plast Reconstr Surg 1992;89(4):591–603, discussion 604–605
8. Ozgur Z, Govsa F, Ozgur T. Anatomic evaluation of the carotid artery bifurcation in cadavers: implications for open and endovascular therapy. Surg Radiol Anat 2008;30(6):475–480
9. Ozgur Z, Govsa F, Ozgur T. Assessment of origin characteristics of the front branches of the external carotid artery. J Craniofac Surg 2008;19(4):1159–1166
10. Vasilic D, Barker JH, Blagg R, Whitaker I, Kon M, Gossman MD. Facial transplantation: an anatomic and surgical analysis of the periorbital functional unit. Plast Reconstr Surg 2010;125(1):125–134
11. Standring S. Gray's Anatomy, 40th ed. New York: Churchill Livingstone; 2009
12. Ozgur Z, Govsa F, Celik S, Ozgur T. Clinically relevant variations of the superior thyroid artery: an anatomic guide for surgical neck dissection. Surg Radiol Anat 2009;31(3):151–159
13. Fukuta K, Potparic Z, Sugihara T, Rachmiel A, Forté RA, Jackson IT. A cadaver investigation of the blood supply of the galeal frontalis flap. Plast Reconstr Surg 1994;94(6):794–800
14. Potparić Z, Fukuta K, Colen LB, Jackson IT, Carraway JH. Galeo-pericranial flaps in the forehead: a study of blood supply and volumes. Br J Plast Surg 1996;49(8):519–528
15. Kierner AC, Aigner M, Zelenka I, Riedl G, Burian M. The blood supply of the sternocleidomastoid muscle and its clinical implications. Arch Surg 1999;134(2):144–147
16. Cordova A, Pirrello R, D'Arpa S, Moschella F. Superior pedicle retroauricular island flap for ear and temporal region reconstruction:

anatomic investigation and 52 cases series. Ann Plast Surg 2008; 60(6):652–657
17. Ulkür E, Açikel C, Eren F, Celiköz B. Use of axial pattern cervico-occipital flaps in restoration of beard defects. Plast Reconstr Surg 2005;115(6):1689–1695
18. Al-Hoqail RA, Meguid EM. Anatomic dissection of the arterial supply of the lips: an anatomical and analytical approach. J Craniofac Surg 2008;19(3):785–794
19. Higashino T, Sawamoto N, Hirai R, Arikawa M. Zygomatico-orbital artery as a recipient vessel for microsurgical head and neck reconstruction. J Craniofac Surg 2013;24(4):e385–e387
20. Pinar YA, Bilge O, Govsa F. Anatomic study of the blood supply of perioral region. Clin Anat 2005;18(5):330–339
21. Atamaz Pinar Y, Govsa F, Bilge O. The anatomical features and surgical usage of the submental artery. Surg Radiol Anat 2005;27(3): 201–205
22. Erdogmus S, Govsa F. The arterial anatomy of the eyelid: importance for reconstructive and aesthetic surgery. J Plast Reconstr Aesthet Surg 2007;60(3):241–245
23. Pinar YA, Ikiz ZA, Bilge O. Arterial anatomy of the auricle: its importance for reconstructive surgery. Surg Radiol Anat 2003;25 (3-4):175–179
24. Hwang K, Kim DH, Huan F, Nam YS, Han SH. The anatomy of the palpebral branch of the infraorbital artery relating to midface lift. J Craniofac Surg 2011;22(4):1489–1490
25. Veyssiere A, Rod J, Leprovost N, et al. Split temporalis muscle flap anatomy, vascularization and clinical applications. Surg Radiol Anat 2013;35(7):573–578
26. Nakajima H, Imanishi N, Minabe T. The arterial anatomy of the temporal region and the vascular basis of various temporal flaps. Br J Plast Surg 1995;48(7):439–450
27. Pinar YA, Govsa F. Anatomy of the superficial temporal artery and its branches: its importance for surgery. Surg Radiol Anat 2006; 28(3):248–253
28. Chen TH, Chen CH, Shyu JF, Wu CW, Lui WY, Liu JC. Distribution of the superficial temporal artery in the Chinese adult. Plast Reconstr Surg 1999;104(5):1276–1279
29. Yu D, Weng R, Wang H, Mu X, Li Q. Anatomical study of forehead flap with its pedicle based on cutaneous branch of supratrochlear artery and its application in nasal reconstruction. Ann Plast Surg 2010;65(2):183–187
30. Erdogmus S, Govsa F. Anatomy of the supraorbital region and the evaluation of it for the reconstruction of facial defects. J Craniofac Surg 2007;18(1):104–112
31. Turgut G, Ozcan A, Yeşiloğlu N, Baş L. A new glabellar flap modification for the reconstruction of medial canthal and nasal dorsal defects: "flap in flap" technique. J Craniofac Surg 2009;20(1):198–200
32. Park SS. The single-stage forehead flap in nasal reconstruction: an alternative with advantages. Arch Facial Plast Surg 2002;4(1): 32–36
33. Onishi K, Maruyama Y, Okada E, Ogino A. Medial canthal reconstruction with glabellar combined Rintala flaps. Plast Reconstr Surg 2007;119(2):537–541

7 Veins of the Face and Neck

Yusuke Shimizu

Introduction

In this chapter, the venous system of the head and neck is categorized into the veins of the face, scalp, and neck. The main venous drainage pathway of the face is through the hemiloop-like vein that surrounds the orbit. The vein can be formed by the supraorbital, angular, or facial veins, depending on its location. It collects most of the blood from the face and connects mainly to the zygomatico-temporal, superior ophthalmic, deep facial, and internal jugular veins. The main venous drainage pathway of the superficial parts of the scalp is through the superficial temporal, middle temporal, occipital, and posterior auricular veins. These veins drain into the external jugular vein. The internal jugular vein is the main venous drainage pathway of the head and neck; the external and anterior jugular veins are the pathways from the superficial layers of the region. The vertebral vein collects blood from the prevertebral muscles and drains into the brachiocephalic vein.

Veins of the Face

The main venous drainage pathway of the face is primarily the facial vein. In the middle of the face, the hemiloop-like vein surrounds the orbit.[1] This vein can be contributed to by the supraorbital, angular, or facial veins, depending on its location (**Fig. 7.1**). These veins are connected to the zygomatico-temporal vein in the upper lateral region of the orbit, to the superior ophthalmic vein in the medial canthal area, to the deep facial vein in the nasolabial area, and to the internal or external jugular veins in the lower lateral area (**Fig. 7.2**). As with most superficial veins, these veins have many variations. Common patterns are discussed here (**Fig. 7.3**).

Supraorbital Vein

The supraorbital vein passes medially above the orbital rim under the orbicularis oculi muscle to connect to the angular vein in the medial canthal area. A branch of the supraorbital vein also connects to the superior ophthalmic vein at the supraorbital notch or foramen. Laterally, it connects to the zygomatico-temporal vein arising from the middle temporal vein near the zygomatic process of the frontal bone. There, it also connects with radicles of the superficial temporal veins.

Surgical Annotations

The zygomatico-temporal vein is known as a *sentinel vein*. The vein is located in a 10-mm zone above which the temporal branch of the facial nerve passes.[2]

Supratrochlear Vein

Basically, one or two large veins arise from the medial canthal area and run toward the forehead. The supratrochlear vein connects to the tributaries of the superficial temporal veins to form a large venous network in the forehead. Both the deep veins from the pericranial layer and the superficial veins from the galea frontalis layer empty into the vein.[3] The supratrochlear vein finally joins the angular or nasal root vein near the medial canthus.[1]

Nasal Root Vein

Arising superficially from the angular vein, the nasal root vein pierces the procerus muscle and anastomoses with its contralateral counterpart to form a large communicating vein under the skin of the nasal root.[1] The nasal root vein is convex toward the nasal tip. It is a bridge of the bilateral hemiloop-like veins. Several tributaries from the external nose connect to the nasal root vein (**Fig. 7.4**).

Angular Vein

The angular vein is formed by the union of the supratrochlear and supraorbital veins. It runs inferiorly across the medial margin of the medial canthal tendon approximately 8 mm from the medial canthus of the eye.[4] It becomes the facial vein at its

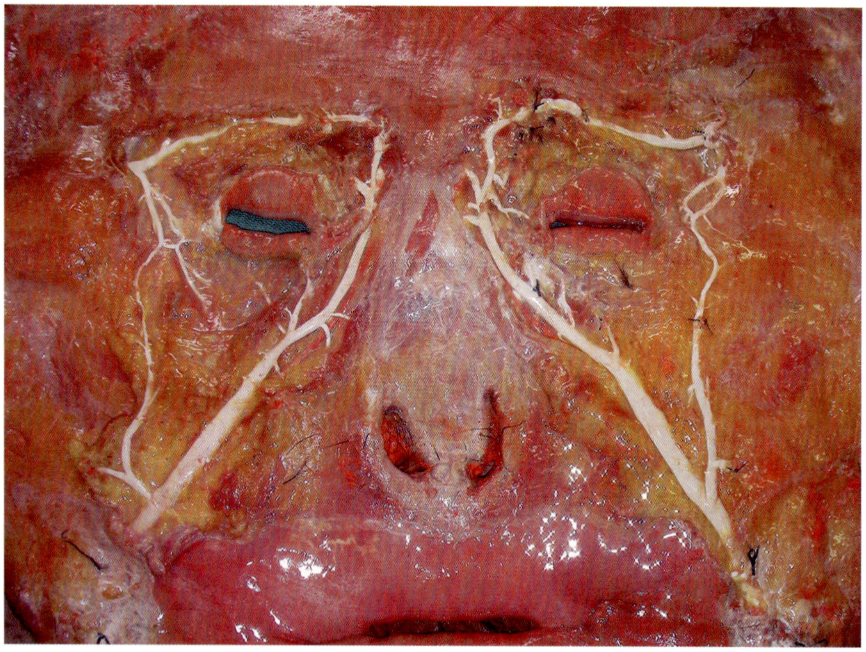

Fig. 7.1 Fresh cadaver specimen with white contrast medium inside the veins. The hemiloop-like vein surrounds the orbit. The vein can be formed by the supraorbital, angular, or facial injected into veins, depending on its location.

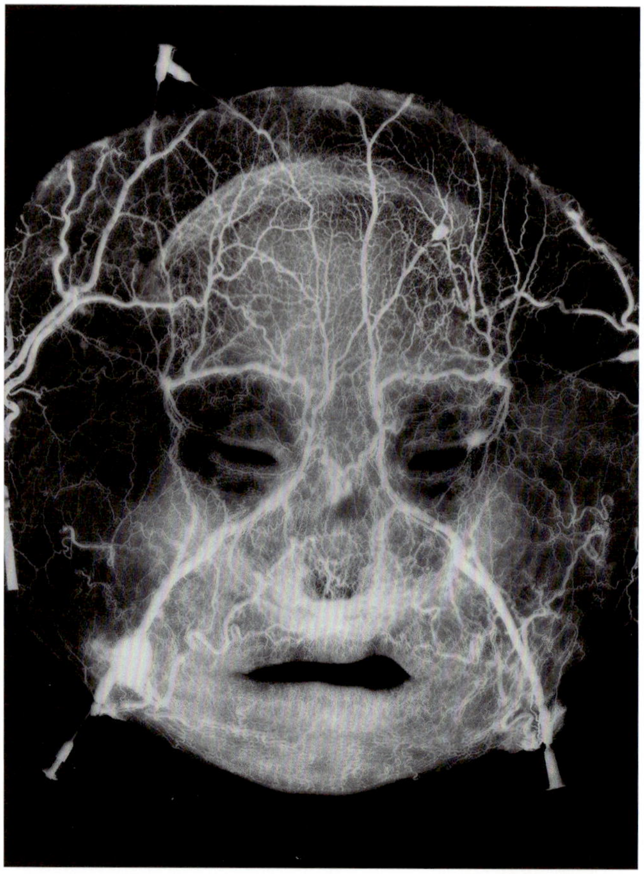

Fig. 7.2 Arteriovenogram of the face. The hemiloop-like vein surrounds the orbit. The tributaries of the superficial temporal vein connect to the vein in the forehead area. The supratrochlear vein connects to the vein in the medial canthal area. The vein drains into the facial vein.

junction with the superior labial vein.[5] The two major veins arise from it, namely, the transverse nasal root vein (superficial) and a branch to form the inferior root of the superior ophthalmic vein (deep). Several tributaries from the external nose and lower eyelid also connect to the angular vein (**Fig. 7.5**).

Superior Ophthalmic Vein

The superior ophthalmic vein is formed at the superomedial margin of the orbit immediately posterior to the trochlea by the union of two contributing roots, namely, a superior root from the supraorbital vein and an inferior root from a branch of the angular vein. It runs with the ophthalmic artery and links the facial and intracranial veins. It traverses the superior orbital fissure to end in the cavernous sinus. The superior ophthalmic vein has venous valves; the blood flows toward the cavernous sinus.[6]

Inferior Ophthalmic Vein

The inferior ophthalmic venous plexus is formed by veins with abundant interconnections.[7] It originates in a network of minute veins in the anterior region of the orbital floor and receives veins from the inferior rectus muscle, inferior oblique muscle, lacrimal sac, and eyelids. It usually joins the superior ophthalmic vein. Rarely, the vein can drain directly into the cavernous sinus.[8] It connects with the pterygoid venous plexus by a small branch that passes through the inferior orbital fissure.

Facial Vein

The facial vein is the main venous drainage pathway of the face. It starts from the angular vein and descends obliquely near the

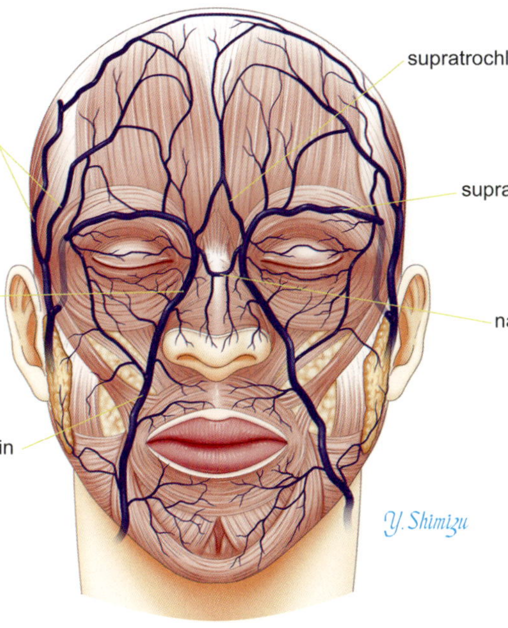

Fig. 7.3 A common pattern of the facial veins. The facial vein begins at the angular vein and descends obliquely near the nasolabial fold.

side of the nasolabial fold. The facial vein and artery lie in close proximity at the level of the lower edge of the mandible. Thereafter, however, the artery takes a tortuous course among the facial muscles, whereas the vein has a direct path from the angular vein to the lower mandibular border.[9] It passes under the facial muscles and crosses the body of the mandible and runs obliquely back under the platysma but superficial to the submandibular gland and digastric and stylohyoid muscles. The facial vein is joined by the anterior division of the retromandibular vein near the mandibular angle and finally drains directly or indirectly into the internal jugular vein.

Cranial to the mandible, the deep facial vein from the pterygoid venous plexus and the inferior palpebral, superior and inferior labial, buccinator, parotid, and masseteric veins join the facial vein. Caudal to the mandible, the submental, tonsillar, external palatine, and submandibular veins join the facial vein.

The facial vein has valves, particularly around the level of the mandible (**Fig. 7.6**).[10] The distribution of venous valves indicates that the blood flow is caudal toward the internal jugular vein in the lower part of the facial vein and normally toward the cavernous sinus in the superior ophthalmic vein.[6]

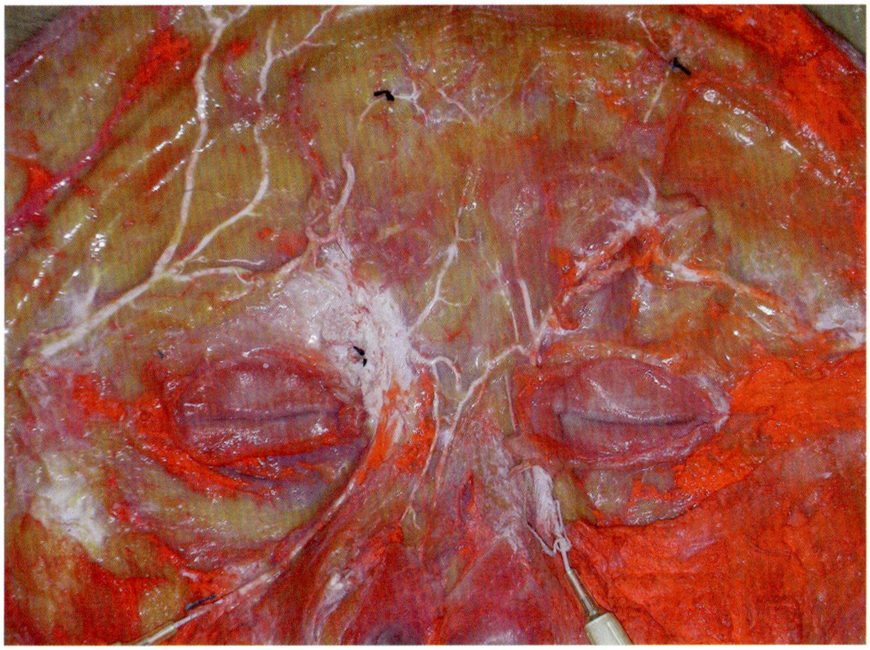

Fig. 7.4 The nasal root vein. The nasal root vein connects the bilateral hemiloop-like veins at the nasal root. Several tributaries from the external nose connect to the vein.

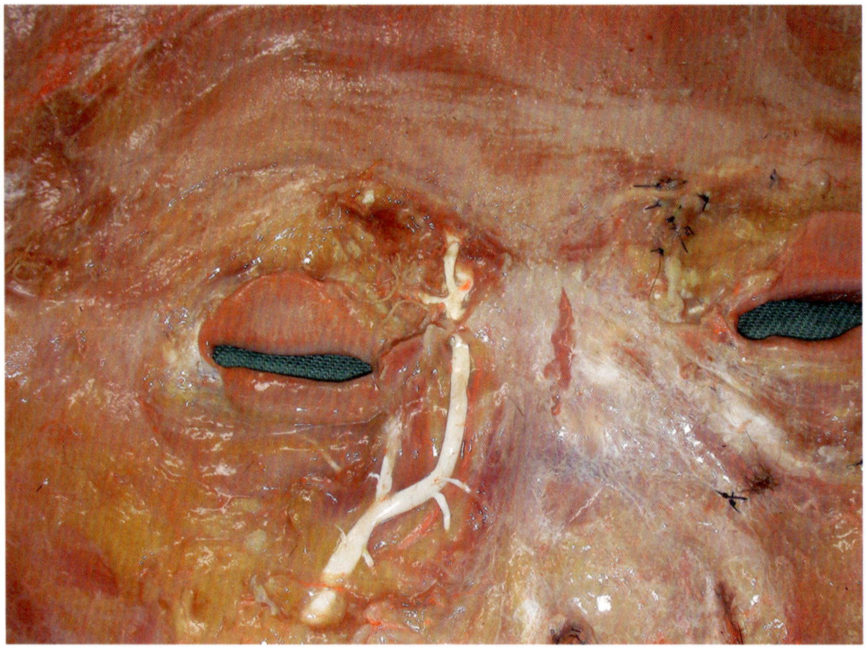

Fig. 7.5 The angular vein. Several tributaries from the external nose and lower eyelid connect to this vein.

Surgical Annotations

The facial vein connects with the cavernous sinus by two major routes, that is, through the superior ophthalmic vein or through the deep facial vein to the pterygoid plexus and, finally, the cavernous sinus. Thus, infection may spread from the face to the intracranial venous sinuses.

Pterygoid Venous Plexus

The pterygoid venous plexus is an extensive network of small vascular channels that are located between the temporalis and lateral pterygoid muscles (**Fig. 7.7**). The sphenopalatine, deep temporal, pterygoid, masseteric, buccal, alveolar, greater palatine, and middle meningeal veins and a branch from the inferior ophthalmic vein join the plexus. The plexus connects with the facial vein through the deep facial vein and with the cavernous sinus through the sphenoidal emissary foramen, foramen ovale, and foramen lacerum. Its deep temporal branch often connects with tributaries of the anterior diploic vein and thus with the middle meningeal veins.

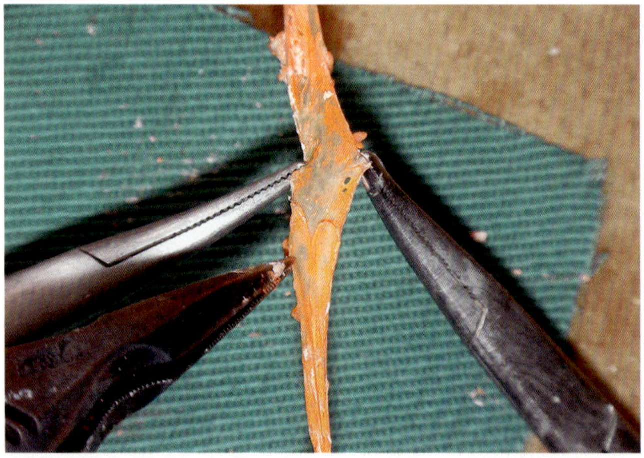

Fig. 7.6 The valve in the facial vein. The facial vein commonly has valves around the level of the mandible.

Surgical Annotations

In reduction malarplasty, which is common in Asian patients, osteotomy should be performed cautiously and not too deep in reaching the periosteum of the posterior side of the maxillary sinus to avoid injuring the deep facial vein, which lies just behind the posterior side of the maxillary sinus.[11]

Maxillary Vein

The maxillary vein consists of a short trunk that serves as the main drainage pathway of the pterygoid venous plexus. It passes backward between the sphenomandibular ligament and neck of the mandible with the mandibular segment of the maxillary artery.[12] It forms the retromandibular vein by connecting with the superficial temporal vein.

Retromandibular Vein

The retromandibular vein is a deep drainage pathway of the face formed by the union of the superficial temporal and maxillary veins. It runs caudally in the parotid gland. It divides into two major branches: (1) an anterior branch that passes forward to join the facial vein to form the common facial vein and a (2) posterior branch that joins the posterior auricular vein to form the external jugular vein.

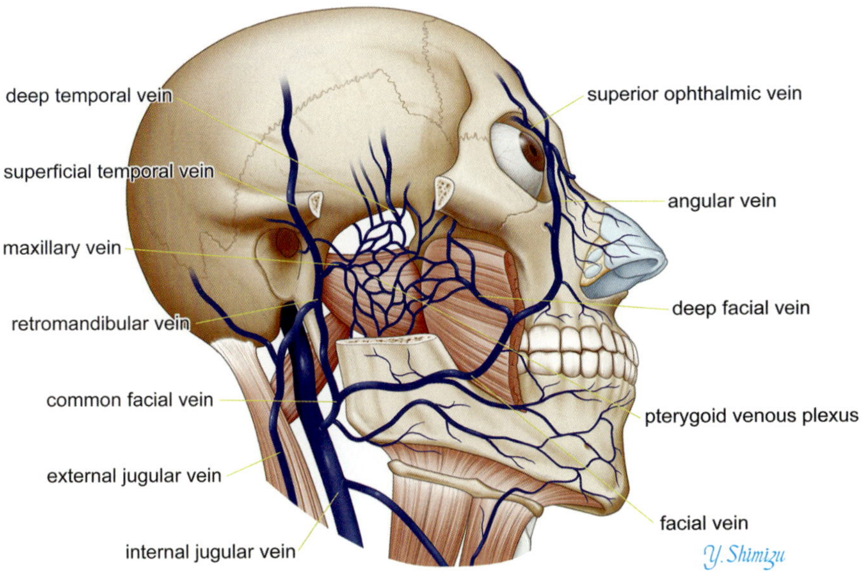

Fig. 7.7 The pterygoid venous plexus. The pterygoid venous plexus is an extensive network of small vascular channels that are located between the temporalis and lateral pterygoid muscles. The sphenopalatine, deep temporal, pterygoid, masseteric, buccal, alveolar, greater palatine, and middle meningeal veins and a branch from the inferior ophthalmic vein join the plexus.

Veins of the Scalp

The main venous drainage pathway of the superficial part of the scalp is through the superficial temporal, middle temporal, occipital, and posterior auricular veins (**Fig. 7.8**).

Superficial Temporal Vein

The superficial temporal vein begins in a widespread network of the scalp. It joins the corresponding vein of the contralateral side, the ipsilateral supratrochlear, supraorbital, posterior auricular, and occipital veins. The vein divides into one, two, or three major branches in the scalp. The pathways are basically independent from the frontal and parietal branches of the superficial temporal artery, except for its proximal portion.[13] The proximal portion of the vein crosses the zygomatic arch and enters the parotid gland to unite with the maxillary vein to form the retromandibular vein. The superficial temporal vein receives blood from the parotid veins, articular veins from the temporomandibular joint, anterior auricular veins, and the transverse facial vein from the side of the face.

Middle Temporal Vein

The middle temporal vein lies beneath the superficial layer of the deep temporal fascia and is distributed in the superficial temporal fat pad between the superficial and deep layers of the deep temporal fascia.[14] The vein connects the supraorbital vein

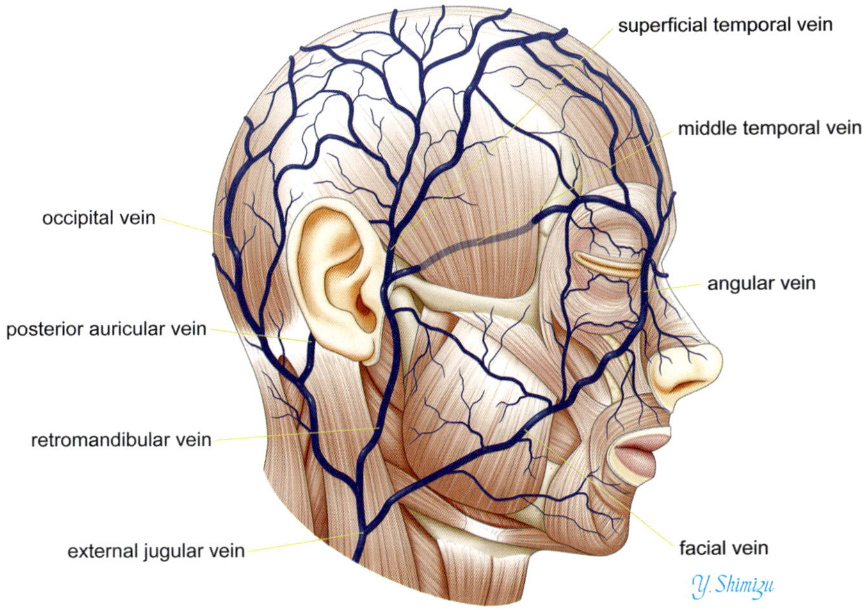

Fig. 7.8 The veins of the scalp. The main venous drainage pathway of the superficial part of the scalp is through the superficial temporal, middle temporal, occipital, and posterior auricular veins.

through the zygomatic temporal vein near the zygomatic process of the frontal bone. As the vein passes back to the proximal side, it pierces and runs several millimeters over the surface of the superficial layer of the deep temporal fascia. Finally, the vein joins the superficial temporal vein approximately 1 cm below the upper aspect of the zygomatic root.

Surgical Annotations

The caliber of the middle temporal vein is significantly greater than that of the superficial temporal vein.[14] The vein can be safely used as a recipient vessel in case of free-tissue transfer.

Occipital Vein

The vein begins as a plexus in the posterior scalp at the external occipital protuberance. It pierces the cranial attachment of the trapezius muscle, turns into a venous plexus in the suboccipital triangle, and joins the deep cervical and vertebral veins. It finally joins the posterior auricular vein. Occasionally, it accompanies the occipital artery and ends in the internal jugular vein. The parietal and mastoid emissary veins link it with the superior sagittal and transverse sinuses.

Posterior Auricular Vein

The posterior auricular vein begins from the parieto-occipital venous network, which communicates with the occipital and superficial temporal veins. It descends behind the auricle to join the posterior branch of the retromandibular vein to form the external jugular vein. It collects the blood from the stylomastoid vein and some tributaries from the cranial surface of the auricle and also often receives a mastoid emissary vein from the sigmoid sinus.

Surgical Annotations

Inadvertent injury of the mastoid emissary vein poses a significant problem not only because of difficulty with hemostasis but also because of its bidirectional flow and close proximity to the sigmoid sinus.[15]

Veins of the Neck

Basically, the internal jugular vein collects most of the blood from the head and neck (**Fig. 7.9, Fig. 7.10**). It drains all but the subcutaneous structures. The external and anterior jugular veins collect blood from the superficial layer of the head and neck. They drain a much smaller volume of tissue than do the deep veins.[16] Some veins connect directly to the subclavian veins, which collect blood from the upper limbs. The internal jugular and subclavian veins connect to form the brachiocephalic vein. The bilateral brachiocephalic veins drain into the superior vena cava.

Subclavian Vein

The subclavian vein is a continuation of the axillary vein that runs from the outer border of the first rib to the medial border of the anterior scalene muscle. From here, it connects with the internal jugular vein to form the brachiocephalic vein. The vein follows the subclavian artery and is separated from the artery by the insertion of the anterior scalene muscle. Hence, the vein

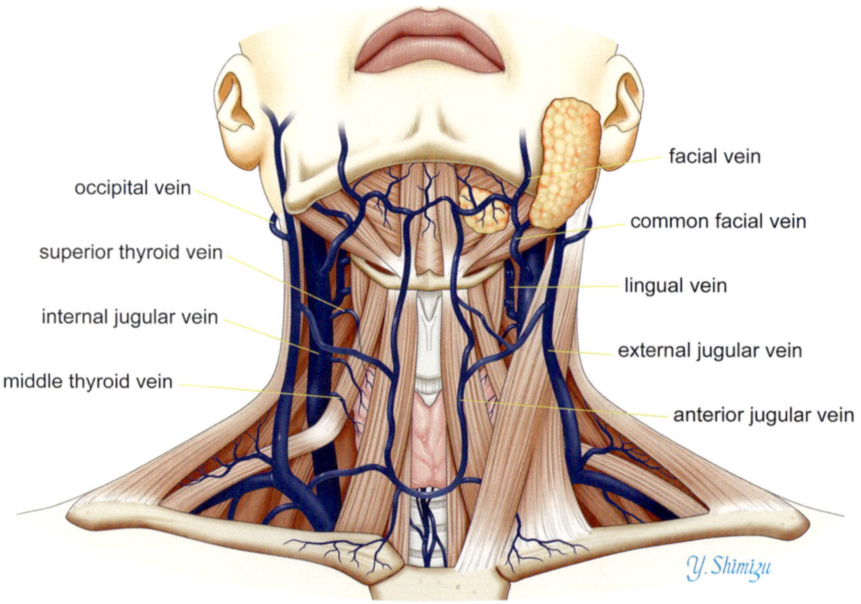

Fig. 7.9 The veins of the neck (anterior view). The internal jugular vein basically collects most of the blood from the head and neck. The external and anterior jugular veins collect blood from the superficial layer of the head and neck. Some veins connect directly to the subclavian veins.

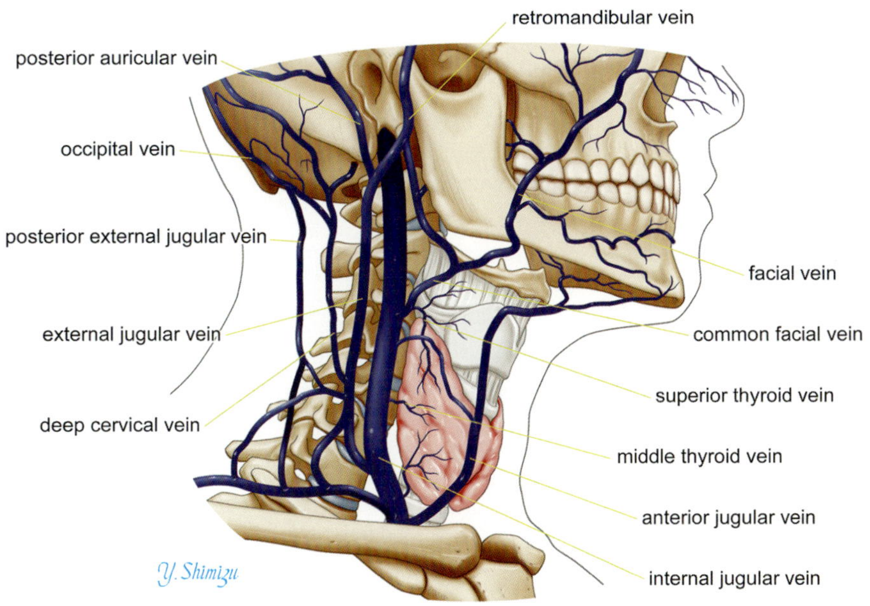

Fig. 7.10 The veins of the neck (lateral view).

lies anterior to the muscle, whereas the artery lies posterior to the muscle. The thoracic duct drains into the left subclavian vein near its junction with the left internal jugular vein (i.e., venous angle), and the right lymphatic duct drains into the junction of the right internal jugular and right subclavian veins.

Internal Jugular Vein

The internal jugular vein collects blood from the skull, brain, face, and most of the neck. The inferior petrosal and sigmoid sinuses unite to form the internal jugular vein, which begins in the jugular foramen at the cranial base. At its origin, there is the so-called superior bulb. The vein runs caudally in the carotid sheath, lying just lateral to the arteries, uniting with the subclavian vein to form the brachiocephalic vein near the sternal end of the clavicle. At its end, there is the so-called inferior bulb, which contains a pair of valves above it. Generally, the left vein is thinner than the right vein.

The posterior aspect of the vein consists of the rectus capitis lateralis muscle, transverse process of the atlas, levator scapulae muscle, middle scalene muscle, cervical plexus, anterior scalene muscles, phrenic nerve, thyrocervical trunk, vertebral vein, and first part of subclavian artery. The medial aspect of the vein is bordered by the the internal and common carotid arteries and vagus nerve. The vagus nerve is usually found between the artery and vein. Superficially, the vein is overlapped above and then covered below by the sternocleidomastoid muscle and crossed by the posterior belly of the digastric muscle and superior belly of the omohyoid muscle. The deep cervical lymph nodes lie along the vein, mainly on its superficial aspect. At the root of the neck, the right internal jugular vein is separated from the common carotid artery; the left usually overlaps its artery. At the cranial base, the internal carotid artery is anterior and is separated from the vein by the ninth to the twelfth cranial nerves. The facial, lingual, pharyngeal, superior, and middle thyroid veins, and sometimes the occipital veins, join the internal jugular vein. It may communicate with the external jugular vein.

Lingual Veins

The lingual veins begin on the dorsum, sides, and undersurface of the tongue and pass back along the course of the lingual artery and end in the internal jugular vein. The dorsal lingual veins drain the dorsum and sides of the tongue and join the lingual veins between the hyoglossus and genioglossus muscles. The deep lingual vein begins near the tip and passes back near the mucous membrane on the inferior surface of the tongue. Near the anterior border of the hyoglossus muscle, it joins a sublingual vein that drains the salivary gland to form the vena comitans of the hypoglossal nerve, which passes back between the mylohyoid and hyoglossus muscles to join the facial, internal jugular, or lingual vein.

Pharyngeal Veins

The pharyngeal veins begin in a pharyngeal plexus posterolateral to the pharynx. After communicating with the pterygoid venous plexus and receiving meningeal veins, they end in the internal jugular vein

Superior Thyroid Vein

The superior thyroid vein begins in the substance of the thyroid gland and passes cranially along with the superior thyroid artery. The vein receives the superior laryngeal and cricothyroid veins and ends in the upper part of the internal jugular vein.

Middle Thyroid Vein

The middle thyroid vein drains the lower part of the thyroid gland, the larynx, and the trachea. It crosses anterior to the common carotid artery to join the lower part of the internal jugular vein.

External Jugular Vein

The external jugular vein largely drains the scalp and face. It lies superficial to the sternocleidomastoid muscle and can be represented by a line that starts just below and behind the angle of the mandible and descends to the clavicle near the posterior border of the sternocleidomastoid muscle. The union of the posterior division of the retromandibular and posterior auricular veins begins near the mandibular angle. It runs caudally in the direction of a line drawn from the angle of the mandible to the middle of the clavicle at the posterior border of the sternocleidomastoid muscle. It is covered by the platysma, superficial fascia, and skin, separated from the sternocleidomastoid muscle by deep cervical fascia. The external jugular vein varies in size, bearing an inverse proportion to the other veins in the neck. The vein is occasionally doubled.[16] It has valves at its entrance into the subclavian vein approximately 4 cm above the clavicle between which it is often dilated. The external jugular vein receives the posterior external jugular vein and, near its end, the transverse cervical, suprascapular, and anterior jugular veins. In the parotid gland, it is often joined by a branch from the internal jugular vein. The occipital vein occasionally joins it.

Anterior Jugular Vein

The anterior jugular vein begins near the hyoid bone by the confluence of the superficial veins from the submaxillary region. It descends between the midline and anterior border of the sternocleidomastoid muscle and turns laterally in the lower part of the neck. It joins the end of the external jugular or subclavian vein directly. The size of the vein is usually in inverse proportion to that of the external jugular vein. It communicates with the internal jugular veins and receives the laryngeal veins and sometimes a small thyroid vein. There are usually two anterior jugular veins and they are united by a large transverse jugular arch above the sternum. The arch receives tributaries from the inferior thyroid veins.

Posterior External Jugular Vein

The posterior external jugular vein begins in the occipital scalp and drains the skin and superficial muscles in the upper and back parts of the neck, lying between the splenius and trapezius muscles. It descends at the back part of the neck and usually joins the middle part of the external jugular vein.

Deep Cervical Vein

The deep cervical vein accompanies its artery between the semispinalis capitis and colli muscles. It starts from veins from the occipital and suboccipital muscles and from the plexuses around the cervical spine. It passes forward between the seventh cervical transverse process and neck of the first rib to join the lower part of the vertebral vein. It receives tributaries from the plexuses around the spinous processes of the cervical vertebrae.

Vertebral Vein

The vertebral vein is formed in the suboccipital triangle by numerous small tributaries from the internal vertebral venous plexuses, which leave the vertebral canal above the posterior arch of the atlas. They unite with small veins from the local deep muscles to form a vessel that enters the foramen in the transverse process of the atlas to descend around the vertebral artery as a plexus. This plexus ends as the single vertebral vein, emerging from the sixth cervical transverse foramen. It descends to join the brachiocephalic vein. A small accessory vertebral vein usually descends from the vertebral plexus. It traverses the seventh cervical transverse foramen and turns forward between the subclavian artery and cervical pleura to also join the brachiocephalic vein. The vertebral vein receives branches from the occipital vein, prevertebral muscles, and internal and external vertebral plexuses. It receives the anterior vertebral and deep cervical veins and sometimes the first intercostal vein.

Anterior Vertebral Vein

The anterior vertebral vein begins as a plexus around the upper cervical transverse processes. It descends with the ascending cervical artery between the attachments of the anterior scalenus and capitis longus muscles and connects with the vertebral vein.

References

1. Shimizu Y, Imanishi N, Nakajima T, Nakajima H, Aiso S, Kishi K. Venous architecture of the glabellar to the forehead region. Clin Anat 2013;26(2):183–195
2. Trinei FA, Januszkiewicz J, Nahai F. The sentinel vein: an important reference point for surgery in the temporal region. Plast Reconstr Surg 1998;101(1):27–32
3. Yoshioka N, Rhoton AL Jr. Vascular anatomy of the anteriorly based pericranial flap. Neurosurgery 2005;57(1, Suppl)11–16
4. Wolff E. Anatomy of the Eye and Orbit. 6th ed. London: H.K. Lewis & Co. Ltd.; 1968
5. Standring S, ed. Gray's Anatomy: The Anatomical Basis of Clinical Practice. 40th ed. Edinburgh: Churchill Livingstone; 2008
6. Zhang J, Stringer MD. Ophthalmic and facial veins are not valveless. Clin Experiment Ophthalmol 2010;38(5):502–510
7. Cheung N, McNab AA. Venous anatomy of the orbit. Invest Ophthalmol Vis Sci 2003;44(3):988–995
8. Natori Y, Rhoton ALJ Jr. Microsurgical anatomy of the superior orbital fissure. Neurosurgery 1995;36(4):762–775
9. Houseman ND, Taylor GI, Pan WR. The angiosomes of the head and neck: anatomic study and clinical applications. Plast Reconstr Surg 2000;105(7):2287–2313
10. Nishihara J, Takeuchi Y, Miki T, Itoh M, Nagahata S. Anatomical study on valves of human facial veins. J Craniomaxillofac Surg 1995; 23(3):182–186

11. Choi BK, Lee KT, Oh KS, Yang EJ. Preservation of the deep facial vein in reduction malarplasty. J Craniofac Surg 2012;23(3):e254–e257
12. Joo W, Funaki T, Yoshioka F, Rhoton AL Jr. Microsurgical anatomy of the infratemporal fossa. Clin Anat 2013;26(4):455–469
13. Imanishi N, Nakajima H, Minabe T, Chang H, Aiso S. Venous drainage architecture of the temporal and parietal regions: anatomy of the superficial temporal artery and vein. Plast Reconstr Surg 2002; 109(7):2197–2203
14. Yano T, Tanaka K, Iida H, Kishimoto S, Okazaki M. Usability of the middle temporal vein as a recipient vessel for free tissue transfer in skull-base reconstruction. Ann Plast Surg 2012;68(3):286–289
15. Kim LK, Ahn CS, Fernandes AE. Mastoid emissary vein: anatomy and clinical relevance in plastic & reconstructive surgery. J Plast Reconstr Aesthet Surg 2014;67(6):775–780
16. Shenoy V, Saraswathi P, Raghunath G, Karthik JS. Double external jugular vein and other rare venous variations of the head and neck. Singapore Med J 2012;53(12):e251–e253

8 Facial Nerve and Temporal Bone

Orlando Guntinas-Lichius

Introduction

The facial nerve has a complex course from the brainstem to the periphery. The nerve crosses critical and frequently accessed surgical structures in cranial-base surgery, otoneurologic surgery, head and neck surgery, and cosmetic surgery. During transtemporal approaches, the surgeon has to drill the temporal bone to avoid injury to the facial nerve. When performing approaches to the regions involving the facial nerve, it is mandatory to understand the topographic anatomy of the facial nerve from different surgical perspectives. This chapter provides an overview of the facial nerve from the brainstem through the temporal bone. The extratemporal course of the facial nerve is presented in Chapter 9. All portions and segments of the facial nerve, its blood supply, surrounding structures, radiologic anatomy, and relation to typical surgical approaches are presented in detail to guide the surgical management of this important structure.

Segments of the Facial Nerve

Because of the intricate course of the facial nerve from the brainstem to the periphery, the course is divided into three different portions. Topographically, the portions of the facial nerve are divided into segments. The portions and segments are summarized in **Table 8.1**. The facial nerve is composed of branchiomotor, parasympathetic, visceroafferent, and somatic-efferent fibers. Facial-nerve branches with different fiber qualities are leaving or entering the nerve during its course to the periphery. The facial nerve has internal branches leaving and entering the nerve in the temporal bone, and all external branches leave the nerve after its exit from the stylomastoid foramen.[1] **Table 8.2** gives an overview of the facial nerve branches.

Intracranial Portion

Three primary brainstem nuclei contribute to the function of the facial nerve: (1) the facial motor nucleus for somatic motor function (in a stricter sense, the facial nerve is an exclusive motor nerve), (2) the superior salivatory nucleus for secretomotor (autonomic) function, and (3) the nucleus of the tractus solitarius for taste. All three nuclei are located in the brainstem (**Fig. 8.1**): (1) the facial motor nucleus in the lower third of the pons in the floor of the fourth ventricle, (2) the superficial salivary nucleus directly next to the facial motor nucleus, and (3) the nucleus of the tractus solitarius lateral to the dorsal vagus nucleus in the medulla oblongata. It is important, when treating a patient with a brainstem lesion and facial palsy, to differentiate the localization of the nuclei of the facial nerve. Depending on the lesion site, the patient can have a supranuclear, nuclear, or infranuclear (peripheral) facial-nerve palsy or a combined lesion; this consideration is important in the prognosis of the palsy and valuable in planning facial-nerve reconstruction surgery. Moreover, a lesion of the superior salivatory nucleus or of the nucleus of tractus solitarius can explain nonmotor deficits of the patient related to the facial nerve.

Medullary Segment

The facial motor nucleus contains the facial motoneuron soma, the axons of which form the facial motor nerve. Here the medullary segment begins. The axons leave the nucleus first in a dorsomedial direction, pass around the nucleus of the abducens nerve to form the internal facial genu (knee) (cf. **Fig. 8.1b**), and leave the brainstem from the anterior pons lateral to the abducens nerve and medial to the vestibulocochlear nerve. The facial motor nerve is joined by the intermediate nervus (nervus intermedius, nerve of Wrisberg) containing sensory and parasympathetic fibers. The parasympathetic fibers of the nervus intermedius arise from the salivatory nuclei, and the taste fibers terminate in the nucleus tractus solitarius. The nervus intermedius is lateral to the facial motor nerve when both leave the brainstem in the cerebellopontine angle (CPA). The medullary segment of the facial nerve ends here, and the cisternal segment begins.

Cisternal Segment

Within the CPA cistern, the facial nerve is most anterior and superior, the vestibulocochlear nerve most posterior, and the nervus intermedius— giving the nerve its name—between the two. This is important when orientating for vestibular schwannoma surgery or facial-nerve repair should be performed in the CPA. The cisternal segment ends when the facial nerve enters the porus acusticus of the internal acoustic meatus. The facial nerve and the nervus intermedius resemble the nerve roots of the spinal cord within the cistern.[2]

Table 8.1 Classification of the course of the facial nerve

Portion/segment	Length (mm)
Intracranial portion	
Medullary segment	3.5–6
Cisternal segment	18–21
Intratemporal portion	
Meatal segment	8–12
Labyrinthine Segment	3–5
Geniculate ganglion segment	3–3
Tympanic segment	8–11
Mastoid segment	13–14
Extratemporal portion (see Chapter 9 for details)	15–20

Intratemporal Portion

Meatal Segment

The facial nerve enters the temporal bone via the internal acoustic meatus. The meatal segment is congruent with the internal acoustic meatus. The facial and vestibulocochlear nerves pass through the internal acoustic meatus on the posteromedial surface of the petrous ridge. The facial nerve is joined by the nervus intermedius. Both are located in the anterior superior quadrant of the internal acoustic meatus above the falciform crest and anterior to Bill's bar. These are important landmarks when approaching the facial nerve via a translabyrinthine, transcochlear, or middle cranial fossa approach.

Labyrinthine Segment

As the facial nerve enters the fallopian canal, the labyrinthine segment begins (**Fig. 8.2**). The fallopian canal houses the labyrinthine, tympanic, and mastoid segments. The nerve takes an anterolateral course between and superior to the cochlea (anterior) and vestibule (posterior). Then the nerve turns back posteriorly at the geniculate ganglion. The labyrinthine segment is short and is the narrowest segment. The facial nerve occupies up to 83% of the labyrinthine canal cross-sectional area compared with only 64% of the more distal mastoid segment.[3] Therefore, it is said that the labyrinthine segment is especially susceptible to vascular compression, which might play a role in treating patients with idiopathic facial palsy (Bell's palsy).

Geniculate Ganglion Segment

The geniculate ganglion segment is equated to the geniculate ganglion (**Fig. 8.3, Fig. 8.4**). Some authorities include the geniculate ganglion with the labyrinthine segment. Following this definition, the geniculate ganglion would reside within the distal part of the labyrinthine segment. The ganglion consists of first-order pseudounipolar nerve cells related to taste sensation from the anterior tongue via the chorda tympani and the greater petrosal nerve. The latter reaches the ganglion from the greater petrosal canal. At the ganglion, the nerve has to bend down to reach the tympanic segment; this bend is called the external genu.

Tympanic Segment

After the geniculate ganglion, the nerve becomes the tympanic segment. The junction to the tympanic segment is formed by an

Table 8.2 Major branches of the facial nerve

Branch	Location	Function
Greater petrosal nerve	Geniculate ganglion segment	Parasympathetic fibers for lacrimal gland and salivary glands and visceroafferent fibers for sensation of palate
Nerve branch to the stapedius muscle	Mastoid segment	Branchiomotor fibers innervating stapedius muscle
Chorda tympani	Mastoid segment	Visceroafferent taste fibers from the anterior third of the tongue
Posterior auricular nerve	Mastoid segment or extratemporal portion	Branchiomotor fibers innervating ear muscle, may contain also sensory fibers
Nerve branch to stylohyoid muscle	Mastoid segment or extratemporal portion	Branchiomotor fibers innervating stylohyoid muscle
Nerve branch to posterior belly of digastric muscle	Mastoid segment or extratemporal portion	Branchiomotor fibers innervating posterior belly of digastric muscle
Parotid plexus	Extratemporal portion	Branchiomotor fibers innervating muscles of facial expression (details in Chapter 9)

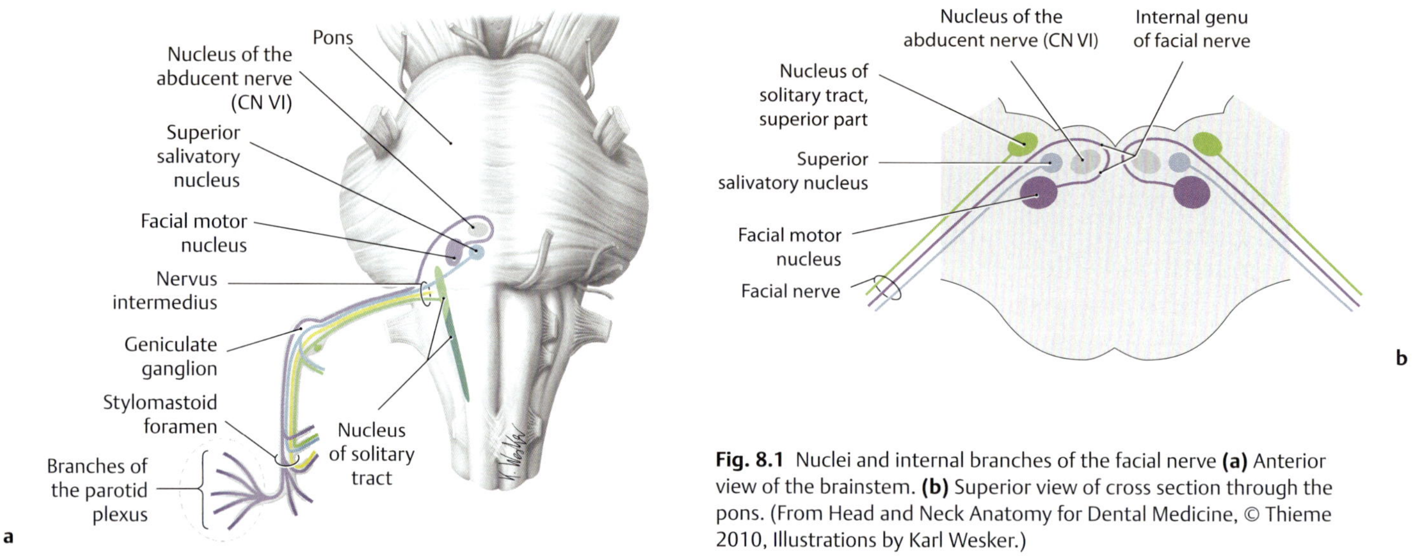

Fig. 8.1 Nuclei and internal branches of the facial nerve **(a)** Anterior view of the brainstem. **(b)** Superior view of cross section through the pons. (From Head and Neck Anatomy for Dental Medicine, © Thieme 2010, Illustrations by Karl Wesker.)

acute angle, and shearing of the facial nerve commonly occurs as the nerve traverses this genu.[4] The facial nerve runs posteriorly beneath the lateral semicircular canal in the medial wall of the middle ear cavity (**Fig. 8.5**). The fallopian canal is often dehiscent, especially in the area near the oval window.[5] This is important during middle ear surgery because the absent bony protection can allow for direct invasion of the facial nerve by chronic infection and because the nerve is at greater risk for iatrogenic injury in such situations. Duplication of the facial

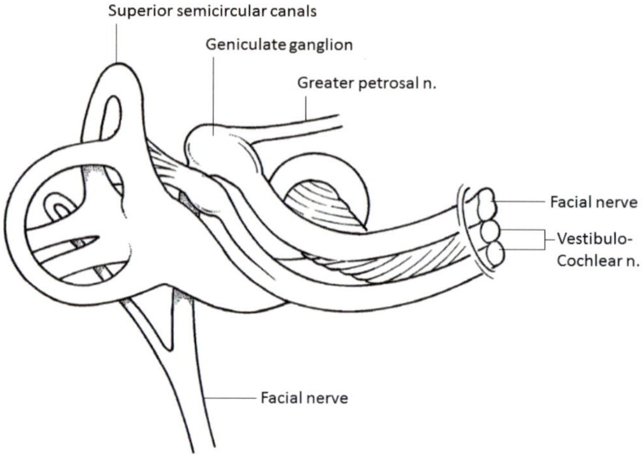

Fig. 8.2 Relation of the meatal, labyrinthine, and geniculate ganglion segments to the inner ear. As the facial nerve exits the internal acoustic meatus at the fundus, it turns gently anteriorly and runs in the otic capsule for 3 to 6 mm between the cochlea and superior semicircular canal.

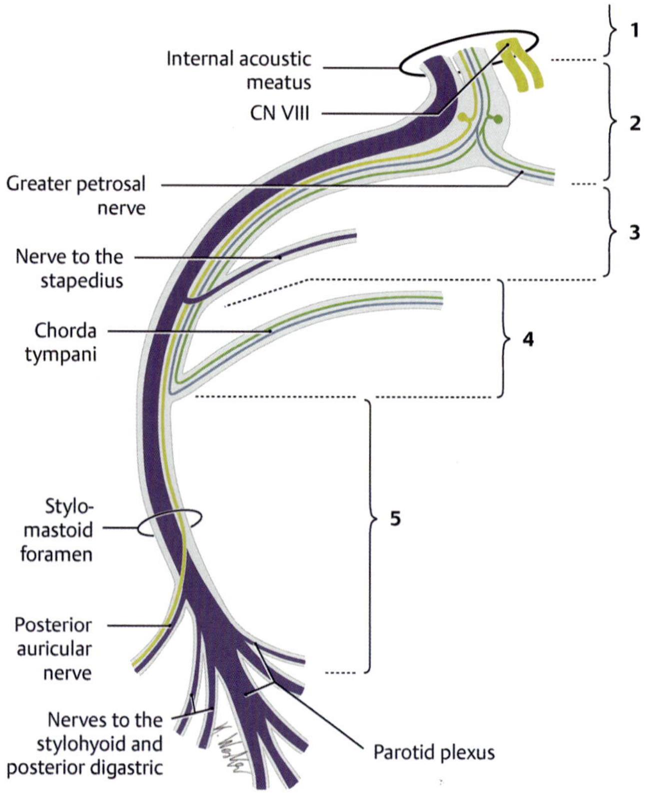

Fig. 8.3 Course and branches of the facial nerve. (1) Internal acoustic meatus. (2) External genu of facial nerve. (3) Proximal mastoid segment. (4) Distal mastoid segment. (5) Extratemporal portion. (Reproduced from Head and Neck Anatomy for Dental Medicine, © Thieme 2010, Illustration by Karl Wesker.)

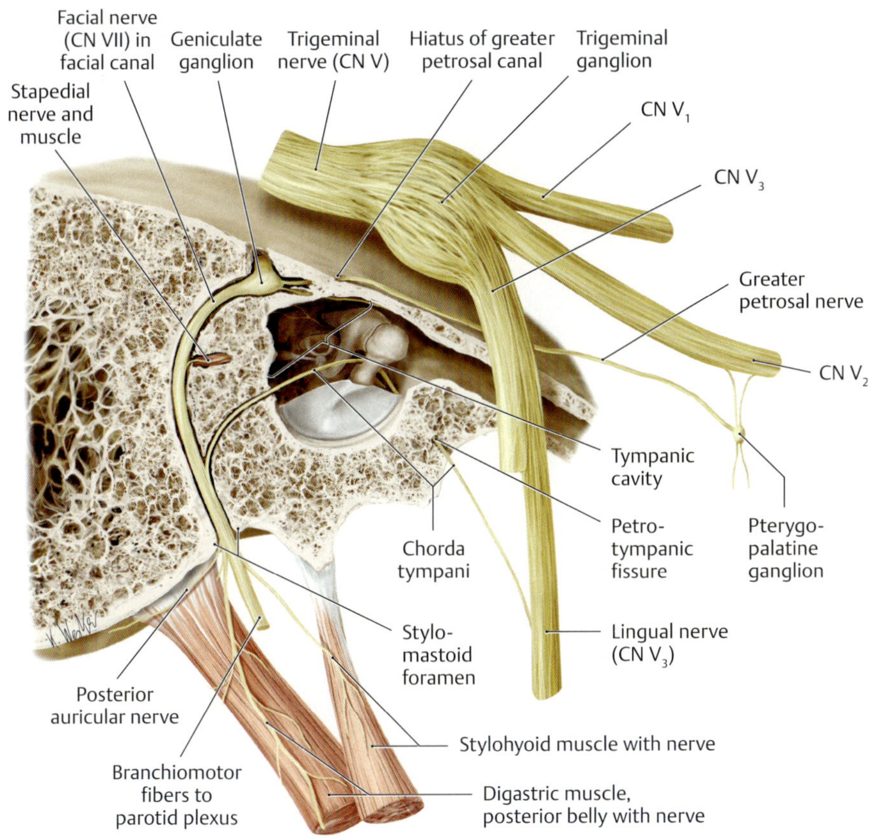

Fig. 8.4 Relation of the intratemporal course of the facial nerve to the middle ear cavity. Lateral view of right temporal bone (petrous part). Both the facial and vestibulocochlear nerves (CN VIII, not shown) pass through the internal acoustic meatus on the posterior surface of the petrous part of the temporal bone. The facial nerve courses laterally in the bone to the external genu, which contains the geniculate ganglion. At the genu, CN VII bends and descends in the facial canal. It gives off three branches between the geniculate ganglion and the stylomastoid foramen. (From Head and Neck Anatomy for Dental Medicine, © Thieme 2010, Illustration by Karl Wesker.)

nerve is rare and seen most often at its tympanic segment and associated with middle and inner ear anomalies.[6] Next, the nerve passes posterior to the cochleariform process, tensor tympani, and oval window. Distal to the pyramidal eminence, the facial nerve makes a second turn, the so-called second genu, which passes downward. Here the mastoid segment of the facial nerve begins. The tympanic segment of the facial nerve has no branches.

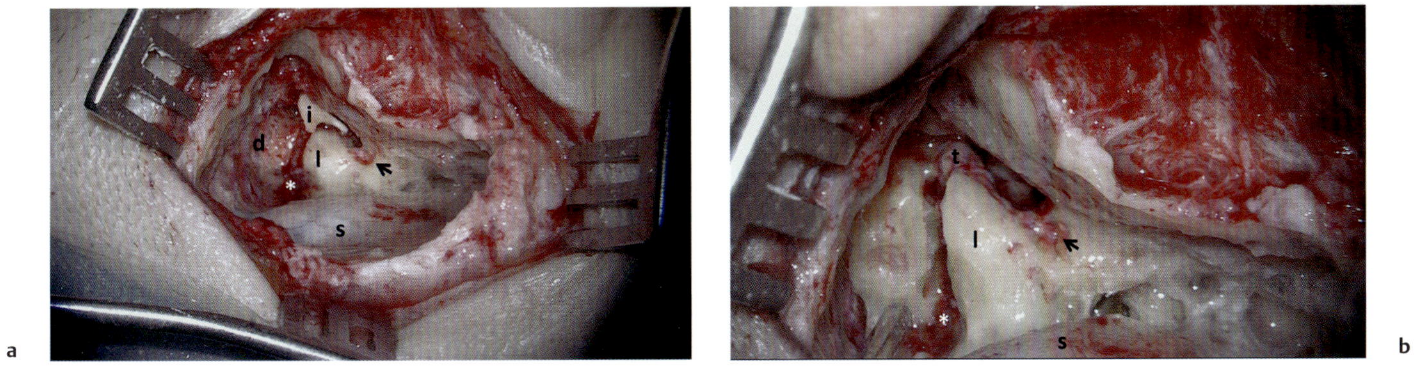

Fig. 8.5 Intraoperative view of extended mastoidectomy in patient with right temporal bone fracture (*). Before **(a)** and after **(b)** extirpation of the incus (i) in order to explore the tympanic segment (t) of the facial nerve. The fracture has exposed and injured the facial nerve in the tympanic segment. Decompressed part of the mastoid segment of the facial nerve (arrow), dura mater of middle cranial fossa (d), lateral semicircular canal (l), and sigmoid sinus (s).

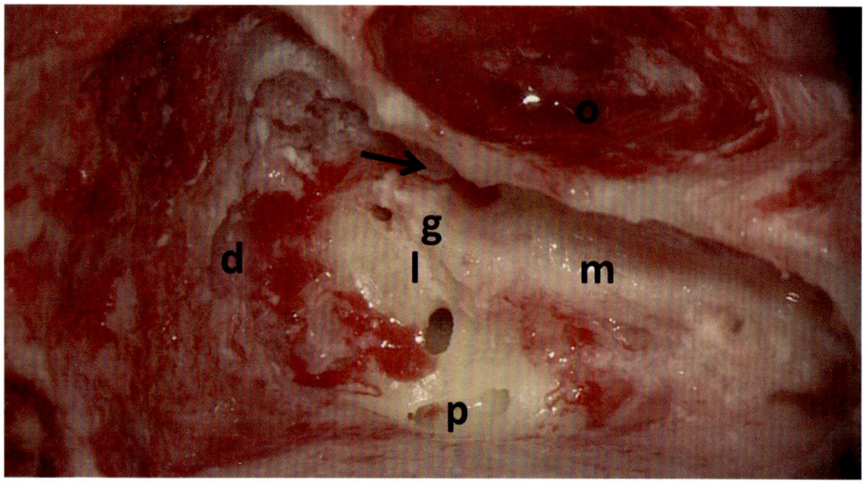

Fig. 8.6 Intraoperative view, translabyrinthine approach during vestibular schwannoma surgery of the right ear showing the relation of the second genu (g) and the mastoid segment (m) of the facial nerve to the lateral semicircular canal (l), the posterior semicircular canal (p), and the incus (*arrow*); dura mater of middle cranial fossa (d); external acoustic meatus (o).

Mastoid Segment

The mastoid segment begins at the second genu of the facial nerve and ends at the stylomastoid foramen (**Fig. 8.6**). Rarely, the second genu is considered separately as the pyramidal segment. The facial nerve gives off three branches from its mastoid segment. These are, from proximal to distal: the branch to the stapedius muscle, the chorda tympani, and the posterior auricular nerve. The chorda tympani passes through the tympanic cavity and the petrotympanic fissure to reach the infratemporal fossa. The chorda tympani is an important landmark when a posterior tympanotomy is being performed so as to define the level of the mastoid facial nerve and the distal limit of the tympanotomy window to the middle ear cavity. The posterior auricular nerve usually arises from the mastoid segment and leaves the temporal bone together with the facial nerve at the stylomastoid foramen. The nerve provides branches to the stylohyoid and posterior digastric muscles normally distal to the stylomastoid foramen (i.e., beyond the mastoid segment but before the extratemporal part of the facial nerve enters the parotid gland).

For facial nerve reconstruction surgery, it is sometimes necessary to access the mastoid segment of the nerve. For example, if a tumor has destroyed parts of the extratemporal facial nerve plexus, it might be that surgical exploration shows that the facial nerve is infiltrated by the tumor up to the stylomastoid foramen. In such a situation, mastoidectomy is performed and the mastoid segment of the facial nerve exposed step-by-step until tumor-free margins of the proximal facial nerve stump are achieved.

Blood Supply of the Intracranial and Intratemporal Portions

The blood supply to the intracranial and intratemporal parts of the facial nerve is provided by three main arteries. During temporal bone and middle cranial fossa surgery, these vessels should be protected to ensure optimal blood supply to the intratemporal portion of the facial nerve. A branch of the anterior inferior cerebellar artery (AICA), the labyrinthine artery, supplies the meatal segment. It may be additionally supplemented directly by small branches from the AICA. Furthermore, a branch of the middle meningeal artery, the superficial petrosal artery, runs in a retrograde fashion along the greater petrosal nerve and supplies this area. The petrosal artery is at risk of being damaged during the middle cranial fossa approach when the dura is elevated from the floor of the fossa.[7] Finally, a branch of the posterior auricular artery, the stylomastoid artery, runs retrograde into the stylomastoid foramen to supply the facial nerve. The labyrinthine segment of the facial nerve is supplied only by thin connections between the labyrinthine artery and superficial petrosal artery as end arteries. Therefore, the labyrinthine segment is the most vulnerable to ischemia, which might be why it is frequently affected in cases of idiopathic facial nerve palsy.

Radiologic Anatomy

The method of choice to depict the typical course of the facial nerve from the brainstem with its first genu (medullary segment) is by magnetic resonance imaging (MRI). With MRI, the facial nerve is also identified in the CPA anterior to the vestibulocochlear nerve within the CPA cistern. The nervus intermedius cannot always be differentiated from the facial motor nerve using standard MRI. Nowadays, 3 Tesla magnetic MRI (3T MRI) allows reliable depiction of the nervus intermedius in most cases.[8] MRI can show that both nerves and the vestibulocochlear nerve are covered by a common dural sheath.[9] Most neuroradiologists and facial nerve surgeons are familiar with computed tomography (CT) as a modality of studying the intratemporal portion of the facial nerve, especially with high-resolution CT (HRCT).[9,10] Using HRCT, the labyrinthine segment is identified on coronal and axial planes as lying between the internal acoustic meatus and the geniculate fossa. It is located between the cochlea and vestibule. Normally, this segment can always be seen when looking at the same axial plane as the lateral semicircular canal. Here the labyrinthine segment is concave on its anteromedial side as it bends around the cochlea. The tympanic segment is located between the lateral semicircular canal and

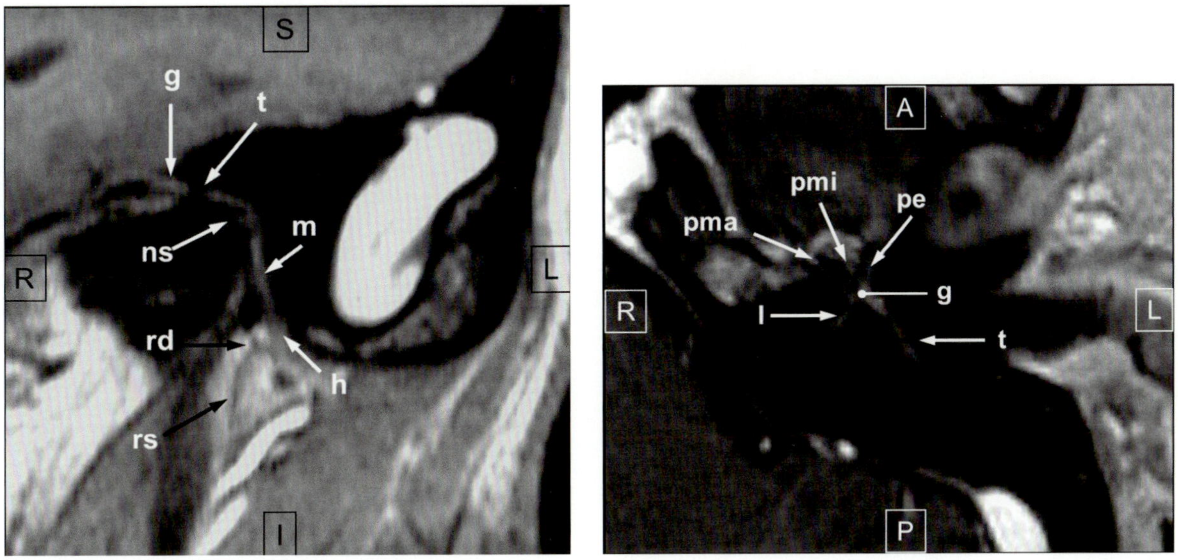

Fig. 8.7 Magnetic resonance imaging (MRI) anatomy of the normal intratemporal facial nerve. **(a)** parasagittal T1-weighted view with gadolinium contrast; **(b)** axial T1-weighter view with gadolinium contrast. A, Anterior; g, geniculate ganglion; h, main trunk at the stylomastoid foramen; I, inferior; L, left; m, mastoid segment; NS, stapedius nerve; P, posterior; pe, external petrosal nerve; pma, greater petrosal; pmi, lesser petrosal nerve; R, right; rd, digastric branch; rs, stylohyoid branch; S, superior; t , tympanic segment. (Reproduced courtesy of Dr. Hartmut Peter Burmeister, Institut für Radiologie, Klinikum Bremerhaven-Reinkenheide, Bremerhaven, Germany.)

the tympanic cavity. Its position is 1–2 mm inferior to the lateral semicircular canal. The tympanic segment is better visualized on axial CT sections. The second genu defining the beginning of the mastoid segment is identified by looking for the posterior semicircular canal. The genu normally courses about 6 mm lateral to the most inferior part of the posterior semicircular canal. Distal to the genu, the mastoid segment can be identified in the mastoid and is seen well on transaxial sections. Alternatively, this most distal intratemporal segment of the facial nerve can be found by following the canal up from the stylomastoid foramen on coronal sections.[10]

MRI, especially high-resolution 3 T MRI with contrast-enhancement, can depict the intratemporal segments of the facial nerve and even small branches like the nerve to the stapes, the posterior auricular branch, the digastric branch, and stylohyoid branch (**Fig. 8.7**).[11]

Surgical Approaches to the Intracranial and Intratemporal Portions of the Facial Nerve

The most common approaches to the facial nerve are via anterior petrosectomies (middle cranial fossa and extended middle cranial fossa approaches), posterior petrosectomies (translabyrinthine [cf. (**Fig. 7.6**)], retrolabyrinthine, and transcochlear approaches), the retrosigmoid approach, the far lateral approach, and anterior transfacial approaches (extended maxillectomy and mandibular swing approaches).[12,13] To examine the facial nerve in the CPA and meatal segment superiorly, anterior petrosal approaches offer good exposures. The posterior petrosectomies provide more direct visualization without the need for cerebellar retraction. The lateral approach exposes parts of the posterior and the entire inferior quadrants of the cisternal segment in the CPA. The retrosigmoid approach best exposes parts of the superior and inferior quadrants and the entire posterior quadrant in the CPA. Anterior and anteroinferior exposures of the facial nerve can be achieved using transfacial approaches.[13] During a middle cranial fossa approach, identification of the greater petrosal nerve is an important step. Mean distances from the arcuate eminence to the hiatus of the greater petrosal nerve in the middle cranial fossa measure about 17.5 mm. The length of this nerve within the middle cranial fossa is approximately 10 mm. From the lateral wall of the middle cranial fossa to a midpoint of the greater petrosal nerve, the mean distance is 39 mm.[14]

The facial recess approach via a posterior tympanotomy is commonly performed to facilitate cochlear implantation. The facial recess approach also allows access to the round window for insertion of middle ear implants in patients with congenital ear atresia. Even in patients with normal ears, access through the superior opening of the facial recess is limited by the presence of both the mastoid segment of the facial nerve and the chorda tympani.[15] Atresia surgery is challenging because of the altered anatomy of the facial nerve.[16] The mastoid segment of the facial nerve is more anteriorly positioned in deformed ears, on average 3 to 7 mm more anteriorly, than in ears with normal anatomy. Furthermore, most facial nerves are located above the round window in the deformed ears.[16] Hence, opening the atretic plate to obtain subfacial access to the round window is recommended in deformed ears to protect the facial nerve.

References

1. Baker EW. Head and Neck Anatomy for Dental Medicine. New York: Thieme; 2010
2. Myckatyn TM, Mackinnon SE. A review of facial nerve anatomy. Semin Plast Surg 2004;18(1):5–12
3. Fisch U, Esslen E. Total intratemporal exposure of the facial nerve. Pathologic findings in Bell's palsy. Arch Otolaryngol 1972;95(4): 335–341
4. May M. Anatomy for the Clinician. In: May M, Schaitkin BM, Hrsg. The Facial Nerve. New York: Thieme; 2000
5. Di Martino E, Sellhaus B, Haensel J, Schlegel JG, Westhofen M, Prescher A. Fallopian canal dehiscences: a survey of clinical and anatomical findings. Eur Arch Otorhinolaryngol 2005;262(2):120–126
6. Glastonbury CM, Fischbein NJ, Harnsberger HR, Dillon WP, Kertesz TR. Congenital bifurcation of the intratemporal facial nerve. AJNR Am J Neuroradiol 2003;24(7):1334–1337
7. El-Khouly H, Fernandez-Miranda J, Rhoton AL Jr. Blood supply of the facial nerve in the middle fossa: the petrosal artery. Neurosurgery 2008; 62(5, Suppl 2)ONS297–ONS303, discussion ONS303–ONS304
8. Burmeister HP, Baltzer PA, Dietzel M, et al. Identification of the nervus intermedius using 3T MR imaging. AJNR Am J Neuroradiol 2011;32(3):460–464
9. Phillips CD, Bubash LA. The facial nerve: anatomy and common pathology. Semin Ultrasound CT MR 2002;23(3):202–217
10. Tüccar E, Tekdemir I, Aslan A, Elhan A, Deda H. Radiological anatomy of the intratemporal course of facial nerve. Clin Anat 2000; 13(2):83–87
11. Burmeister HP, Hause F, Baltzer PA, et al. Improvement of visualization of the intermediofacial nerve in the temporal bone using 3T magnetic resonance imaging: part 1: the facial nerve. J Comput Assist Tomogr 2009;33(5):782–788
12. Sanna M, Khrais T, Mancini F, et al. The Facial Nerve in Temporal Bone and Lateral Skull Base Microsurgery. Stuttgart: Thieme; 2006.
13. Bernardo A, Evins AI, Visca A, Stieg PE. The intracranial facial nerve as seen through different surgical windows: an extensive anatomosurgical study. Neurosurgery 2013; **72**(2, Suppl Operative) ons194–ons207, discussion ons207
14. Tubbs RS, Custis JW, Salter EG, Sheetz J, Zehren SJ, Oakes WJ. Landmarks for the greater petrosal nerve. Clin Anat 2005;18(3):210–214
15. Hamamoto M, Murakami G, Kataura A. Topographical relationships among the facial nerve, chorda tympani nerve and round window with special reference to the approach route for cochlear implant surgery. Clin Anat 2000;13(4):251–256
16. Fu Y, Dai P, Zhang T. The location of the mastoid portion of the facial nerve in patients with congenital aural atresia. Eur Arch Otorhinolaryngol 2014;271(6):1451–1455

9 Peripheral Branches of the Facial Nerve

Andrew P. Trussler

Introduction

Navigation around the facial nerve is important in any facial procedure, invasive or noninvasive. With the advent of a "less is more" trend in facial aesthetics, attention toward avoidance of the facial nerve has been falsely perpetuated. Less attention to educating medical residents on deeper-plane facelift techniques has developed an "out of sight, out of mind" attitude toward the facial nerve and its branches. Attention is gained when an inadvertent facial nerve injury happens, without the knowledge of how or where it could have occurred. It is hoped that this chapter on facial nerve anatomy will shed light on the anatomical landmarks and fascial boundaries of the nerve, as well as highlight danger zones of facial nerve injury (**Fig. 9.1**).

Facial nerve injury during facelift surgery is a relatively rare but real occurrence, with an incidence ranging between 0.5 and 2.6%. This risk may be acceptably low in a primary superficial facelift, where the risk of injury to the facial nerve may be considered less, although the actual risk may be the introduction of scarring around the nerve and risk of contorting the nerve position, which makes it prone to injury in a secondary facelift procedure after a superficial facelift has failed. The more superficial facelift techniques have been subjected to longevity issues, although this topic has been subjectively debated. A 2- to 5-year longevity of a superficial lift is well documented. If the continued superficial plane is used, the risk for injury may be with superficial musculoaponeurotic system (SMAS)plication or SMASectomy, although if the deeper plane is entered, scarring may distort the facial nerve branches, making them susceptible to injury. Even injectables can cause enough irritation and scarring whereby care should be taken to maintain the fascial boundaries of the facial nerve during SMAS dissection.

A sub-SMAS dissection is safe, and the facial nerve does have a predictable location, which makes navigating around it easy for the experienced facelift surgeon. There are predictable locations that the nerve is tethered either in fascia or with a neurovascular ligamentous adhesion. These are the areas where caution is warranted when elevating the facelift flap.

Understanding of the facial nerve in three dimensions is beneficial when elevating the SMAS. Knowledge about the cutaneous landmarks, the bony landmarks, and the depth of the nerve as it traverses the face from posterior to anterior makes the ability to alter and customize the SMAS flap to meet each individual's rejuvenation goals. The thickness of the face and SMAS does vary in different patients, and a thin-faced patient will likely have a thin SMAS flap; therefore, numerical depth is less clinically applicable where anatomical boundaries with fascial planes are more relevant in facelift surgery.

Facial Nerve

The facial nerve is a motor nerve as it exits through the stylomastoid foramen at the skull base. The main trunk is anterior to the midportion of the earlobe and lies approximately 2 cm below the skin; it is surrounded by dense fascia. The nerve ascends from the stylomastoid foramen into the parotid gland at an approximate 45-degree angle. The main trunk branches within 1 cm of entering the parotid gland as two main trunks superior and inferior. The nerve trunks bifurcate the parotid gland's two lobes and travel superficial to the deep lobe at a depth of 1 cm (**Fig. 9.2a,b**). The two main trunks of the facial nerve split into the formal trunks of the named branches of the face as they exit the parotid gland (**Fig. 9.2c**).

Frontal Branch

The subcutaneous course of the frontal (temporal) branch was initially described in 1966 by Ramos and Pitanguy (**Fig. 9.3**).[1] Their findings of an anatomical study showed that the frontal branch coursed from 0.5 cm from the tragus to 1.5 cm lateral to the supraorbital rim. Their findings have provided a topographic map for the nerve, although its depth in three dimensions continues to be confusing. Numerous studies have described its location, but consensus has not been attained as to the depth or its fascial boundaries.

The fascial relationships of the frontal branch of the facial nerve vary remarkably within the literature. It remains ambiguous in part because of the lack of a standardized nomenclature and in part because of the considerable variation in the described depth of the nerve at various levels across the zygomatic temporal region. As shown by the works of Furnas, Gosain et al, and Stuzin et al, no consistency exists as to the exact fascial plane and safe plane of dissection in and across the zygomatic arch.[2–5] Confounding the issue further are the numerous names attributed to the various fascial layers. The temporoparietal fascia, which is a continuation of the SMAS, has multiple names and has been referred to as the superficial temporal fascia and or the galea aponeurotica. The deep temporal fascia envelops the temporalis muscle and extends down to the zygomatic arch, fusing with the periosteum anteriorly and posteriorly. This layer is often broken down into superficial and deep portions, which are separated by the temporal fat pad as described by Stuzin et al.[4,5] With regard to the superficial deep temporal fascia, several names exist in the literature and include the intermediate fascia and the innominate fascia.[4–6] Finally, there are descriptions of the loose areolar plane between the temporoparietal fascia and

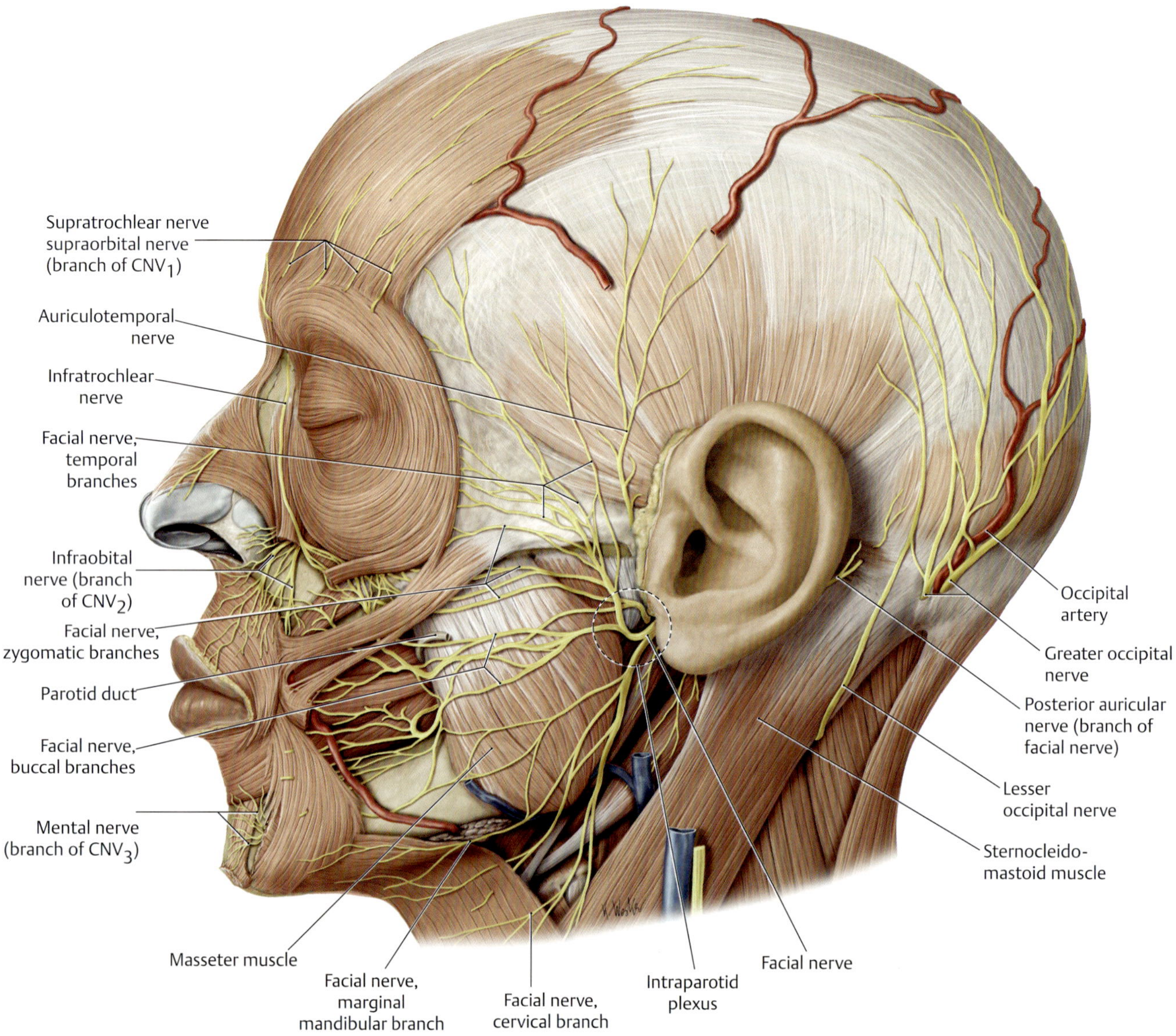

Fig. 9.1 Overview of the facial nerve (left lateral view). (Reproduced from THIEME Atlas of Anatomy, Head and Neuroanatomy, © Thieme 2010, Illustration by Karl Wesker.)

the deep temporal fascia, and some authors refer to this area as a separate fascial plane and have referred to it as the innominate fascia or subaponeurotic plane. These variations and discrepancies are partly to blame for the lack of consistency with respect to the depth and location of the frontal branch of the facial nerve across the zygomatic temporal region.

The thought that the nerve branch travels within the SMAS has clinically correlated with the alteration of facelift technique. Stuzin et al. describe a lateral low SMAS fasciotomy to protect the frontal branch with a superior extension to the lateral canthus.[7] In the high SAMS technique, the SMAS is incised transversely at a level above the zygomatic arch. The advantage of this technique would be to provide a vertical vector to the facelift with a composite flap containing SMAS and subcutaneous cheek tissue.[8,9] Based on previous studies, one might expect a 100% incidence of frontal branch injury, but in reality the author has not had any permanent nerve injury. The technique to prevent nerve injury in this technique includes a subcutaneous temporal dissection superficial to the frontal branch 2 cm above the arch at the level of the lateral canthus. The nerve is isolated on a temporal mesentery with deep dissection on the deep temporal fascia. After the SMAS has been elevated, the level of SMAS transection is then incised with a push cut across the arch to the orbicularis oculi while maintaining the temporal mesentery.

The high SMAS facelift uses a multiplanar sub-SMAS and subcutaneous dissection to mobilize the cheek and then a transverse SMAS fasciotomy above the zygomatic arch to allow for a vertical vector of repositioning. This direction of facelift replaces the facial soft tissue as a composite unit to a youthful and natural position. The transverse SMAS incision has been one point of

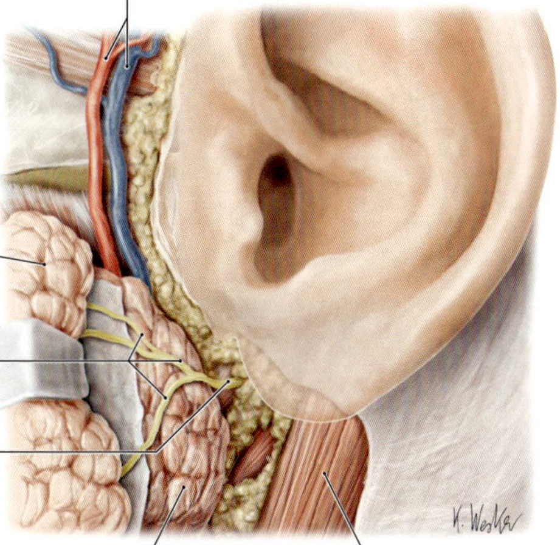

a

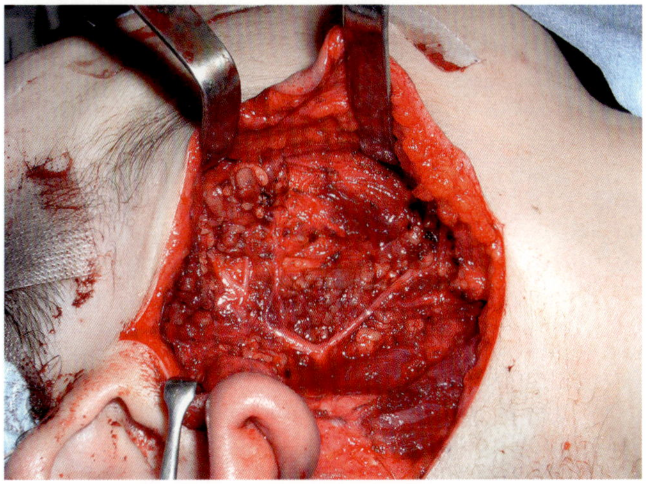

b

Fig. 9.2 The facial nerve in the parotid gland **(a)** Main trunk of the facial nerve and parotid plexus (left lateral view). The nerve ascends from the stylomastoid foramen into the parotid gland and bifurcates into two main trunks: superior and inferior. (From THIEME Atlas of Anatomy, Head and Neuroanatomy, Thieme 2010, Illustration by Karl Wesker.) **(b)** Operation findings of a right parotid tumor. The superficial layer of the right parotid gland was resected and parotid plexus of the facial nerve was exposed.

contention in gaining acceptance of this procedure secondary to the lack of consensus of the course of the frontal branch and the inherent risk of frontal branch injury. The study by Trussler et al has demonstrated that if the procedure is performed appropriately, the frontal branch is deep to the SMAS above the zygomatic arch and has an additional layer of fascia, the parotid temporal fascia, covering it.[10] This fascia was first described in 1965 by Furnas as a laminated areolar tissue continuous with the galea.[3] Additional descriptions have included a superficial temporal fascia, temporoparietal fascia, and innominate fascia. I propose that the fascia be named by its origin and insertion, like that of the parotid masseteric fascia and temporaparietal fascia, so that the terminology is uniform in this region. The parotid temporal fascia is not a novel fascia, as demonstrated by previous descriptions, although this term is a plea for consistency so that the course of the frontal branch can be easily related to the fascial boundaries over the zygomatic arch. This study employs both gross dissections under loop magnification as well as histologic evaluation of 1 cm intervals over the arch. The frontal branch of the fascial nerve can be easily identified by its sub-

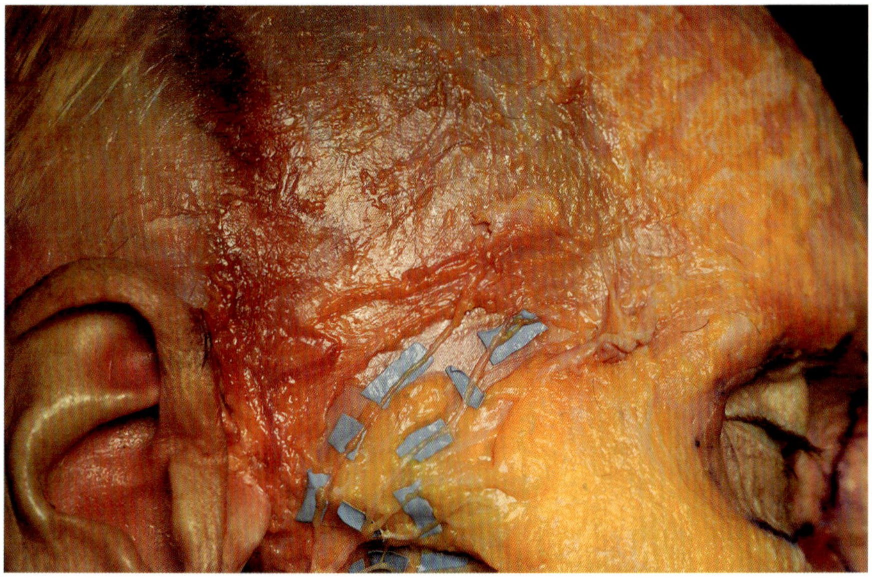

Fig. 9.3 Dissection of the right temporal branch of the facial nerve.

cutaneous course over from the tragus to the lateral brow. The cutaneous landmarks defined by Pitanguy were confirmed to be accurate in this study,[1] although this was not the focus of the study. The frontal branch was identified in all cadaver dissections via a pretragal incision and a sub-SMAS dissection with elevation of the parotid and identification of the zygomatico-frontal trunk of the facial nerve. This trunk was uniformly covered by the investing fascia of the parotid, which then extended superiorly as the parotid temporal fascia where the nerve traveled in a heterogeneous fat pad. The SMAS was easily elevated off this fascia as there was an areolar plane between them. This plane was easily elevated to above the arch, with the SMAS maintaining its integrity; the parotid temporal fascia can be elevated off of the nerve to above the zygomatic arch as demonstrated in the dissection video accompanying this chapter.

The histologic evaluation reinforces the dissection findings and demonstrates that there are two independent fascial planes below the arch; these planes are maintained to approximately 2 cm above the arch when the frontal branch penetrates the temporal-parietal fascia and travels with the anterior branch of the superficial temporal artery.

The findings of the study by Trussler et al showed that the frontal branch has a defined anatomical course and uniform fascial plane within which it travels (**Fig. 9.4**).[10] The nerve does not travel within the SMAS, which is the thought and teaching that have been passed on in the anatomical teaching in this area. This inaccurate description imposes a false sense of security when approaching the arch and midface from a superior and deep plane and is echoed in past descriptions of the subperiosteal facelift having a high number of frontal branch palsies. In evaluating the histologic specimens, the nerve closely abuts the periosteum of the arch, and if the arch is to be accessed, it should be done so by bilaminating the deep temporal fascia, elevating the periosteum off of the arch, or both. Additionally, the SMAS can be elevated above the arch and exists as a layer on histologic evaluation, which contradicts a previous study demonstrating that the SMAS does not cross the arch.

All these findings are clinically supported by the fact that I have performed more than 1,000 high SMAS facelifts without any permanent nerve injuries. This clinical finding demonstrates that the high SMAS facelift is safe and the frontal branch of the facial nerve is protected by the parotid temporal fascia at the zygomatic arch.

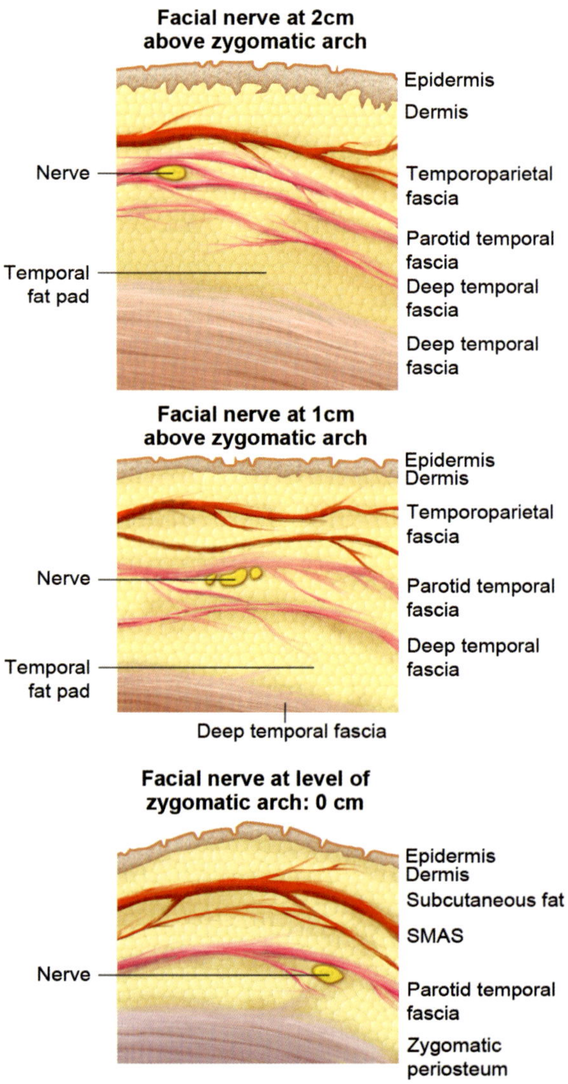

Fig. 9.4 The fascia plane where the temporal branch travels.

Zygomatic Branch

The zygomatic branch of the facial nerve has clinical implications in lower eyelid function and midface movement. It is at risk as it exits the parotid gland, although it travels within similar bounds as the frontal branch. Its terminal branches can be injured in lower eyelid and midface procedures. This type of injury is clinically less severe secondary to its multiple rami. The zygomatic branch of the facial nerve travels within the superior portion of the parotid gland. The nerve branches from the superior trunk in the parotid gland and lies deep to the parotid masseteric temporal fascia. It runs with the transverse facial artery in line with the parotid duct as it travels anteriorly into the buccal space. The nerve travels beneath the zygomatic as major muscle but may give a branch superficial to the muscle, which innervates the orbicularis oculi laterally. The zygomatic branch of the facial nerve gives off rami to innervate the deep surface of the levator and orbicularis oculi. There is medial cross-innervation of the buccal and zygomatic medial branches, which has significance in the blink response, lower eyelid position, and tone. Injury to these rami during open lower eyelid procedures may result in an ectropion, which can correct as these small branches reinnervate the muscle (**Fig. 9.5**).

In the cheek, the zygomatic branch is covered by the parotid gland. The area of vulnerability exists at the origin of the zygomaticus muscle or McGregor's patch, where there is a dense ligamentous adhesion with the neurovascular bundle, which indicates the transition from deep to superficial planes of the nerve.[11] Scissor spreading in the superficial plane, as well as pressure instead of cautery for hemostasis, can help eliminate injury to the branch. The perforator vessels from the transverse facial artery are typically encountered as well as the zygomatico-orbital sensory branch.

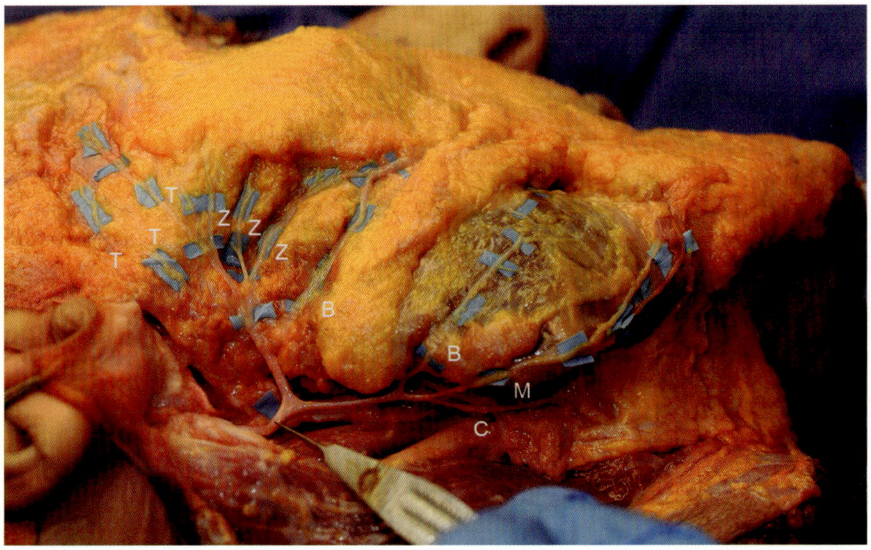

Fig. 9.5 Dissection of the right facial nerve. B, buccal branch; C, cervical branch; M, marginal mandibular branch; T, temporal branch; Z, zygomatic branch.

Buccal Branch

The buccal branch rami travel within the midportion of the parotid gland. The rami exit the nerve more posteriorly than the superior trunk rami because the parotid gland is narrower as it descends into the tail. The buccal rami travel anteriorly on the masseter muscle and below the parotid masseteric fascia. At the anterior border of the masseter, the nerve branches traverse from the deep fascia to perforate into the more superficial buccal fat compartment. The end point is the undersurface of the facial levator muscles (**Fig. 9.6**).

Elevation of the SMAS flap off of the parotid is relatively easy as the dissection progresses anteriorly. The dissection off of the parotid and onto the parotid masseteric fascia is a landmark to prevent damage to the buccal branches, which are seen below the transparent fascia in an avascular plane. Dissection into the masseter muscle is indicative of too deep of a dissection and possible injury to the buccal branches. Vertical scissor spreading is all that is needed to elevate the SMAS off the parotid masseteric fascia. Previous surgery and injections may make this plane adherent and difficult to elevate.

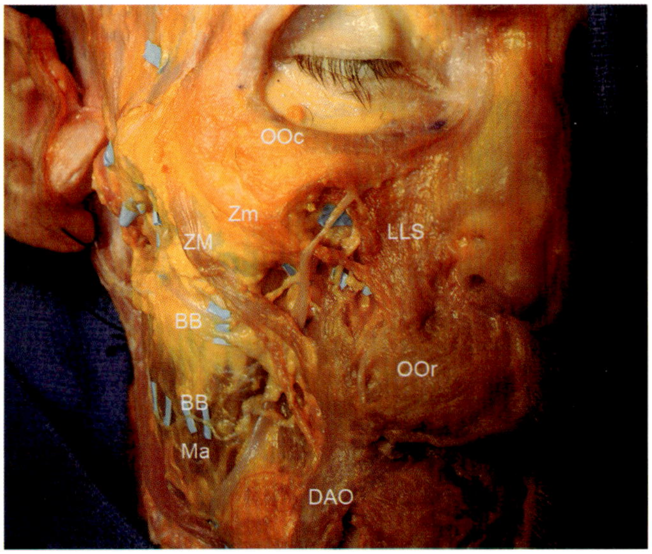

Fig. 9.6 Dissection of the right buccal branch. BB, buccal branch of the facial nerve; DAO, depressor anguli oris; LLS, levator labii superioris; Ma, masseter; OOc, orbicularis occuli; OOr, orbicularis oris; ZM, zygomatic major; Zm, zygomatic minor.

Mandibular Branch

The mandibular gland exits the parotid at the angle of the mandible. It is covered with the transitional fascia of the parotid masseteric and deep cervical fasciae. The nerve travels anteriorly above the mandibular border in most patients (**Fig. 9.7**). In 19% of cases, the nerve is located below the border of the mandible and can be found 1 to 3 cm below the border before it crosses the anterior to the facial vessels.[12] In cases in which the nerve is below the mandible, it runs anteriorly and crosses the surface of the posterior digastric muscle and then the capsule of the submandibular gland, lying deep to the investing cervical fascia and curving a variable distance below the mandible. The nerve perforates through the deep cervical fascia at the inferior border of the midmandible near the anterior margin of the masseter muscle, where it then crosses superficial to the facial artery to enter the buccal space lying beneath the platysma, ultimately innervating the major lip depressors and mentalis muscle.

The marginal mandibular nerve can be injured in the cheek and in the neck. Inadvertent injury can occur with subcutaneous dissection along the mid-mandibular border with push-cut scissor dissection, blunt injury with liposuction or injection, as well as electrocautery after bleeding occurs in this area after blind dissection. Injury to the nerve in the neck can occur if the dissection traverses the platysma and enters the deep cervical fascia. Dissection of the neck platysma should start several centimeters below the angle of the mandible in a relatively loose,

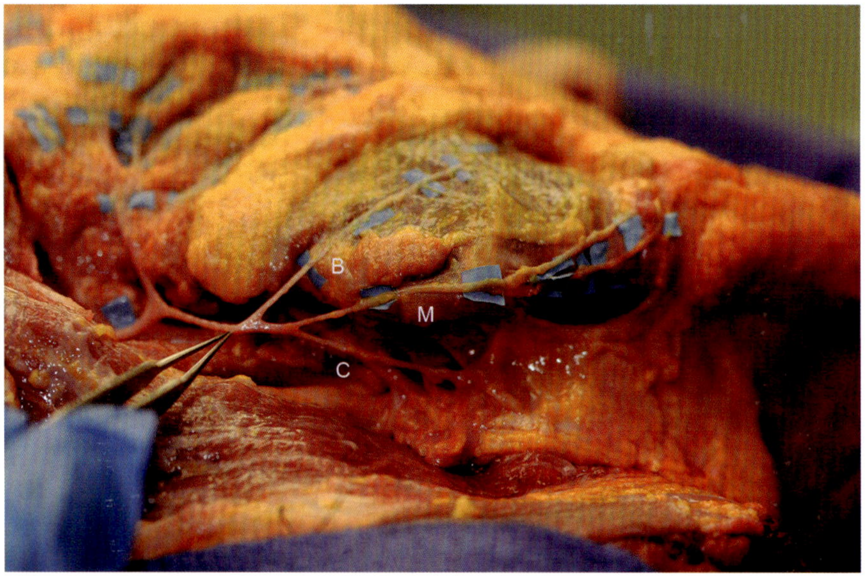

Fig. 9.7 Dissection of the right buccal, mandibular and cervical branches. B, buccal branch; C, cervical branch; M, marginal mandibular branch.

avascular areolar plane. In a revision neck-lift procedure, adherence of the platysma to the skin may direct the dissection through the platysma and inadvertent injury to the nerve if this dissection plane is continued.

In a sub-SMAS cheek dissection, the greatest risk of injury for the marginal mandibular nerve is in the lower anterior cheek as the buccal space is approached. Vertical spreading and blunt dissection over the parotid masseteric fascia adequately elevate the SMAS flap, with care taken to avoid the lower anterior border of the mandible where the nerve crosses the facial vessels. Hemostasis under the extended SMAS flap in the lower cheek should be attained with pressure and not electrocautery.

Cervical Branch

The cervical branch exits the parotid gland at its caudal border below the angle of the mandible. It immediately perforates through fibrous adhesions at the tail of the parotid and travels above the deep cervical fascia. The nerve travels within the fibroareolar connective tissue to the undersurface of the platysma, where it divides and sends rami anteriorly and inferiorly.

Dissection beneath the SMAS and platysma can risk injuring the cervical branch anterior to the angle of the mandible, where it emerges from the parotid gland. Dissection in front of the angle at a level deep to the platysma should be performed with blunt dissection to elevate the SMAS flap. This dissection can be difficult secondary to the dense fascial adhesions over this area; freeing the SMAS and platysma enough for movement should be the goal rather than an extensive dissection.

The danger zones for the cervical branch and the mandibular branch are adjacent to each other and can be treated as a single zone during a SMAS-platysma facelift, 1 cm above the border of the mandible to 2 cm below the mandible from the angle to the oral commissure (**Fig. 9.7**). Adequate mobilization of the SMAS-platysma flap may entail the release of the fascial attachments in this area. A dissection plane above this danger zone in the cheek and below in the neck can be connected with blunt dissection and spreading, which can create a mobile mesentery of soft tissue to help protect the path of the mandibular and cervical nerve branches.

Conclusions

- Know the variations of the nerve branches.
- Understand the fascial boundaries of the nerve branches.
- Use safe dissection techniques in the areas of fascial adherence.
- Hold pressure rather than cauterize bleeding in the anterior cheek.

References

1. Pitanguy I, Ramos AS. The frontal branch of the facial nerve: the importance of its variations in face lifting. Plast Reconstr Surg 1966;38(4):352–356
2. Furnas DW. Landmarks for the trunk and the temporofacial division of the facial nerve. Br J Surg 1965;52(9):694–696
3. Gosain AK, Sewall SR, Yousif NJ. The temporal branch of the facial nerve: how reliably can we predict its path? Plast Reconstr Surg 1997;99(5):1224–1236
4. Stuzin JM, Wagstrom L, Kawamoto HK, Wolfe SA. Anatomy of the frontal branch of the facial nerve: the significance of the temporal fat pad. Plast Reconstr Surg 1989;83(2):265–271
5. Stuzin JM, Baker TJ, Gordon HL. The relationship of the superficial and deep facial fascias: relevance to rhytidectomy and aging. Plast Reconstr Surg 1992;89(3):441–451
6. Abul-Hassan HS, von Drasek Ascher G, Acland RD. Surgical anatomy and blood supply of the fascial layers of the temporal region. Plast Reconstr Surg 1986;77(1):17–28
7. Stuzin JM, Baker TJ, Gordon HL, Baker TM. Extended SMAS dissection as an approach to midface rejuvenation. Clin Plast Surg 1995; 22(2):295–311
8. Barton FE Jr. The SMAS and the nasolabial fold. Plast Reconstr Surg 1992;89(6):1054–1059

9. Barton FE Jr, Hunt J. The high-superficial musculoaponeurotic system technique in facial rejuvenation: an update. Plast Reconstr Surg 2003;112(7):1910–1917
10. Trussler AP, Stephan P, Hatef D, Schaverien M, Meade R, Barton FE. The frontal branch of the facial nerve across the zygomatic arch: anatomical relevance of the high-SMAS technique. Plast Reconstr Surg 2010;125(4):1221–1229
11. Furnas DW. The retaining ligaments of the cheek. Plast Reconstr Surg 1989;83(1):11–16
12. Dingman RO, Grabb WC. Surgical anatomy of the mandibular ramus of the facial nerve based on the dissection of 100 facial halves. Plast Reconstr Surg Transplant Bull 1962;29(3):266–272

10 Sensory Nerves of the Head and Neck

Ibrahim Khansa, Jenny C. Barker, and Jeffrey E. Janis

Introduction

In the past two decades, significant advances have been made in the description of the sensory anatomy of the head and neck, mostly in the cosmetic surgery literature. This progress was driven in large part by the discovery that compression of sensory nerves in the head and neck may contribute to the pathogenesis of migraine headaches.

Migraine headaches are a robust clinical challenge that affects 17.1% of women and 5.6% of men in the United States.[1] Traditional pharmacologic treatment is often insufficient. New surgical options for the treatment of migraine headache have been developed based on the finding that extracranial sensory branches of the trigeminal and cervical spinal nerves can be irritated, entrapped, or compressed at multiple points along their anatomical course, ultimately leading to a cascade of physiologic events that results in migraine headaches.[2–5]

In addition to the abundant clinical studies that have been published in support of the surgical treatment of migraine headaches, complementary anatomical studies have been performed that describe the detailed anatomy of the sensory nerves involved, as well as the compression points along their course. These include the frontal trigger point (supraorbital and supratrochlear nerves, or STNs), the temporal trigger point (zygomaticotemporal nerve [ZTN] and auriculotemporal nerve [ATN]), the occipital trigger point (greater occipital, third occipital, and lesser occipital nerves [LONs]), and the nasoseptal trigger point. In this chapter, we begin by summarizing the hypotheses on the pathogenesis of migraine headaches and then describe the detailed anatomy of the sensory nerves involved, along with their compression points.

Pathogenesis of Migraine Headaches

The final common pathway in the pathogenesis of migraine headaches appears to be hyperexcitability of cerebral neurons resulting from lower than normal threshold to excitation of the neuronal membrane,[6] which is believed to be due to localized dural inflammation and vasodilation of meningeal vessels that are supplied by the trigeminal nerve. The mechanism of aura is believed to be cortical spreading depression, characterized by cortical neuronal excitation, followed by depression of normal neuronal activity.[6]

Irritation of the trigeminal nerve, from either a central[7] or peripheral source, causes inflammation and vasodilation in the region of the dura mater supplied by the trigeminal nerve via release of nociceptive mediators such as calcitonin gene-related peptide, substance P, and neurokinin A.[6,8] The central trigger theory of migraine headache postulates that central neurovascular events cause irritation of the trigeminal nerve, leading to the release of nociceptive substances from the nerve, triggering dural inflammation and the migraine pain cascade. This theory ascribes the proven ability of botulinum toxin A to reduce the frequency and severity of migraine headaches[9,10] to its ability to be taken up by the trigeminal nerve peripherally, travel downstream through the axon, and block the release of nociceptive substances at the synaptic interface of the trigeminal nerve with the dura. In an in vitro study, Durham et al found that botulinum toxin A decreased the amount of calcitonin gene-related peptide released from activated rat trigeminal neurons.[11]

In contrast, the peripheral trigger theory of migraine headache postulates that irritation of the trigeminal nerve occurs peripherally via compression of one of the sensory branches of the trigeminal or cervical nerves by muscle, fascia, bone, artery, or mucosa. This theory attributes the efficacy of botulinum toxin A to its ability to weaken temporarily the muscles by blocking acetylcholine release at the neuromuscular junction, thus reducing muscular compression of branches of the trigeminal nerve.[12] This theory is also validated by the efficacy of surgical trigger-point decompression. Indeed, surgical release of branches of the trigeminal nerve entrapped in muscle, fascia, bone, artery, and mucosa has been shown to be effective at reducing the frequency, intensity, and severity of migraine headaches in most patients who have been refractory to medical management through retrospective chart reviews,[5,13] prospective cohort studies,[2,3] and a prospective randomized trial using sham surgery as a placebo control.[4] In addition, patients with migraine headaches often have tenderness to palpation that precisely localizes to their trigger points, which further lends credence to the peripheral trigger theory.[14]

The central and peripheral theories of the pathogenesis of migraine headaches may not, in fact, be incompatible. A combination of peripheral and central sensitization may act in synergy to produce migraine headaches,[15] and current therapeutic strategies—including medications, botulinum, and surgical decompression—may prove to be multimodal in their mechanism of action.

Peripheral Trigger Points in Migraine Headaches

Frontal Trigger Point

Supraorbital Nerve

Origin and Course

The supraorbital nerve (SON) is one of the two terminal cutaneous branches of the frontal nerve, which is a branch of the ophthalmic division of the trigeminal nerve (V1). The frontal nerve

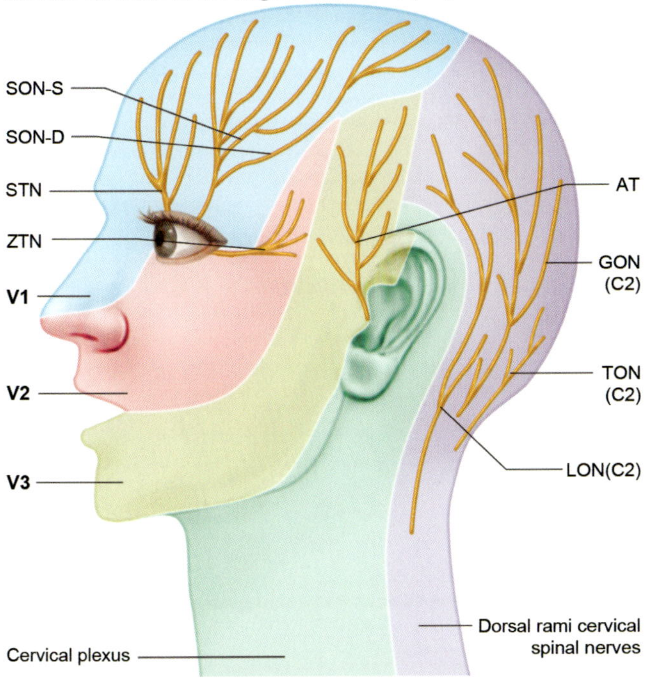

Fig. 10.1 Sensory distributions of nerves involved in migraine trigger points: AT, auriculotemporal nerve; GON, greater occipital nerve; LON, lesser occipital nerve; SON-D, deep branch of the supraorbital nerve; STN, supratrochlear nerve; TON, third occipital nerve; SON-S, superficial branch of the supraorbital nerve; V1, ophthalmic branch of the trigeminal nerve; V2, maxillary branch of the trigeminal nerve; V3, mandibular branch of the trigeminal nerve; ZTN, zygomaticotemporal nerve.

passes through the superior orbital fissure and divides into two branches: the SSTN and the SON, both of which run beneath the orbital roof. The SON proceeds laterally and most commonly exits the orbit through a supraorbital notch located on the supraorbital rim, but it can also exit through a foramen located cephalad to the supraorbital rim.

After exiting the orbit, the SON divides into a deep (lateral) branch and a superficial (medial) branch. The deep branch has a more consistent course and runs between the galea aponeurotica and the periosteum toward the temporal fusion line laterally[16] and provides sensation to the frontoparietal scalp (**Fig. 10.1**). Cuzalina and Holmes described the reproducible location of the deep branch of the SON in a study that examined 75 patients undergoing endoscopic browlift[17] and found the deep branch of the SON to be located an average of 0.56 mm from a vertical line drawn tangentially to the medial limbus of the iris. The superficial branch of the SON is more variable in location. It pierces the frontalis muscle in a fanlike pattern with numerous branches and provides sensory innervation to the forehead skin and anterior scalp.[16]

Points of Compression and External Landmarks

The first compression point of the SON consists of either the supraorbital notch or foramen (**Fig. 10.2, Table 10.1**). When a supraorbital notch is present as the SON exits from the superior orbital rim, there is frequently a fascial band that completes the circular shape of the notch and can compress the SON against the frontal bone, as observed by Janis et al[18] and then studied extensively by Fallucco et al,[19] who found that a supraorbital notch was present 83% of the time and a foramen 27% of the time (10% of specimens had both a notch and a foramen). They found that 86% of supraorbital notches had a fascial band. The fascial bands were further divided into three classifications. Type 1 bands, which occurred in 51.2% of specimens, were described as “simple” and consisted of a single fascial band. Type 2 bands, occurring in 30.2% of specimens, consisted of bony spicules with a fascial band completing the bridge overlying the supraorbital notch. Type 3 bands, occurring in 18.6% of specimens, contained a septum that allowed for more than a single passageway for the neurovascular bundle through the supraorbital notch.

These were further divided into types 3A and 3B classification, depending on whether the septum was horizontal or vertical, with each occurring 9.3% of the time (**Fig. 10.2**).[19] When present, a supraorbital foramen can act as a bony compression point.[20] Beer et al described the SON exit from 507 European skulls and discovered that in 74% of cases, the location of the exit was asymmetric between sides in the same person.[21] The average distance from the nasion to either a supraorbital notch or foramen was 31 mm. A single exit point exists in most circumstances, but in approximately 10 to 15% of people, more than one exit point exists.[21,22] Agthong et al examined specimens from 70 men and 40 women in an Asian population and noted that when measured from the midline, the nerve exit trended toward a more lateral location in men (25.1 mm) than in women (24.1 mm).[22] Interestingly, this study demonstrated an equal rate of supraorbital notch versus foramen in this population. Conversely, Cutright et al examined 20 specimens each from white versus black and male versus female populations and found that a notch was present 92.5% of the time and a foramen present in the remaining specimens.[23] They also noted a more lateral location in men versus women and in blacks versus whites (24.1 mm in white men, 26.1 mm in black men, 22.3 mm in white women, and 25.5 mm in black women). Saylam et al described the presence of a supraorbital notch in 71.6% of specimens, with an average distance of 25.2 mm from the midline.[24] Webster et al examined the variability in nerve exit patterns between sides within the same person in a study with 111 skulls.[25] In approximately 50% of specimens, a bilateral supraorbital notch was found, in 25% a bilateral supraorbital foramen, and in 25%, a notch on one side with a foramen on the contralateral side. Extrapolating definitive conclusions about the presence of a notch versus a foramen as well as a precise location of nerve exit from the data reviewed here is limited by the fact that no two studies examined comparable populations in sufficient numbers with comparable reference points to measure nerve exit; however, the data highlight the importance of appreciating the frequent variability within different people and even within the same patient.

The second compression point of the SON is the corrugator supercilii muscle (CSM), where branches of the nerve course directly through the muscle in 78% of people.[18,26] In an anatomical study of 25 cadavers, Janis et al described the branching patterns of the SON in relation to the CSM and discovered four unique patterns.[18] In a type I branching pattern, which occurred in 40% of specimens, the deep branch of the SON interacted with the CSM. In a type 2 pattern, occurring in 34% of specimens, a

b

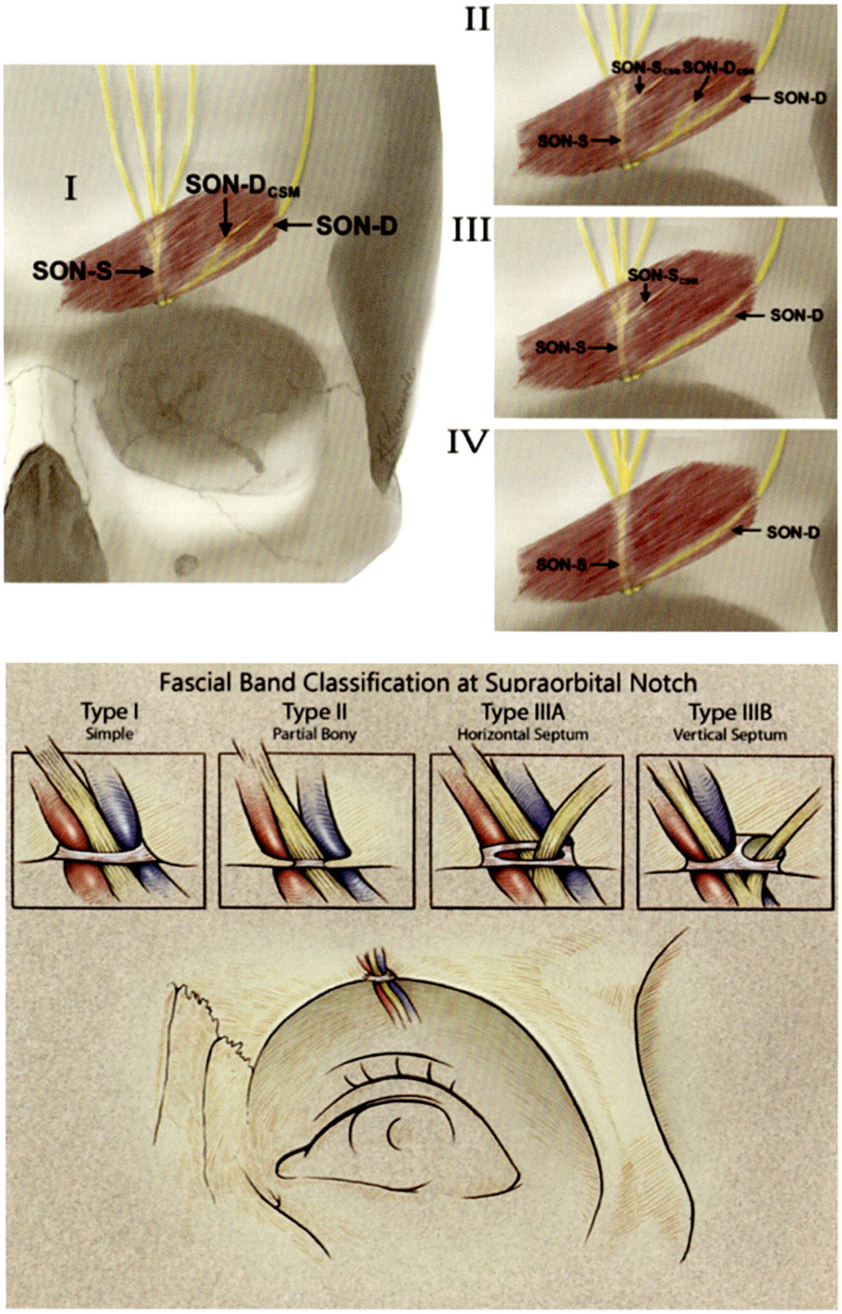

Fig. 10.2 **(a)** Compression points of the supraorbital nerve. (Reproduced with permission from Bindingnavele VK1, Bresnick SD, Urata MM, et al. Superior results using the islandized hemipalatal flap in palatoplasty: experience with 500 cases. Reproduced from Plast Reconstr Surg 2008; 122(1):232.) **(b)** Supraorbital nerve course through the corrugator supercilii muscle. Fascial band classification at the supraorbital notch. (Reproduced with permission from Fallucco M1, Janis JE, Hagan RR. The anatomical morphology of the supraorbital notch: clinical relevance to the surgical treatment of migraine headaches. (Reproduced with permission from Plast Reconstr Surg 2012;130(6):1227–1233.)

branches of both the superficial and deep branches of the SON interacted with the CSM. In a type 3 pattern, which occurred in 4% of specimens, only the superficial branch of the SON interacted with the CSM. Lastly, in a type IV pattern, occurring in 22% of specimens, the branching of the SON occurred more cephalad to the CSM, without any interaction with the muscle (**Fig. 10.2, *lower left***).

Clinical Correlation

The supraorbital and STNs constitute the frontal trigger point, the most commonly described trigger point among migraine patients. Patients with a frontal trigger point typically have a strong CSM, as indicated by deep frown lines. They often have tenderness over the SON, and they experience headaches that are "imploding" and are worse in the afternoon and with stress.[27]

The first compression point is decompressed via a supraorbital foraminotomy (for a foramen) or fasciotomy (for a notch). The second trigger point is addressed by resection of the corrugator myofascial unit through either subtotal resection of the CSMs or more effectively by resection of the entire glabellar muscle group, including the CSM and portions of the depressor supercilii and procerus muscles. This resection is achieved through either a transpalpebral approach or with an endoscopic approach through small hairline incisions,[2] although the endoscopic approach has been shown to visualize more of the muscle and therefore may lead to more successful complete resection and better decompression.[28,29]

Table 10.1 Compression points of the supraorbital nerve

Compression point	Name	Type	Frequency	Horizontal location (from midline)	Craniocaudal location	Reference
1	Supraorbital notch	Fascial/ bony	83.3%[a] (51.2% fascial band, 30.2% partial bony band, 9.3% horizontal septum, 9.3% vertical septum)		At the superior orbital rim	Fallucco et al[19]
	Supraorbital foramen	Bony	26.7%[a]	31 mm		Beer et al[21]
				25.1 mm in men, 24.1 mm in women		Agthong et al[22]
				24.1 mm in white men, 26.1 mm in black men, 22.3 mm in white women, and 25.5 mm in black women		Cutright et al[23]
				25.2 mm		Saylam et al[24]
2	Corrugator supercilii	Muscular	78% (40% deep branch, 34% deep and superficial branch, 4% superficial branch)	2.9 –43.3 mm[b]	9.8–32.6 mm cranial to nasion[b]	Janis et al[18]

[a]10% of specimens had both a supraorbital notch and a foramen.
[b]These measurements indicate the extent of the corrugator supercilii muscle.

Multiple clinical studies have been completed that address muscular, fascial or bony release of the frontal trigger point.[5,13,30] Success rates of migraine headache improvement or migraine headache elimination have been high when performed independently or concurrently with decompression of other trigger points. Interestingly, the proportion of patients who benefit from surgical decompression (79.2%)[5] closely mirrors the percentage of patients who have interaction between the SON and the CSM (78%).[18]

Supratrochlear Nerve

Origin and Course

The STN is one of the two terminal cutaneous branches of the frontal branch of the ophthalmic division of the trigeminal nerve (V1). It provides sensory innervation to the midline forehead (**Fig. 10.1**). Much less has been published about the anatomy of the smaller STN compared with the larger SON. The STN proceeds medially to exit the superior orbital rim via a notch or a foramen, then travels cranially through the CSM. Miller et al examined the anatomy of the STN in 10 cadavers and found that the nerve coursed between 1.6 and 2.3 cm lateral to the midline at the level of the superior orbital rim.[31] After exiting the orbital rim, the STN courses through the CSM as it travels cephalad.

Points of Compression and External Landmarks

The first compression point of the STN occurs as it exits the orbit via either a notch or a foramen (**Table 10.2**). In a dissection of 50 cadaver hemiheads by Janis et al, the STN was found to exit the orbit via a notch in 72% of specimens, located an average of 1.75 cm from the midline.[32] The floor of the notch consisted of a fibrous band in all cases. In 68% of specimens, the nerve was observed to pass directly through the notch; however, in 8%, the nerve pierced the fascial band and coursed directly through the connective tissue. In another 8%, the fascial band was very broad and flattened the nerve against the bony surroundings. A true bony foramen occurred in 18% of specimens and was located an average of 4 mm cranial to the superior orbital rim.

The second compression point occurs as the STN interacts with the CSM. Janis et al found that 84% of the time, the STN

Table 10.2 Compression points of the supratrochlear nerve

Compression Point	Name	Type	Frequency	Horizontal location (from midline)	Craniocaudal location	Reference
1	Frontal notch	Fascial/bony	72%	17.5 mm	At the superior orbital rim	Janis et al[32]
	Frontal foramen	Bony	18%		4 mm cranial to superior orbital rim	Janis et al[32]
2	Corrugator supercilii	Muscular	88% (84% two branches, 4% one branch)	Enters muscle 18.7 mm, exits muscle 19.6 mm	15 mm cranial to superior orbital rim	Janis et al[32]

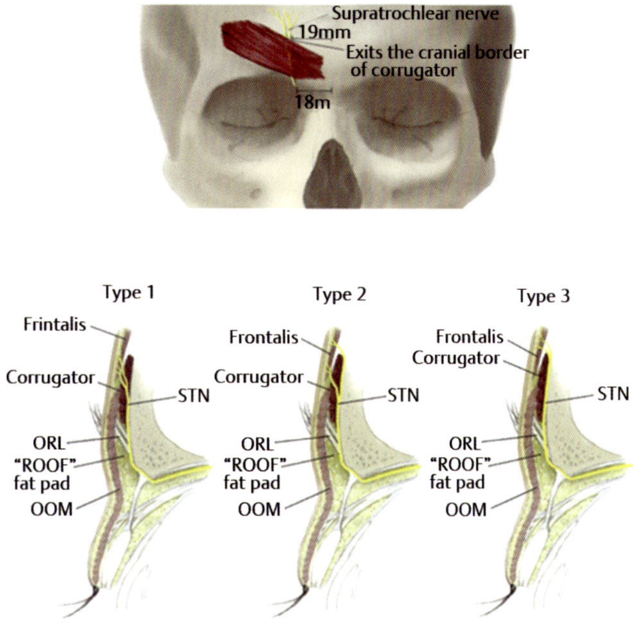

Fig. 10.3 Compression points of the supratrochlear nerve. (Reproduced with permission from Janis JE1, Hatef DA, Hagan R, et al. Anatomy of the supratrochlear nerve: implications for the surgical treatment of migraine headaches. Plast Reconstr Surg 2013;131(4): 743–750.)

divided into two branches within the retro-orbicularis fat, which then both entered the CSM at an average of 18.7 mm lateral to the midline, and exited it 19.6 mm lateral to the midline and 15 mm cranial to the superior orbital rim (**Fig. 10.3**).[32] In 4% of specimens, only one STN branch entered the CSM, and the other one stayed deep; in 12% of specimens, neither branch traveled through the CSM, but rather both remained deep to the muscle.

Clinical Correlation

The STN and the SON constitute the frontal trigger point, and release of both nerves is usually achieved simultaneously. Anatomical studies involving the STN have highlighted the importance of extending surgical dissection medially to fully decompress it. It has been hypothesized that failure to fully decompress the most medial aspect of the frontal trigger site may have resulted in early clinical failures.[32]

Temporal Trigger Point

Zygomaticotemporal Nerve

Origin and Course

The ZTN is one of the two terminal branches of the zygomatic nerve, which is a branch of the maxillary division of the trigeminal nerve (V2).[33] The zygomatic nerve enters the orbit via the inferior orbital fissure, travels along the lateral orbital wall,[34] then divides into the zygomaticofacial nerve (ZFN) and ZTN. The ZTN provides sensation to the skin of the temple (**Fig. 10.1**), as well as parasympathetic innervation to the lacrimal gland.[34]

In a study by Janis et al, 30% of subjects were found to have two ZTN branches.[33] Among those, 20% had branching of the ZTN within the orbit, with the two branches exiting via two separate zygomaticotemporal foramina. In the remaining 80%, the ZTN branched after exiting the orbit. Accessory branches of the ZTN were found in 50 to 55% of patients. Among those with accessory ZTN branches, the ZTN branches were cranial to the main branch in 30% on the left (located an average of 16mm lateral and 12.2 mm cranial to the lateral palpebral commissure) and in 55% on the right (located an average of 15.7 mm lateral and 16.5 mm cranial to the lateral palpebral commissure). The ZTN branches were immediately adjacent to the main branch in 30% on the left (located an average of 17.7 mm lateral and 6 mm cranial to the lateral palpebral fissure) and in 9% on the right (located an average of 19.0 mm lateral and 5.0 mm cranial to the lateral palpebral commissure). The ZTN branches were lateral to the main branch in 40%, on the left (located an average of 34.2 mm lateral and 6.7 mm cranial to the lateral palpebral commissure), and in 36% on the right (located an average of 28.7 mm lateral and 6.0 mm cranial to the lateral palpebral commissure). In all cases with a lateral branch, this branch travelled horizontally to join the ATN. Tubbs et al have confirmed this communication with the ATN in 13% of hemiheads.[35] In addition, Odobescu et al found that 82% of individuals had small connections between the ZTN and the frontal division of the facial nerve.[36]

Points of Compression and External Landmarks

The first compression point occurs as the ZTN enters the temporal fossa. The nerve exits the lateral orbit via a bony canal and emerges in the temporal fossa via a bony foramen (**Fig. 10.4, Table 10.3**)[34]; 94% of individuals have one zygomaticotemporal foramen, and the remaining 6% have two foramina.[33] The foramen is located in the frontal bone within the temporal fossa and is found an average of 6.7 ± 6.12 mm lateral to the lateral orbital rim and 7.88 ± 6.9 mm cranial to the nasion. In an anatomical study of 400 hemiskulls, Loukas et al found that the location of the zygomaticotemporal foramen varied widely depending on ethnic background and that up to 50% of individuals lacked a zygomaticotemporal foramen.[37]

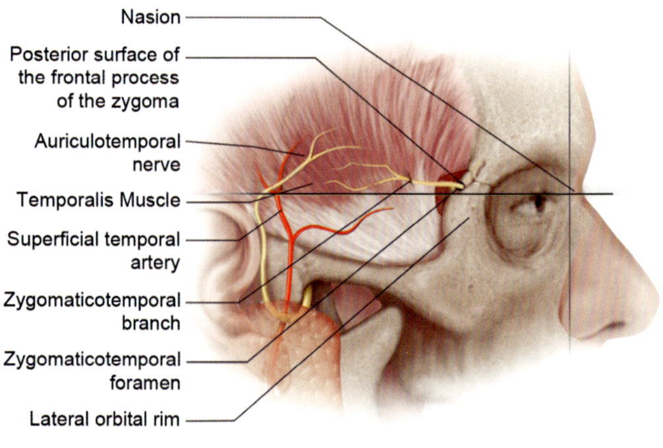

Fig. 10.4 Compression points of the zygomaticotemporal nerve.

Table 10.3 Compression points of the zygomaticotemporal nerve

Compression point	Name	Type	Frequency	Horizontal location	Craniocaudal location	Reference
1	Zygomaticotemporal foramen	Bony	100%	6.7 ± 6.12 mm lateral to the lateral orbital rim	7.88 ± 6.9 mm superior to the nasion	Janis et al[33]
2	Temporalis muscle	Muscular	50%			Janis et al[33]
	Deep temporal fascia	Fascial	50%	16.9 mm lateral to the lateral ocular commissure	6.5 mm superior to the lateral ocular commissure	Janis et al[33] Totonchi et al[34]
				10.1 ±1.5 mm lateral to the zygomatico-frontal suture	22.2 ± 3.1 mm superior to upper margin of zygomatic arch	Jeong et al[38]
					23 mm cranial to the zygomatic arch	Tubbs et al[35]

The second compression point is the temporalis muscle/deep temporal fascia. After exiting the orbit, the ZTN enters the deep aspect temporalis muscle and travels intramuscularly in 50% of individuals.[33] Among those whose ZTN has an intramuscular course, this course is short and direct in 44% and long and tortuous in 56%. In the 50% of individuals who have no intramuscular course, the ZTN travels between the temporal periosteum and the temporalis muscle before piercing the deep temporal fascia. In an intraoperative endoscopic anatomical study of 20 patients, Totonchi et al found that the ZTN pierced the deep temporal fascia 16.9 mm lateral and 6.5 mm cranial to the lateral palpebral commissure,[34] whereas Jeong et al found that it pierced the deep temporal fascia 10.1 ± 1.5 mm lateral to the zygomaticofrontal suture and 22.2 ± 3.1 mm cranial to the upper margin of the zygomatic arch.[38] This was confirmed by Tubbs et al, who found that the ZTN pierced the deep temporal fascia an average of 23 mm cranial to the zygomatic arch.[35]

Clinical Correlation

Patients with migraine headaches originating from the ZTN tend to have temporal pain, usually in the morning, associated with stress, grinding, clenching, or temporomandibular joint dysfunction.[27] Murillo first described open resection of the ZTN and of the superficial temporal artery (STA) for temporal migraine headaches in 34 patients in 1968[39]; results were positive in 88.2% of patients. The technique for ZTN decompression has since been refined by Guyuron and is now usually performed via an endoscopic approach. Dissection is performed just superficial to the deep temporal fascia until the ZTN is identified. It is then avulsed, with resection of approximately 3 cm of the nerve, allowing the proximal end of the nerve to retract and get buried into the temporalis muscle.[40] Avulsion of the ZTN may cause temporary paresthesia and anesthesia in the temporal region, which are usually temporary.[41] The method of ZTN decompression has been examined by Chim et al.[42] In an animal study on rat sural nerves, they found that nerve avulsion and burying in muscle led to the lowest rate of neuroma formation.

In a study of 246 patients undergoing endoscopic decompression of the ZTN, Kurlander et al found that at 1 year postoperatively 55% of patients had complete elimination of temporal migraine headaches, with an additional 30% of patients having significant improvement.[41] In a prospective evaluation of 71 patients with a temporal trigger site undergoing surgical avulsion of the ZTN, with a mean 396-day follow-up, Guyuron et al demonstrated complete migraine elimination in 63%, with at least 50% improvement in migraine severity, duration, and frequency in an additional 35%.[3] In a single-blinded, randomized controlled trial comparing actual decompression of the ZTN in 19 patients with sham surgery in nine patients, those undergoing actual decompression had significant improvements in migraine intensity, frequency, and duration from baseline, which was not the case for those undergoing sham surgery.[4] In a review of 19 patients undergoing ZTN avulsion for the treatment of migraine headaches from a temporal trigger site, with a mean follow-up of 661 days, Janis et al demonstrated complete migraine elimination in 52.6% of patients, with an additional 36.8% having at least 50% improvement.[5]

Auriculotemporal Nerve

Origin and Course

The ATN is a branch of the mandibular division of the trigeminal nerve (V3). It is a sensory nerve that provides sensation to the tragus and anterior ear, as well as to the posterior temporal region (**Fig. 10.1**). It also carries autonomic nervous fibers, providing sympathetic innervation to the scalp and parasympathetic innervation to the parotid gland.

The ATN emerges within the superficial parotid gland along the posteromedial aspect of the temporomandibular joint[43] and travels cranially within the temporoparietal fascia, crossing the posterior aspect of the zygomatic arch.[44] It travels as a single branch in 50% of people, and up to four branches in the remainder.[45] As the nerve travels cephalad, it parallels and runs lateral to the STA.[44] In the upper temporal area, the nerve becomes more superficial, lying superficial to the temporoparietal fascia.

Points of Compression and External Landmarks

In an anatomical study of 10 cadavers, Chim et al found that in all specimens the ATN traveled under a fascial compression

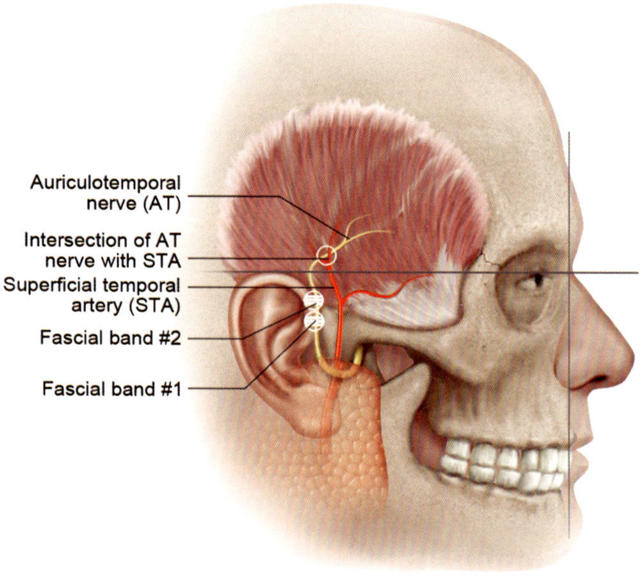

Fig. 10.5 Compression points of the auriculotemporal nerve.

band (compression point 1), present an average of 13.1 ± 5.9 mm anterior and 5.0 ± 7.0 mm cranial to the most anterosuperior point of the external acoustic meatus (**Fig. 10.5, Table 10.4**).[46]

They also showed that in 85% of specimens, a second, more cranial, fascial compression band (compression point 2) was present an average of 11.9 ± 6.0 mm anterior and 17.2 ± 10.4 mm cranial to the most anterosuperior point of the external acoustic meatus.

The third potential compression point consists of the intersection with the STA, found in up to 80% of specimens; 81.2% of those specimens demonstrated a simple intersection. Most commonly in this situation, the artery crossed superficial to the nerve (62.5%), at a point 19.2 ± 10.0 mm anterior and 39.5 ± 16.6 mm superior to the most anterosuperior point of the external acoustic meatus. In the remaining 18.8% of the simple intersection specimens, multiple branches of the nerve crossed superficial to the artery at multiple points, with variable anatomy among the specimens. In 18.8% of the specimens with an AT-STA intersection, helical intertwining over an average distance of 10.3 ± 0.4 mm was noted to extend between 20.0 ± 15.6 mm and 24.7 ± 17.9 mm anterior and 53.7 ± 4.7 mm and 62.7 ± 3.8 mm cranial to the most anterosuperior point of the external acoustic meatus.[46] In a study of 25 fresh cadavers, Janis et al also described the third compression point of the ATN in detail[44]: it was present in 34% of specimens at a point located an average of 107.88 ± 17.73 mm lateral to the facial midline and 37.53 ± 15.29 mm cranial to a horizontal line passing through the nasion. Among the specimens that demonstrated an intersection between the ATN and STA, the intersection consisted of a simple crossing in 88.2% and a helical intertwining in 11.8%. In cases of a helical intertwining, this extended from 123 mm to 117 mm lateral to the midline and from 25 mm to 38 mm cranial to a horizontal line through the nasion.

Table 10.4 Compression points of the auriculotemporal nerve

Compression point	Name	Type	Frequency	Horizontal location	Craniocaudal location	Reference
1	Fascial band 1	Fascial	100%	13.1 ± 5.9 mm anterior to anterosuperior EAC	5.0 ± 7.0 mm superior to anterosuperior EAC	Chim et al[46]
2	Fascial band 2	Fascial	85%	11.9 ± 6.0 mm anterior to anterosuperior EAC	17.2 ± 10.4 mm superior to anterosuperior EAC	Chim et al[46]
3	Superficial temporal artery	Arterial	Simple intersection: 65%	19.2 ± 10.0 mm anterior to anterosuperior EAC	39.5 ± 16.6mm superior to anterosuperior EAC	Chim et al[46]
			Helical intertwining: 15%	20.0 ± 15.6 mm to 24.7 ± 17.9 mm anterior to anterosuperior EAC	53.7 ± 4.7 mm to 62.7 ±3.8 mm superior to anterosuperior EAC	
			Simple intersection: 30%	107.88 ± 17.73 mm lateral to midline	37.53 ± 15.29 mm superior to nasion	Janis et al[44]
			Helical intertwining: 4%	123–117 mm lateral to midline	25–38 mm superior to nasion	

Abbreviations: EAC, external acoustic canal.

Clinical Correlation

The ATN has been hypothesized to be the trigger point in patients with persistent temporal migraine headaches who underwent ZTN release.[44] Patients with an ATN trigger point typically have pain along the course of the ATN in the high temporal region.[27,46] This pain may be pulsatile if nerve compression is due to impingement of the superficial temporal artery on the AT.[44]

Although a surgical technique directly addressing the first two fascial compression points has not been described yet, decompression of the ATN intersection with the STA involves making a short incision overt the point of maximal tenderness[46] or in the temporal hairline[44] and exposing the ATN. If the STA artery is found to be crossing over the nerve, the artery is ligated. If the artery is not crossing over the nerve, the nerve is transected, and its ends are buried in the temporalis muscle.

Nasoseptal Trigger Point

Pathophysiology

Nasoseptal headaches are attributed to intranasal mucomucosal contact points that are present in up to 4% of the population.[47] The contact areas are believed to cause neural irritation, leading to the release of inflammatory mediators, specifically substance P. This causes nociceptive signals to be transmitted along afferent C fibers to the dura mater, which then lead to vasodilation and perivascular inflammation in the dura, generating a migraine headache.

Points of Compression

Intranasal contact points can usually occur between the septum and the superior turbinate, middle turbinate, or medial wall of the ethmoid sinus (**Fig. 10.6**). Causes of these contact points include septal deformities, such as septal deviation and septal spurs; turbinate deformities such as turbinate hypertrophy; and concha bullosa,[48] which refers to a pneumatized turbinate that may impinge on the nasal septum.[49]

In patients with migraine headaches attributed to a nasoseptal trigger point, Ferrero et al found that the frequency of intranasal mucosal contact points was the following: septum-middle turbinate plus septum-superior turbinate in 42.8%, septum-middle turbinate in 36%, septal spur in 7.1%, septal spur plus septum-middle turbinate in 7.1%, septal spur plus septum-middle turbinate plus septum-superior turbinate in 7.1%.[50]

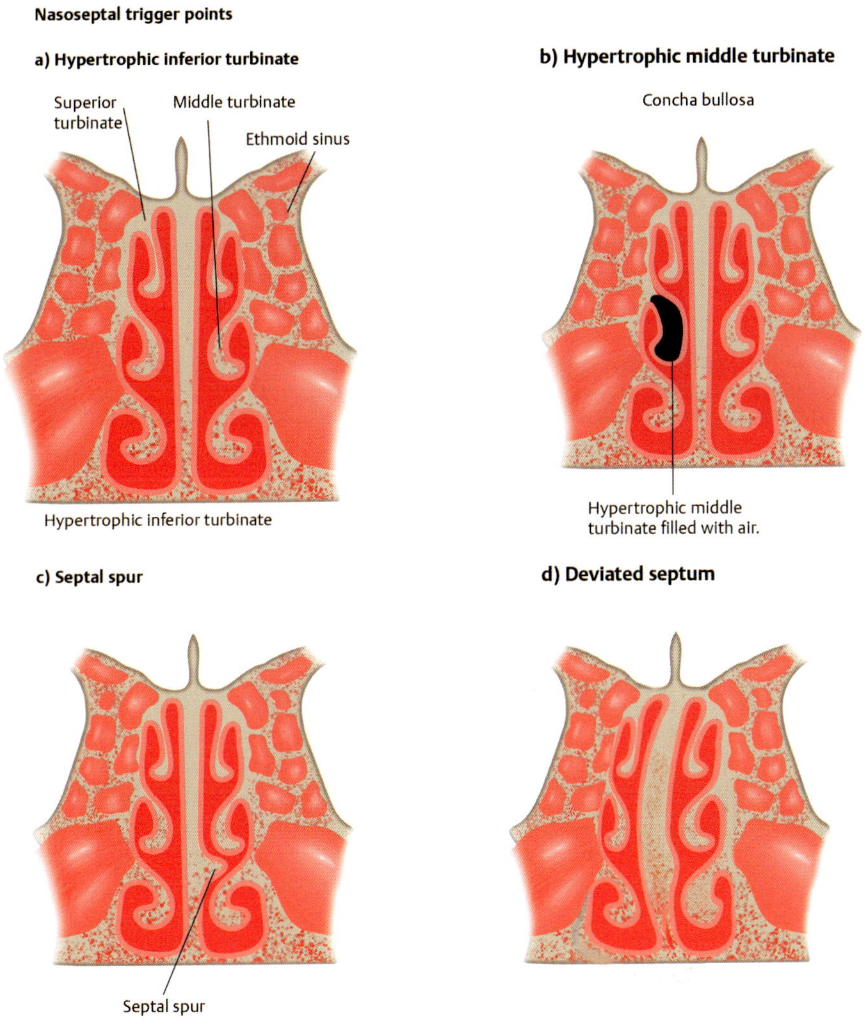

Fig. 10.6 Nasoseptal trigger points: **(a)** Hypertrophic inferior turbinate. **(b)** Hypertrophic middle turbinate with concha bullosa. **(c)** Septal spur. **(d)** Deviated septum.

Clinical Correlation

Patients with a nasoseptal migraine trigger point typically complain of retrobulbar pain, usually worse in the early morning, and related to weather, allergies, and hormonal cycles and associated with rhinorrhea.[27] Confirmation of the nasoseptal trigger point as the causative agent in migraine may take the form of application of topical local anesthetic or injection of local anesthetic into the contact point during an active headache. Improvement or elimination of the headache confirms the contact point as a trigger.[51] Another modality for diagnosis would be a combination of constellation of symptoms (as above) combined with computed tomographic scan findings of anatomical contact points (usually most easily seen on coronal images). Rhinosinusitis must also be excluded.[47]

Surgical techniques to address nasoseptal trigger points must address the underlying anatomical abnormality to eliminate the mucosal contact point and include septoplasty, middle turbinectomy, and medial ethmoidectomy.

In a study of 12 patients with migraine headaches attributed to the nasoseptal trigger point, Behin et al found that surgery reduced headache frequency from 17.7 days per month to 7.7 days per month and mean headache severity from 7.8 to 3.6.[47] Headache severity improved by 50% or more in 76.2% of subjects and was eliminated in 42.9%. In a study of 30 patients with migraine headaches from a nasoseptal trigger point, endoscopic nasal surgery achieved complete headache relief in 43% and significant improvement in 47%.[52] Welge-Luessen followed up on 20 patients with migraine headaches from a nasoseptal trigger point for a period of 10 years after endoscopic septoplasty, partial ethmoidectomy, and turbinectomy (if indicated) and found that 30% had complete headache resolution and an additional 35% had significant improvement.[53] In a study of eight patients with a nasoseptal trigger point who underwent septoplasty or inferior and/or middle turbinectomies, either alone or in conjunction with other trigger sites, with a follow-up of 661 days, Janis et al demonstrated significant overall improvement in 100%, with 62.5% having complete elimination of migraine headaches.[5] In a prospective evaluation of 62 patients with a nasoseptal trigger point undergoing surgical treatment, with a mean follow-up of 396 days, Guyuron et al demonstrated complete migraine elimination in 34% of patients, with an additional 55% experiencing at least 50% improvement.[3]

Occipital Trigger Point

Greater Occipital Nerve

Origin and Course

The greater occipital nerve (GON) is the medial branch of the dorsal ramus of the C2 spinal nerve. It measures approximately 5 mm in diameter as it enters the semispinalis capitis muscle.[54] The GON initially travels in a caudal, posterior, and lateral direction until it reaches the lower border of the obliquus capitis inferior muscle. It then hooks around this muscle and travels cranially, superficial to the obliquus capitis inferior muscle, and deep to the semispinalis capitis muscle. The nerve then crosses the semispinalis capitis muscle from deep to superficial and runs cranially deep to the trapezius muscle. It then pierces the trapezius muscle to become subcutaneous and provides sensory innervation to the posterior scalp (**Fig. 10.1**).

Points of Compression and External Landmarks

Janis et al studied the potential compression points of the GON in 50 cadaver hemiheads.[55] They identified six potential points of compression of the GON as it traveled cranially through the posterior neck (**Fig. 10.7**, **Table 10.5**). The first compression point occurred as the GON crossed tight fascial bands between the obliquus capitis inferior and semispinalis muscles before continuing its cranial course. This point occurred at an average 20.13 mm lateral and 77.38 mm caudal to the external occipital protuberance (EOP).

The second compression point occurred when the GON entered the deep surface of the semispinalis capitis 17.46 mm lateral and 59.71 mm caudal to the EOP. The GON pierced the semispinalis capitis muscle in 90% of specimens by Bovim et al.[56]

The third compression point occurred when the GON emerged from the superficial surface of the semispinalis capitis 15.52 mm lateral and 34.52 mm caudal to the EOP. This point of compression has been studied extensively and confirmed by several other authors. Mosser et al conducted an anatomical study and found that point of emergence of the GON from the semispinalis capitis muscle could be found 29.1 mm (right) to 28.7 mm (left) caudal to the EOP and 14.1 mm (right) to 13.8 mm (left) lateral to the EOP.[54] This was also confirmed by Ducic et al,[57] who found the point of emergence to be 14.9 mm lateral and 30.2 mm inferior to the EOP and who also noted that the course of the GON was asymmetric in 43.9% of individuals. Tubbs et al found that the GON pierced the semispinalis capitis muscle 2 cm cranial to the intermastoid line.[58] The mean intramuscular course in the semispinalis capitis muscle was 7.6 mm (right) and 8.9 mm (left).

The fourth compression point, as demonstrated by Janis et al,[55] occurred as the GON entered the trapezius muscle, 24.0 mm lateral and 21.0 mm caudal to the EOP. The fifth compression point occurred as the GON pierced the tendinous insertion of the trapezius into the nuchal line, 37.07 mm lateral and 4.36 mm caudal to the EOP.

The sixth compression point consisted of the interaction of the GON with the occipital artery,[59] identified in 54% of specimens. This took the form of a simple intersection in 29.6% (with the nerve always crossing superficial to the artery) and of helical intertwining in 70.4%. In cases where there was a single point of intersection, this occurred 30.27 mm ± 6.83 mm lateral and 10.67 mm ± 8.25 mm caudal to the EOP. In cases where there was a helical intertwining, this occurred between 25.34 mm ± 12.16 mm and 42.09 mm ± 25.61 mm lateral and between 24.91 mm ± 12.87 mm and 0.97 mm ± 8.34 mm caudal to the EOP, with a total length of helical intertwining of 37.6 mm ± 14.5 mm. The location of the interaction between the GON and the occipital artery is quite variable, as evidenced by the high standard deviations reported. In fact, although it is referred to as the sixth compression point, it often occurs proximal to point 5 along the course of the GON. It may be superficial or deep to the trapezius muscle. In a review of 272 patients undergoing GON decompression, Junewicz et al noted that the GON branched in 7.4% of patients, most often into two branches.[60] They noted

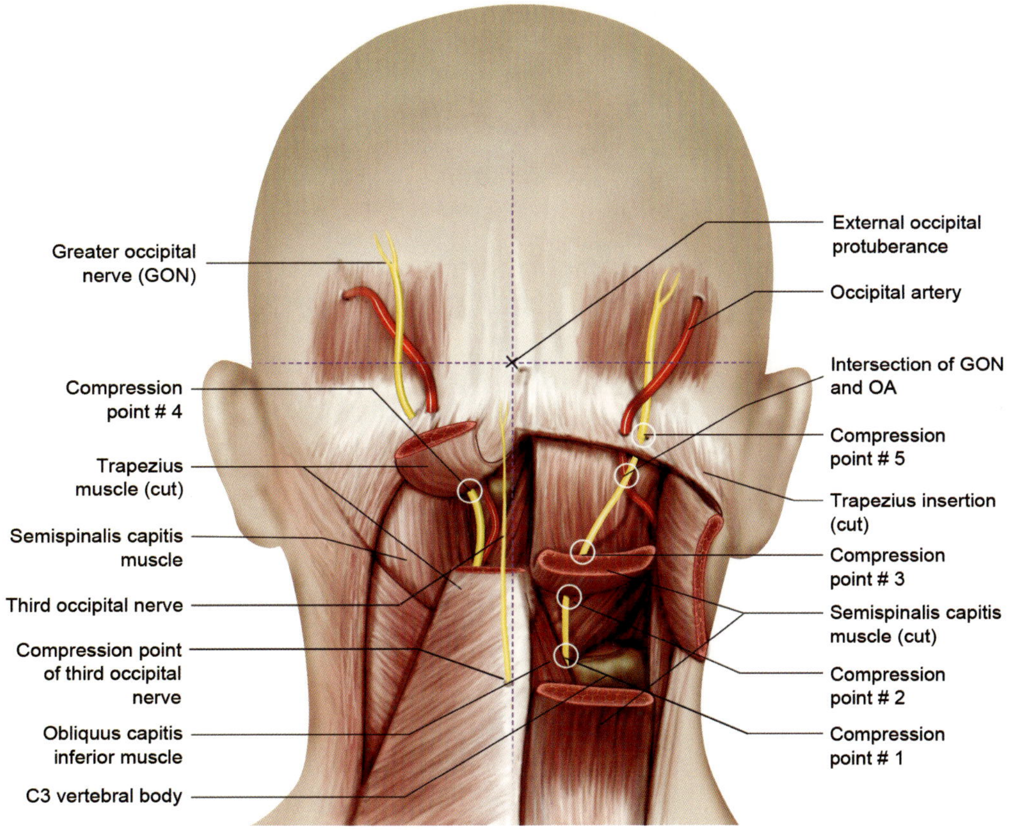

Fig. 10.7 Compression points of greater occipital and third occipital nerves.

Table 10.5 Compression points of the greater occipital nerve

Compression point	Name	Type	Frequency	Horizontal location (from midline)	Craniocaudal location	Reference
1	Bands between obliquus capitis and semispinalis	Fascial		20.1 mm	77.38 mm below EOP	Janis et al[55]
2	Entrance into semispinalis	Muscular	90%	17.46 mm	59.71 mm	Janis et al[55] Bovim et al[56]
3	Exit from semispinalis	Muscular	90%	11.5 mm	37.3 mm below EOP	Vital et al[61]
				14.1 ± 4.4 mm on right, 13.8 ± 4.3 mm on left	29.1 ± 7.8 mm on right, 28.7 ± 6.6 mm on left below EOP	Mosser et al[54]
				14.9 ± 4.5 mm	30.2 ± 5.1 mm	Ducic et al [57]
				15.52 mm	34.52 mm	Janis et al[55]
					2 cm above intermastoid line	Tubbs et al[58]
4	Entrance into trapezius	Muscular		24 mm	21 mm	Janis et al[55]
5	Through trapezius insertion	Musculo-tendinous		37.07 mm	4.36 mm	Janis et al[55]
6	Occipital artery	Arterial	16%	Simple intersection: 30.27 ± 6.83 mm	Simple intersection: 10.67 ± 8.25 mm	Janis et al[55]
			38%	Helical intertwining: 25.34 ± 12.16 mm–42.09 ± 25.61 mm	Helical intertwining: 24.91 ± 12.87 mm–0.97 ± 8.34 mm	

Abbreviations: EOP, external occipital protuberance.

an interaction between the GON and the occipital artery in 64% of patients

Clinical Correlation

Patients with migraine headaches from a GON trigger point usually have upper cervical and occipital pain related to heavy exercise and strain. They may also have cervical muscle tightness and tenderness over the GON.[27]

There are multiple reports of "occipital neuralgia" occurring for various reasons,[58] from whiplash to C2 osteophytes and arthritis causing compression of the GON. GON compression may be static or dynamic, as demonstrated by Vital et al, who demonstrated that the GON may be compressed by its musculofascial surroundings during neck flexion and rotation.[61]

Diagnosis of the occipital trigger point as a cause of migraine headaches has traditionally focused on compression point 3, the point of emergence of the GON from the semispinalis capitis muscle. Anthony found that injection of local anesthetic around the GON 1.5 cm lateral to the midline and 3 cm inferior to the EOP during a migraine attack led to migraine resolution in 88% of patients.[62]

Traditional treatments have focused on nerve ablation, including C2 dorsal rhizotomy, C2 dorsal ganglionectomy, or radiofrequency ablation of the C2 dorsal root. Anthony et al. found that greater occipital neurectomy led to resolution of migraine headaches in 70% of patients for a mean duration of 8.1 months.[62] Such ablative treatment, however, often resulted in significant numbness in the occipital region.

Modern nerve-preserving treatments of migraine headaches with an occipital trigger point revolve around decompression of the six potential compression points. Either a midline vertical or a horizontal incision is performed in the posterior nuchal area through the skin and subcutaneous tissue. The trapezius fascia is exposed and incised just lateral to the midline. The GON is exposed and dissected free from the semispinalis capitis muscle. A segment of semispinalis capitis muscle is removed medial to the nerve, and a triangular segment of trapezius muscle and fascia is removed lateral to the nerve. Fascial bands overlying the GON are released. If the occipital artery crosses the nerve, it is ligated.

Long-term outcomes of GON decompression have been favorable. In a prospective evaluation of 34 patients with an occipital trigger site undergoing GON decompression, with a mean 396-day follow-up, Guyuron et al. achieved at least 50% improvement in migraine intensity, duration, and frequency in 100% of patients, with 62% of them having complete migraine elimination.[3] In a single-blinded, placebo-controlled, randomized trial, Guyuron et al randomized 18 patients with migraine headaches stemming from a GON trigger point to actual or sham surgery.[4] There was a significant improvement in migraine headache frequency, intensity, and duration in the actual surgery group, which was significantly greater than the improvement experienced by the sham surgery group ($P = 0.03$). Janis et al studied 16 patients with migraine headaches from an occipital trigger site who underwent GON decompression, either alone or in combination with other trigger sites.[5] After a follow-up period of 661 days, 93.8% demonstrated significant improvement, with 56.3% having complete migraine elimination. Ducic et al followed up on 202 patients who underwent GON decompression, either alone or in conjunction with CSM excision, with a minimum follow-up of 12 months[15]; 80.5% of the patients had significant improvement, with 43.4% having complete migraine headache relief.

The role of occipital artery ligation is still unclear. Chmielewski et al analyzed 170 patients who underwent GON decompression.[63] Among them, 55 patients underwent occipital artery resection, and 115 did not. Patients undergoing occipital artery resection had significantly lower rates of surgery success, defined as 50% or more reduction in migraine headaches (80.0% vs. 91.3%, $P = 0.047$) and migraine elimination (38.2% vs. 64.3%, $P = 0.002$), which suggests that occipital artery resection may not always be beneficial in patients undergoing GON decompression. Further studies may be needed, but what can be stated is that some patients who have a high suspicion of symptoms related to this area (geographic location, pulsatile nature, positive Doppler signal at the point of maximal pain) likely would benefit from decompression of this trigger point.

Lesser Occipital Nerve

Origin and Course

The LON originates from the ventral ramus of the C2, and sometimes C3, spinal nerves. It is a cutaneous nerve that innervates the superior ear, as well as the postauricular and lateral neck areas (**Fig. 10.1**). It emerges from beneath the posterior border of the sternocleidomastoid (SCM).[64] The LON then travels superolaterally along the posterior border of SCM. Ducic et al found that in 85% of specimens, the LON can be located along the posterior border of the SCM, 3 cm inferior to occipital protuberance.[57] It is more variable in the remaining 15%. It then crosses over the SCM and travels superolaterally to the postauricular region at a point 7 cm lateral to the EOP and 3 cm medial to mastoid.[58] The nerve then branches into a medial and lateral component at the midpoint between the EOP and the intermastoid line.

Points of Compression and External Landmarks

The LON's point of emergence from beneath the posterior border of the SCM is located an average of 61.3 ± 12.3 mm (right) or 68.9 ± 10.1 mm (left) lateral to the posterior midline and 53.2 ± 16.1 mm caudal to a horizontal line drawn through the inferior aspect of the external acoustic meatuses (**Fig. 10.8, Table 10.6**).[64] Most of the time, the nerve simply emerges around the muscle edge, but in 13.3% of specimens, the LON actually pierces it. This is the first potential compression point. Lee et al located this point of emergence from the SCM an average of 64 ± 14 mm lateral to the posterior midline and 50 ± 9 mm caudal to a line drawn through the most anterosuperior aspects of the external acoustic meatuses.[65] Unlike Dash et al, Lee et al found no compression at the point of emergence from the SCM. This muscular compression point can be treated with neuromuscular blockade or nerve block. Dash et al suggest addressing the LON with botulinum toxin in a region approximately 3 cm in diameter centered at a point 6.5 cm from midline and 5.3 cm below the line between the external acoustic meatuses.[64]

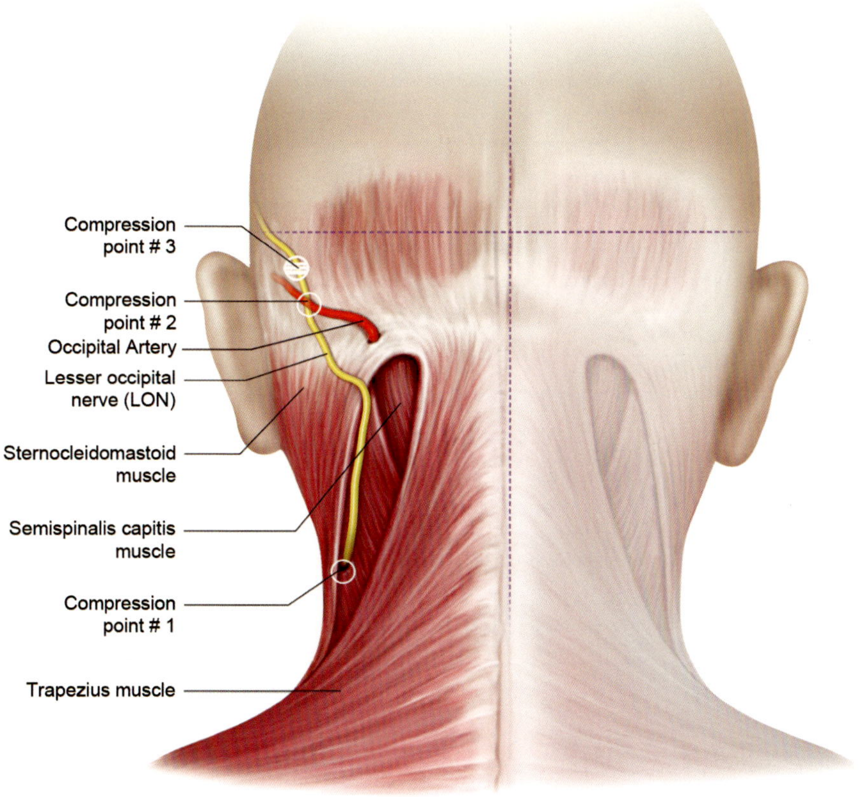

Fig. 10.8 Compression points of lesser occipital nerve.

In 55% of cadavers, the LON had an intersection with the occipital artery, constituting the second potential compression point.[65] This intersection was located 51 ± 9 mm lateral to the midline and 20 ± 14.5 mm inferior to a horizontal line through the most anterosuperior points of the external acoustic meatuses. In 82% of those cases, the intersection was a simple crossing located 50.7 ± 10.9 mm lateral to the midline and 22.5 ± 16.3 caudal to the horizontal line through the most anterosuperior points of the external acoustic meatuses. In the remaining 18%, there was a helical intertwining between the two structures, the midpoint of which was located 52.2 ± 6.8 mm lateral to the midline and 15.7 ± 11.2 mm caudal to the *x*-axis.

The third compression point, observed in 20% of specimens, consisted of a fascial band located 47 ± 8.1 mm lateral to the midline and 13.1 ± 15.2 mm inferior to a horizontal line through the most anterosuperior points of the external acoustic meatuses.[65]

Table 10.6 Compression points of the lesser occipital nerve

Compression point	Name	Type	Frequency	Horizontal location (from midline)	Craniocaudal location	Reference
1	Emergence from SCM	Muscular	13.3%	61.3 ± 12.3 mm (right) or 68.9 ± 10.1 mm	53.2 ± 16.1 mm caudal to inferior EAC	Dash et al[64]
				64 ± 14 mm	50 ± 9 mm caudal to anterosuperior EOP	Lee et al[65a]
2	Occipital artery	Arterial	Simple intersection: 45.1%	50.7 ± 10.9 mm	22.5±16.3 mm caudal to anterosuperior EAC	Lee et al[65]
			Helical intertwining: 9.9%	52.2 ± 6.8 mm	15.7 ± 11.2 mm caudal to anterosuperior EAC	
3	Fascial band	Fascial	20%	47 ± 8.1 mm	13.1 ± 15.2 mm caudal to anterosuperior EAC	Lee[65]

Abbreviations: EAC, external acoustic meatus; EOP, external occipital protuberance; SCM, sternocleidomastoid.
[a]Did not find compression at this point.

Table 10.7 Compression points of the third occipital nerve

Compression point	Name	Type	Frequency	Horizontal location (from midline)	Craniocaudal location	Reference
1	Emergence from semispinalis	Muscular	100%	13.0 ± 5.0 mm (left), 13.3 ± 5.8 mm (right)	60.7 ± 20.2 mm (left), 63.4 ± 20.8 ± mm (right) caudal to inferior external acoustic meatus	Dash et al[64]

Clinical Correlation

Patients with LON compression typically have symptoms similar to those seen with GON compression, but the pain is more lateral along the course of the LON. The LON may be implicated in patients with migraine headaches resulting from an occipital trigger point who undergo GON release without complete relief.[5]

To decompress the LON, it is released from all muscular and fascial attachments, ligated, and its ends are implanted into the SCM muscle. Guyuron et al also recommend injecting triamcinolone in the area intraoperatively in order to minimize the risk of neuroma formation.[30]

Few clinical studies have reported the outcomes of LON release, and most patients in those studies underwent concomitant GON release, which makes quantification of the outcomes of isolated LON release difficult.

Third Occipital Nerve

Origin and Course

The third occipital nerve (TON), also known as the dorsal occipital nerve, originates from the medial branch of the dorsal ramus of the C3 spinal nerve.[64] It is a sensory nerve that innervates the posterior medial scalp and neck (**Fig. 10.1**).

The TON always emerges from the semispinalis capitis muscle by piercing it and then travels cranially in the subcutaneous plane towards the posterior medial scalp. The average diameter of the TON is 1.3 mm.[66] Each TON has multiple interconnections with the ipsilateral GON and the contralateral TON.

Points of Compression and External Landmarks

Dash et al found that the TON pierces the semispinalis capitis muscle at a point 13.0 ± 5.0 mm (left) to 13.3 ± 5.8 mm (right) lateral to the posterior midline and 60.7 ± 20.2 mm (left) to 63.4 ± 20.8 ± mm (right) inferior to a horizontal line drawn through the inferior aspect of the external acoustic meatuses (**Fig. 10.7, Table 10.7**).[64] Tubbs et al found that point approximately 5 to 6 cm caudal to the external occipital protuberance, 3 cm caudal to the intermastoid line, and 3 to 7 mm lateral to the midline.[66]

The vertical location of the TON varies significantly; therefore, to reliably block this nerve, Dash et al suggest performing two injections 1.3 cm lateral to the midline, with one injection 1 cm above a horizontal line drawn through the inferior aspect of the external acoustic meatuses and a second injection 1 cm below.[64]

Clinical Correlation

Similar to the lesser occipital nerve, the third occipital nerve may be implicated in some patients with occipital trigger points who do not fully respond to release of the GON.[5,64] Cervicogenic headaches stemming from third occipital nerve irritation can be due to osteoarthritis of the C2-C3 zygapophysial joint or whiplash. Lord et al found that 27% incidence of TON-induced headaches in post-whiplash patients.[67]

In the past, patients were successfully treated with third occipital nerve blockade,[67,68] radiofrequency ablation,[69] or neurectomy.[66] Recently described surgical release methods of TON release involve releasing it from the surrounding semispinalis capitis muscle and then avulsing the nerve. Avulsion of the TON is performed by applying traction to it and avulsing it, thus allowing it to retract into the musculature instead of being trapped in the scar of the surgical field.[15]

Like the LON, few clinical studies have clearly outlined the outcomes of isolated TON release in migraine decompression surgery. Lee et al conducted a retrospective review of patients undergoing GON release and compared those in whom the TON was encountered and avulsed with those in whom it was not[70]; no difference in outcomes between the two groups was found.

Summary

The peripheral trigger theory postulates that compression of sensory branches of the trigeminal and cervical nerves in the head and neck generates the nociceptive signals responsible for migraine headaches. Surgical decompression of those compression points has been proven, in multiple studies, to be effective at reducing the frequency, severity, and duration of migraine headaches. In a systematic review comparing various nerve decompression modalities in migraine headaches, surgical decompression showed the highest efficacy and the lowest complication rate.[71] To perform adequate and safe surgical decompression, however, a thorough and detailed knowledge of the anatomy of those compression points, their external landmarks, and their anatomical variants is essential. This chapter summarizes the published anatomical data on the known migraine trigger sites.

References

1. Lipton RB, Bigal ME, Diamond M, Freitag F, Reed ML, Stewart WF; AMPP Advisory Group. Migraine prevalence, disease burden, and the need for preventive therapy. Neurology 2007;68(5):343–349
2. Guyuron B, Tucker T, Davis J. Surgical treatment of migraine headaches. Plast Reconstr Surg 2002;109(7):2183–2189
3. Guyuron B, Kriegler JS, Davis J, Amini SB. Comprehensive surgical treatment of migraine headaches. Plast Reconstr Surg 2005;115(1): 1–9
4. Guyuron B, Reed D, Kriegler JS, Davis J, Pashmini N, Amini S. A placebo-controlled surgical trial of the treatment of migraine headaches. Plast Reconstr Surg 2009;124(2):461–468
5. Janis JE, Dhanik A, Howard JH. Validation of the peripheral trigger point theory of migraine headaches: single-surgeon experience using botulinum toxin and surgical decompression. Plast Reconstr Surg 2011;128(1):123–131
6. Welch KMA. Contemporary concepts of migraine pathogenesis. Neurology 2003;61(8, Suppl 4)S2–S8
7. Bolay H, Reuter U, Dunn AK, Huang Z, Boas DA, Moskowitz MA. Intrinsic brain activity triggers trigeminal meningeal afferents in a migraine model. Nat Med 2002;8(2):136–142
8. Moskowitz MA. The neurobiology of vascular head pain. Ann Neurol 1984;16(2):157–168
9. Silberstein S, Mathew N, Saper J, Jenkins S; For the BOTOX Migraine Clinical Research Group. Botulinum toxin type A as a migraine preventive treatment. Headache 2000;40(6):445–450
10. Relja M, Poole AC, Schoenen J, Pascual J, Lei X, Thompson C; European BoNTA Headache Study Group. A multicentre, double-blind, randomized, placebo-controlled, parallel group study of multiple treatments of botulinum toxin type A (BoNTA) for the prophylaxis of episodic migraine headaches. Cephalalgia 2007;27(6):492–503
11. Durham PL, Cady R, Cady R. Regulation of calcitonin gene-related peptide secretion from trigeminal nerve cells by botulinum toxin type A: implications for migraine therapy. Headache 2004;44(1): 35–42, discussion 42–43
12. Kung TA, Guyuron B, Cederna PS. Migraine surgery: a plastic surgery solution for refractory migraine headache. Plast Reconstr Surg 2011;127(1):181–189
13. Guyuron B, Varghai A, Michelow BJ, Thomas T, Davis J. Corrugator supercilii muscle resection and migraine headaches. Plast Reconstr Surg 2000;106(2):429–434, discussion 435–437
14. Calandre EP, Hidalgo J, García-Leiva JM, Rico-Villademoros F. Trigger point evaluation in migraine patients: an indication of peripheral sensitization linked to migraine predisposition? Eur J Neurol 2006;13(3):244–249
15. Ducic I, Hartmann EC, Larson EE. Indications and outcomes for surgical treatment of patients with chronic migraine headaches caused by occipital neuralgia. Plast Reconstr Surg 2009;123(5): 1453–1461
16. Knize DM. Transpalpebral approach to the corrugator supercilii and procerus muscles. Plast Reconstr Surg 1995;95(1):52–60, discussion 61–62
17. Cuzalina AL, Holmes JD. A simple and reliable landmark for identification of the supraorbital nerve in surgery of the forehead: an in vivo anatomical study. J Oral Maxillofac Surg 2005;63(1):25–27
18. Janis JE, Ghavami A, Lemmon JA, Leedy JE, Guyuron B. The anatomy of the corrugator supercilii muscle: part II. Supraorbital nerve branching patterns. Plast Reconstr Surg 2008;121(1):233–240
19. Fallucco M, Janis JE, Hagan RR. The anatomical morphology of the supraorbital notch: clinical relevance to the surgical treatment of migraine headaches. Plast Reconstr Surg 2012;130(6):1227–1233
20. Chepla KJ, Oh E, Guyuron B. Clinical outcomes following supraorbital foraminotomy for treatment of frontal migraine headache. Plast Reconstr Surg 2012;129(4):656e–662e
21. Beer GM, Putz R, Mager K, Schumacher M, Keil W. Variations of the frontal exit of the supraorbital nerve: an anatomic study. Plast Reconstr Surg 1998;102(2):334–341
22. Agthong S, Huanmanop T, Chentanez V. Anatomical variations of the supraorbital, infraorbital, and mental foramina related to gender and side. J Oral Maxillofac Surg 2005;63(6):800–804
23. Cutright B, Quillopa N, Schubert W. An anthropometric analysis of the key foramina for maxillofacial surgery. J Oral Maxillofac Surg 2003;61(3):354–357
24. Saylam C, Ozer MA, Ozek C, Gurler T. Anatomical variations of the frontal and supraorbital transcranial passages. J Craniofac Surg 2003;14(1):10–12
25. Webster RC, Gaunt JM, Hamdan US, Fuleihan NS, Giandello PR, Smith RC. Supraorbital and supratrochlear notches and foramina: anatomical variations and surgical relevance. Laryngoscope 1986; 96(3):311–315
26. Janis JE, Ghavami A, Lemmon JA, Leedy JE, Guyuron B. Anatomy of the corrugator supercilii muscle: part I. Corrugator topography. Plast Reconstr Surg 2007;120(6):1647–1653
27. Liu MT, Armijo BS, Guyuron B. A comparison of outcome of surgical treatment of migraine headaches using a constellation of symptoms versus botulinum toxin type A to identify the trigger sites. Plast Reconstr Surg 2012;129(2):413–419
28. Liu MT, Chim H, Guyuron B. Outcome comparison of endoscopic and transpalpebral decompression for treatment of frontal migraine headaches. Plast Reconstr Surg 2012;129(5):1113–1119
29. Walden JL, Brown CC, Klapper AJ, Chia CT, Aston SJ. An anatomical comparison of transpalpebral, endoscopic, and coronal approaches to demonstrate exposure and extent of brow depressor muscle resection. Plast Reconstr Surg 2005;116(5):1479–1487, discussion 1488–1489
30. Guyuron B, Kriegler JS, Davis J, Amini SB. Five-year outcome of surgical treatment of migraine headaches. Plast Reconstr Surg 2011; 127(2):603–608
31. Miller TA, Rudkin G, Honig M, Elahi M, Adams J. Lateral subcutaneous brow lift and interbrow muscle resection: clinical experience and anatomic studies. Plast Reconstr Surg 2000;105(3):1120–1128
32. Janis JE, Hatef DA, Hagan R, et al. Anatomy of the supratrochlear nerve: implications for the surgical treatment of migraine headaches. Plast Reconstr Surg 2013;131(4):743–750
33. Janis JE, Hatef DA, Thakar H, et al. The zygomaticotemporal branch of the trigeminal nerve: Part II. Anatomical variations. Plast Reconstr Surg 2010;126(2):435–442
34. Totonchi A, Pashmini N, Guyuron B. The zygomaticotemporal branch of the trigeminal nerve: an anatomical study. Plast Reconstr Surg 2005;115(1):273–277
35. Tubbs RS, Mortazavi MM, Shoja MM, Loukas M, Cohen-Gadol AA. The zygomaticotemporal nerve and its relevance to neurosurgery. World Neurosurg 2012;78(5):515–518
36. Odobescu A, Williams HB, Gilardino MS. Description of a communication between the facial and zygomaticotemporal nerves. J Plast Reconstr Aesthet Surg 2012;65(9):1188–1192
37. Loukas M, Owens DG, Tubbs RS, Spentzouris G, Elochukwu A, Jordan R. Zygomaticofacial, zygomaticoorbital and zygomaticotemporal foramina: anatomical study. Anat Sci Int 2008;83(2): 77–82

38. Jeong SM, Park KJ, Kang SH, et al. Anatomical consideration of the anterior and lateral cutaneous nerves in the scalp. J Korean Med Sci 2010;25(4):517–522
39. Murillo CA. Resection of the temporal neurovascular bundle for control of migraine headache. Headache 1968;8(3):112–117
40. Guyuron B, Becker DB. Surgical treatment of migraine headaches. In: Guyuron B, Eriksson E, Persing JA, et al, eds. Plastic Surgery: Indications and Practice. Philadelphia, PA: Saunders Elsevier; 2009:1655–1665
41. Kurlander DE, Punjabi A, Liu MT, Sattar A, Guyuron B. In-depth review of symptoms, triggers, and treatment of temporal migraine headaches (site II). Plast Reconstr Surg 2014;133(4):897–903
42. Chim H, Miller E, Gliniak C, Cohen ML, Guyuron B. The role of different methods of nerve ablation in prevention of neuroma. Plast Reconstr Surg 2013;131(5):1004–1012
43. Schmidt BL, Pogrel MA, Necoechea M, Kearns G. The distribution of the auriculotemporal nerve around the temporomandibular joint. Oral Surg Oral Med Oral Pathol Oral Radiol Endod 1998;86(2): 165–168
44. Janis JE, Hatef DA, Ducic I, et al. Anatomy of the auriculotemporal nerve: variations in its relationship to the superficial temporal artery and implications for the treatment of migraine headaches. Plast Reconstr Surg 2010;125(5):1422–1428
45. Gülekon N, Anil A, Poyraz A, Peker T, Turgut HB, Karaköse M. Variations in the anatomy of the auriculotemporal nerve. Clin Anat 2005;18(1):15–22
46. Chim H, Okada HC, Brown MS, et al. The auriculotemporal nerve in etiology of migraine headaches: compression points and anatomical variations. Plast Reconstr Surg 2012;130(2):336–341
47. Behin F, Behin B, Bigal ME, Lipton RB. Surgical treatment of patients with refractory migraine headaches and intranasal contact points. Cephalalgia 2005;25(6):439–443
48. Harley DH, Powitzky ES, Duncavage J. Clinical outcomes for the surgical treatment of sinonasal headache. Otolaryngol Head Neck Surg 2003;129(3):217–221
49. Clerico DM. Pneumatized superior turbinate as a cause of referred migraine headache. Laryngoscope 1996;106(7):874–879
50. Ferrero V, Allais G, Rolando S, Pozzo T, Allais R, Benedetto C. Endonasal mucosal contact points in chronic migraine. Neurol Sci 2014;35(Suppl 1):83–87
51. Homsioglou E, Balatsouras DG, Alexopoulos G, Kaberos A, Katotomichelakis M, Danielides V. Pneumatized superior turbinate as a cause of headache. Head Face Med 2007;3:3–8
52. Tosun F, Gerek M, Ozkaptan Y. Nasal surgery for contact point headaches. Headache 2000;40(3):237–240
53. Welge-Luessen A, Hauser R, Schmid N, Kappos L, Probst R. Endonasal surgery for contact point headaches: a 10-year longitudinal study. Laryngoscope 2003;113(12):2151–2156
54. Mosser SW, Guyuron B, Janis JE, Rohrich RJ. The anatomy of the greater occipital nerve: implications for the etiology of migraine headaches. Plast Reconstr Surg 2004;113(2):693–700
55. Janis JE, Hatef DA, Ducic I, et al. The anatomy of the greater occipital nerve: Part II. Compression point topography. Plast Reconstr Surg 2010;126(5):1563–1572
56. Bovim G, Bonamico L, Fredriksen TA, Lindboe CF, Stolt-Nielsen A, Sjaastad O. Topographic variations in the peripheral course of the greater occipital nerve. Autopsy study with clinical correlations. Spine 1991;16(4):475–478
57. Ducic I, Moriarty M, Al-Attar A. Anatomical variations of the occipital nerves: implications for the treatment of chronic headaches. Plast Reconstr Surg 2009;123(3):859–863, discussion 864
58. Tubbs RS, Salter EG, Wellons JC III, Blount JP, Oakes WJ. Landmarks for the identification of the cutaneous nerves of the occiput and nuchal regions. Clin Anat 2007;20(3):235–238
59. Janis JE, Hatef DA, Reece EM, McCluskey PD, Schaub TA, Guyuron B. Neurovascular compression of the greater occipital nerve: implications for migraine headaches. Plast Reconstr Surg 2010;126(6): 1996–2001
60. Junewicz A, Katira K, Guyuron B. Intraoperative anatomical variations during greater occipital nerve decompression. J Plast Reconstr Aesthet Surg 2013;66(10):1340–1345
61. Vital JM, Grenier F, Dautheribes M, Baspeyre H, Lavignolle B, Sénégas J. An anatomic and dynamic study of the greater occipital nerve (n. of Arnold). Applications to the treatment of Arnold's neuralgia. Surg Radiol Anat 1989;11(3):205–210
62. Anthony M. Headache and the greater occipital nerve. Clin Neurol Neurosurg 1992;94(4):297–301
63. Chmielewski L, Liu MT, Guyuron B. The role of occipital artery resection in the surgical treatment of occipital migraine headaches. Plast Reconstr Surg 2013;131(3):351e–356e
64. Dash KS, Janis JE, Guyuron B. The lesser and third occipital nerves and migraine headaches. Plast Reconstr Surg 2005;115(6):1752–1758, discussion 1759–1760
65. Lee M, Brown M, Chepla K, et al. An anatomical study of the lesser occipital nerve and its potential compression points: implications for surgical treatment of migraine headaches. Plast Reconstr Surg 2013;132(6):1551–1556
66. Tubbs RS, Mortazavi MM, Loukas M, et al. Anatomical study of the third occipital nerve and its potential role in occipital headache/neck pain following midline dissections of the craniocervical junction. J Neurosurg Spine 2011;15(1):71–75
67. Lord SM, Barnsley L, Wallis BJ, Bogduk N. Third occipital nerve headache: a prevalence study. J Neurol Neurosurg Psychiatry 1994; 57(10):1187–1190
68. Bogduk N, Marsland A. On the concept of third occipital headache. J Neurol Neurosurg Psychiatry 1986;49(7):775–780
69. Hamer JF, Purath TA. Response of cervicogenic headaches and occipital neuralgia to radiofrequency ablation of the C2 dorsal root ganglion and/or third occipital nerve. Headache 2014;54(3):500–510
70. Lee M, Lineberry K, Reed D, Guyuron B. The role of the third occipital nerve in surgical treatment of occipital migraine headaches. J Plast Reconstr Aesthet Surg 2013;66(10):1335–1339
71. Ducic I, Felder JM III, Fantus SA. A systematic review of peripheral nerve interventional treatments for chronic headaches. Ann Plast Surg 2014;72(4):439–445

11 Superficial Musculoaponeurotic System and the Facial Soft Tissues

Yoko Tabira, Joe Iwanaga, Tsuyoshi Saga, and Koichi Watanabe

Introduction

The soft tissue layers of the face from the surface down are generally made up of the skin, subcutaneous fat, superficial fascia (superficial musculoaponeurotic system [SMAS]), mimetic muscles, and deep tissue layers. Structurally, these layers vary among the different regions of the face. For example, the subcutaneous fat layer does not exist in the eyelid, lip, or nose. The deep tissue layer is covered by deep fascia and includes the parotid gland, masseter muscle, buccal fat pad, deep temporal fascia, and temporalis muscle. The structures within the deep tissue layer also vary among the different facial regions. Each layer is connected to adjacent layers and supports proper anatomical positioning of the facial soft tissue against gravity. Among the soft tissue layers of the face, the SMAS is the key structure of the facial fascial system. This chapter describes the basic structure of each layer and presents cadaver dissections and microscopic images.

Subcutaneous Fat Layer

The subcutaneous fat is located beneath the dermis and is present throughout most of the entire body. In body regions other than the face, the subcutaneous fat layer is divided into two layers by the superficial fascia, and each layer exhibits different characteristics. The superficial fat layer contains many fibrous septa and is involved in protection from external forces. Nakajima et al[1] termed this fat layer the protective adipofascial system. In contrast, the deep fat layer provides flexibility to musculoskeletal movement and is termed the lubricant adipofascial system. The facial subcutaneous fat contains many fibrous septa and has a structure similar to that of the protective adipofascial system. The subcutaneous fat layer has an intimate relationship with the SMAS. Many connective tissue fibers rise upward to the dermis and provide a strong connection between the dermis and SMAS. Each lobule of the subcutaneous fat is small and surrounded by dense fibrous septa. In the cheek region, a thick fat tissue layer lies on the SMAS and is distinct from the subcutaneous fat layer. This fat tissue is called the malar fat pad.

Malar Fat Pad

The malar fat pad is the fat tissue that lies superficial to the SMAS in the cheek region. It is triangular shaped and bound medially along the nasolabial crease, superiorly along the orbital rim, and laterally along the convex curved line connecting the lateral canthus and nasolabial crease around the corner of the mouth. At the location of the malar fat pad, the upper half of the SMAS comprises the orbicularis oculi muscle, and the lower half comprises the superficial upper lip elevator muscles. The lower half of the SMAS is quite thin and almost discontinuous and has no mechanical bearing capacity. The malar fat pad is firmly fixed to the dermis and relatively loosely fixed to the SMAS layer in this region. The zygomatic ligament, which is an osteocutaneous ligament located on the zygoma lateral to the origin of the zygomatic minor muscle, inserts in the overlying dermis and pierces and anchors the malar fat pad to connect it to the deeper tissue layers.

Cosmetically, the malar fat pad slides downward and inward over the SMAS with aging, deepening the nasolabial crease. Fat tissue is also present beneath the orbicularis oculi muscle. This fat tissue is called the suborbicularis oculi fat pad and lacks continuity with the malar fat pad.

SMAS

The SMAS is the fascial tissue layer located just beneath the subcutaneous fat layer. It connects the facial muscles with the dermis, transmits contraction of the facial muscles to the skin, and assists in creating facial expression. The SMAS is the key structure in surgical treatment of the face, and an accurate knowledge of its anatomy is extremely important. The existence of superficial fascia in the head and neck region has been discovered in fragments; for example, the superficial temporal fascia and galea aponeurotica were not originally recognized as a continuous layer. The concept of a fascia layer that spreads throughout the entire head and neck region in one sheet and is integrated with the conventional fragmental fascial structures (i.e., the concept of the SMAS) was first advocated by Mitz and Peyronie in 1976.[2] The SMAS is a fascial layer that is connected superiorly to the frontalis muscle and inferiorly to the platysma muscle. Its thickness decreases as it continues to the anterior cheek area. Although some opinions differ, the generally prevailing thoughts regarding the SMAS are almost identical to those proposed by Mitz and Peyronie.[2]

The SMAS lies on the same horizontal plane as the platysma muscle and extends superiorly to the superficial temporal fascia, galea aponeurotica, and frontalis muscle in its upper region (**Fig. 11.1**). However, some authorities have questioned the continuity of the SMAS in the temporal region. Gosain et al[3] reported that the SMAS terminates within 1 cm below the zygomatic arch and is not continuous with the temporoparietal fascia (superficial temporal fascia). Intraoperatively, the area over the zygomatic arch has a complicated structure. The superficial temporal artery passing from the deep plane to the superficial temporal fascia layer and the temporal branch of the facial nerve also passes from the deep layer to the inferior surface of the superficial temporal fascia. The SMAS is also difficult to dissect as a uniform layer. It is quite thick in the parotid–masseteric

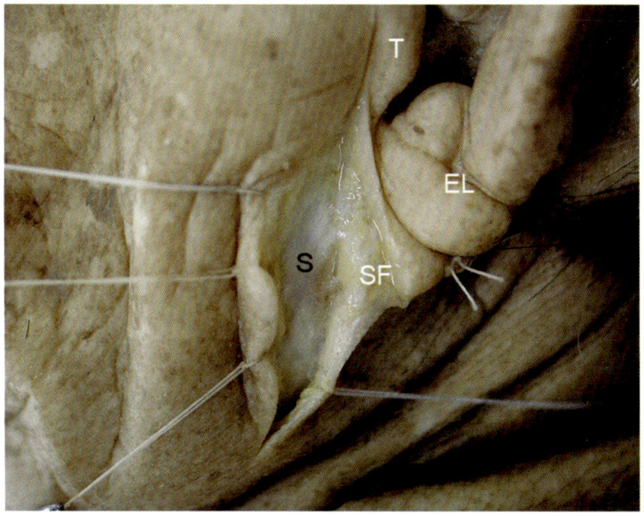

a

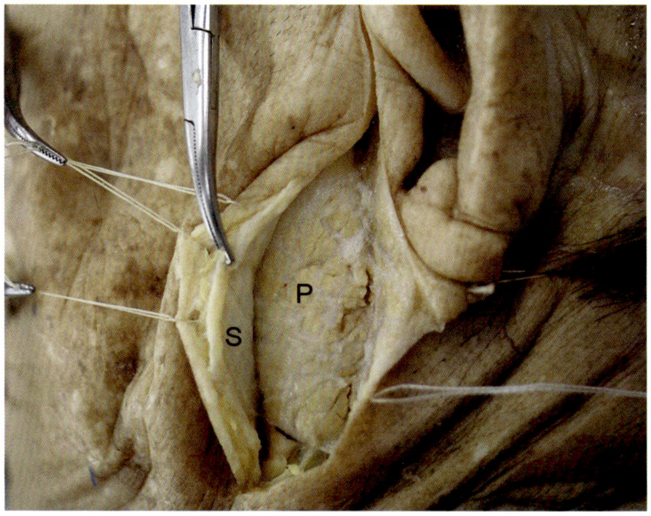

b

Fig. 11.1 Cadaveric dissection of the superficial musculoaponeurotic system (SMAS) in the parotid region. **(a)** The SMAS is seen as a white fibrous layer under the subcutaneous fat. EL, Earlobe; T, tragus; S, SF, subcutaneous fat. **(b)** The SMAS is elevated with Kocher forceps. The parotid gland is observed in the sub-SMAS layer. P, Parotid gland; S, SMAS.

and zygomatic areas and is easily dissected in this region under gross visualization. Beyond the anterior border of the masseter muscle, however, the SMAS becomes quite thin and almost invisible, making it quite difficult to dissect, raising questions about the continuity of the SMAS. Gardetto et al[4] stated that the SMAS cannot be detected in any facial region other than the parotid region. Jost and Levet[5] questioned whether the SMAS actually continues to the orbicularis oculi muscle from an embryologic point of view. The orbicularis oculi originates from the sphincter colli profundus; however, the platysma muscle, which lies on the same plane as does the SMAS, originates from a different layer (i.e., the platysma layer). Thus, confusion results from the histologic differences among the soft tissue layers of the lateral and central facial regions. Ghassemi et al[6] claimed that the SMAS can be histologically classified as type 1 or type 2. Type 1 SMAS describes the common architecture of the posterior part of the face and is observed in the forehead, parotid region, zygomatic region, infraorbital region, and lateral aspect of the nasolabial fold. The subdermal structure comprises a meshwork of fibrous septa enveloping lobules of fat cells. Type 2 SMAS is found in the upper and lower lips, and the subdermal tissue comprises a meshwork of intermingled collagen, elastic fibers, and muscle fibers.

With respect to the relationship of the SMAS with mimetic muscles, Mitz and Peyronie[2] reported that the SMAS invests in and extends into the external part of the superficial facial muscles involving the risorius, frontalis, platysma, and orbicularis oculi muscles. Stuzin et al[7] reported that the SMAS invests in the zygomaticus major and zygomaticus minor, in addition to the muscles described by Mitz and Peyronie.[2] The mimetic muscle layer is three-dimensional, and each of its muscles is located at a different depth from the surface. According to embryologic hypothesis, these facial muscles originate from three layers: the sphincter colli superficialis, sphincter colli profundus, and platysma, the last of which is located between the two sphincters. The sphincter colli profundus differentiates and becomes the buccinators, orbicularis oris, levator anguli oris, levator labii superioris, depressor anguli oris, and similar muscles. The platysma becomes other facial muscles, and the sphincter colli superficialis degenerates in many mammals. Freilinger et al[8] reported the three-dimensional structure of the mimetic muscles as comprising four layers: layer 1, depressor anguli oris, zygomaticus minor, and orbicularis oculi; layer 2, depressor labii inferioris, risorius, platysma, zygomaticus major, and levator labii superioris alaeque nasi; layer 3, orbicularis oris and levator labii superioris; and layer 4, mentalis, levator anguli oris, and buccinator. The SMAS is presumed to have a close relationship with the two superficial layers of the mimetic muscles as described by Freilinger et al.[8] According to Freilinger et al, however, some muscles are superficial to the SMAS (e.g., the platysma). Thus, the descriptions of the SMAS are presumed to be based more on clinical theory than strictly on embryologic theory.

There are many opinions about the embryologic origin of the SMAS.[2,9] For example, some researchers have reported that the superficial fascia (tela subcutanea), which is a loose fibrous layer located just under the skin, is also observed in other parts of the body.[2] Others have described fibrous degeneration of the platysma,[5] a distinct fibromuscular layer comprising the platysma and parotid fascia,[10] a musculoaponeurotic layer continuous with the platysma,[6] and an evolutionary form of the panniculus carnosus.[11] Some reports state that the SMAS contains muscle fibers,[2,8] which indicates the embryologic origin of the SMAS layer. One anatomical textbook also shows that the platysma sometimes extends farther upward than usual, in some cases as high as the zygoma.[12] Such a markedly upward-extending platysma is considered to represent remaining muscle fibers along the platysma layer. Another possibility is that a primitive muscle remains in the SMAS layer.[13] Lei et al[14] termed the muscle that spreads over the parotid gland *the transverse nuchae muscle* and assumed that this muscle is the SMAS muscle fiber described by Mitz and Peyronie.[2] This muscle was found in about 5% of our dissections.

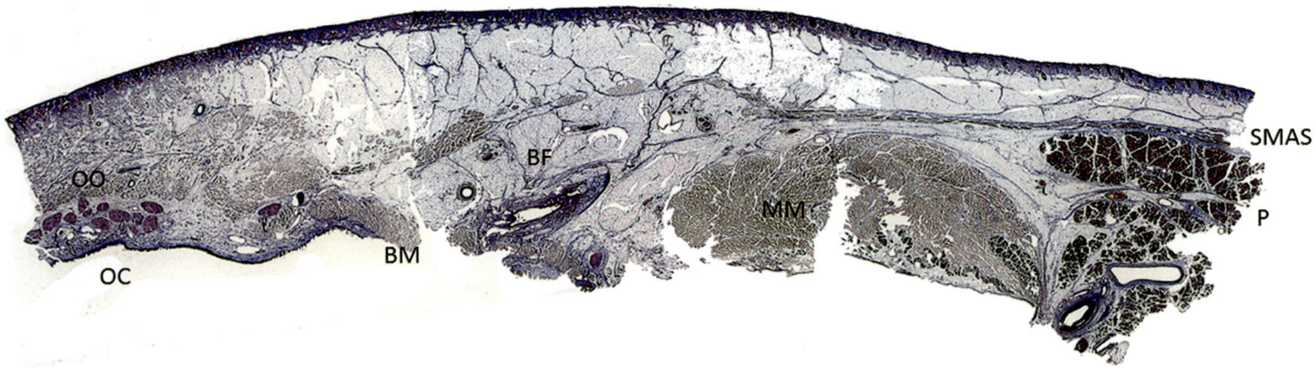

Fig. 11.2 Cross-section from the parotid gland to the upper lip (composite photograph of three preparation specimens; Masson trichrome stain, ×1). BF, Buccal fat pad; BM, buccinator muscle; MF, malar fat pad; MM, masseter muscle; OC, oral cavity; OO, orbicularis oris muscle; P, parotid gland; SMAS, superficial musculoaponeurotic system.

Histologic Findings of the SMAS

Parotid Area to Cheek Region

The SMAS is a thick membranous tissue that lies on the parotid gland and extends anteriorly, maintaining almost the same thickness until reaching the anterior border of the masseter (**Fig. 11.2**). Some branched muscular fibers of the platysma are present within the SMAS layer. The subcutaneous fat tissue layer is relatively thin in this area. The fibrous septa within this layer basically run parallel to the SMAS and delineate long, oval-shaped fat tissue in the horizontal plane. The SMAS becomes dramatically thinner beyond the anterior border of the masseter as it enters the cheek area; it can be barely traced by the position of split peripheral part of the platysma. The thick fat tissue superficial to the SMAS layer is the malar fat pad. This fat tissue contains fibrous septa that run perpendicular to the SMAS toward the dermis and separate the fat tissue into long ovals in the vertical plane. The fat tissue observed anterior to the masseter is the buccal fat pad, which fills the masticatory space.

Temporal Region

In the temporal region, the SMAS meets the superficial temporal fascia (**Fig. 11.3**). The superficial temporal fascia usually comprises fibrous tissue without muscle; however, it sometimes contains visible degenerative facial muscles such as the superior auricular muscle and temporoparietal muscle. The SMAS becomes somewhat ambiguous between these two fasciae, around the region of the zygomatic arch. Toward the temporal region, the SMAS layer separates into fibers containing fat tissue, no longer constituting a sheet of membrane. This finding is in contrast to the idea that the SMAS is continuous. The fibers gradually converge as they course upward. The subcutaneous fat layer above the SMAS also becomes thinner toward the head.

Lower Eyelid

It is generally recognized that the SMAS runs superficial to the zygomaticus major and minor and continues to the orbicularis oculi; however, it is difficult to confirm that the SMAS constitutes one continuous sheet in this area (**Fig. 11.4**). The thick fat

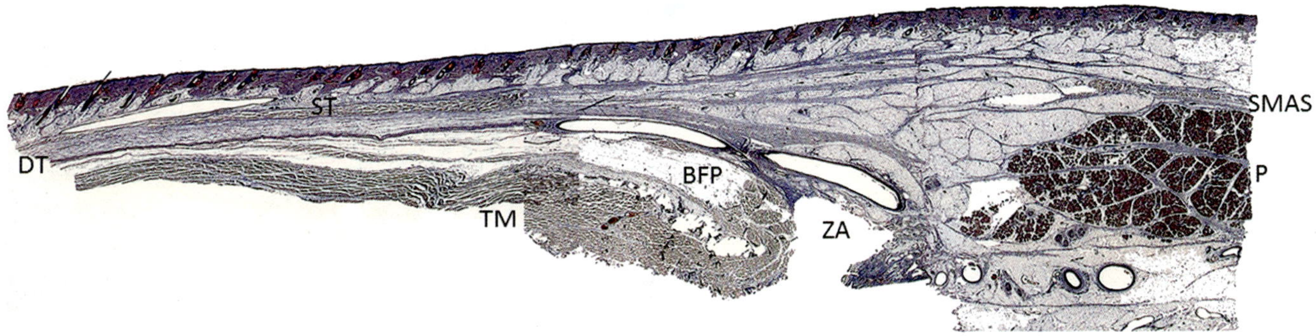

Fig. 11.3 Cross section from the parotid gland to the temporal region (composite photograph of three preparation specimens, Masson trichrome stain, ×1). BF, Buccal fat pad; DT, deep temporal fascia; P, parotid gland; SMAS, superficial musculoaponeurotic system; ST, superficial temporal fascia (in this case, the temporoparietal muscle); TM, temporalis muscle; ZA, zygomatic arch (removed).

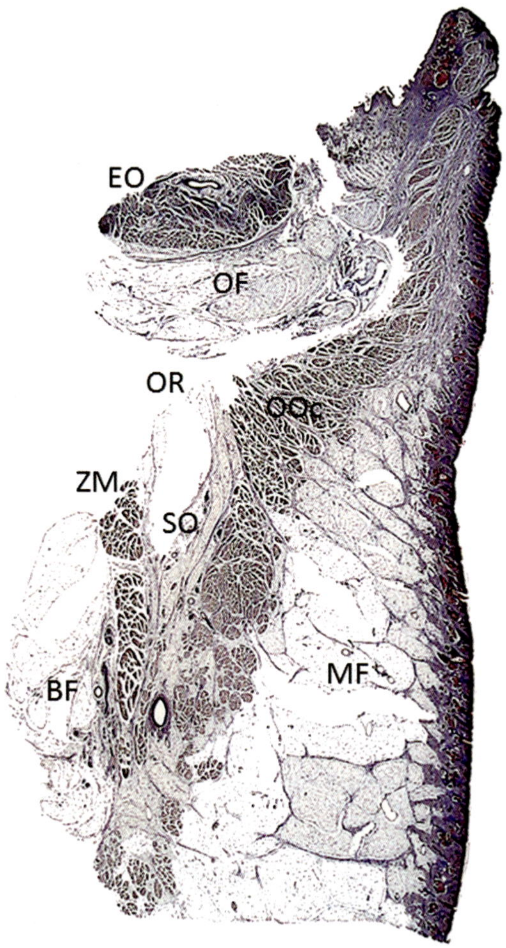

Fig. 11.4 Cross-section of lower eyelid (Masson trichrome stain, ×1). EO, extraocular muscle; MF, malar fat pad; OF, orbital fat; OOc, orbicularis oculi muscle; SO, suborbicularis oculi fat pad; ZM, zygomatic muscles.

tissue overlying the SMAS layer is the malar fat pad. It is thick in the middle region of the cheek and ends at the orbital rim. The fat pad is vertically long and oval in shape, and its fibrous septa are strongly connected as they course toward the dermis. The fat tissue beneath the orbicularis oculi is the suborbicularis oculi fat pad.

Facial Soft Tissue Layer Deep To the SMAS (Mimetic Muscle Layer and Deep Tissue Layer)

Many structures important to facial function are located in the tissue layer deep to the SMAS, including the mimetic muscles, facial nerve, parotid gland, muscles of mastication, and others. When performing surgical procedures involving the sub-SMAS plane, accurate anatomical knowledge is required to prevent damage to these structures. The main structures encountered on the floor of the lateral face during sub-SMAS dissection are the parotid gland and the masseter muscles (**Fig. 11.5a**). The parotid masseteric fascia envelops these structures. A part of the buccal fat pad exposed at the anterior masseteric muscle also constitutes the floor of the plane. In the anterior region of the face, the deep layer of the mimetic muscles includes structures such as the levator labii superioris, levator anguli oris, and buccinator muscles (**Fig. 11.5b**). The most important structures in the sub-SMAS plane are the peripheral branches of the facial nerve. The facial nerve runs through the parotid gland after emerging from the external skull base via the stylomastoid foramen, and the branches of the nerve run along the fascia after emerging from the superior, anterior, and inferior borders of the parotid gland. The peripheral branches of the facial nerve (the temporal, zygomatic, buccal, marginal mandibular, and cervical branches, especially the zygomatic and buccal branches) run along the basal floor. In contrast, the temporal, marginal mandibular, and cervical branches rise up to the SMAS plane from the base. These branches innervate the SMAS muscles, mainly the frontalis muscle, depressor anguli oris, platysma, and some others. The sub-SMAS space also contains some fiber bundles that support the facial skin. These fibers from a structure called the retaining ligament, which divides the sub-SMAS space into small compartments. The next section of this chapter describes the main retaining ligaments of the face and the sub-SMAS spaces related to the ligaments.

Mimetic Muscles and Facial Nerve

The details of the mimetic muscles and facial nerve are addressed in other chapters (Chapters 9 and 12).

Parotid Masseteric Fascia

The parotid masseteric fascia is a deep fascia that envelops the parotid gland and masseter muscle. This fascia also covers the parotid duct, the peripheral branches of the facial nerve, and the surface of the buccal fat pad. In its more anterior part, the fascia extends to the deep layer, reaching the elevator muscles of the upper lip. It continues to the deep cervical fascia inferiorly beyond the margin of mandible. Finally, it continues to the temporal fascia (deep temporal fascia) superiorly over the zygomatic arch.[7]

Retaining Ligaments of the Face

Some fibrous structures arising from the basal floor are observed in the sub-SMAS plane. These structures connect to the dermis and play a role in anchoring the facial skin, resisting gravity, and preventing drooping of the facial soft tissue. Loosening of this system causes aging changes of the facial appearance. This anchoring system is based on the retaining ligaments. McGregor first reported the retaining ligament of the face, termed the zygomatic ligament or McGregor's patch. Furnas subsequently summarized the retaining ligaments in 1989[15] and described four retaining ligaments: the zygomatic (McGregor's patch), mandibular, platysma–auricular, and anterior platysma

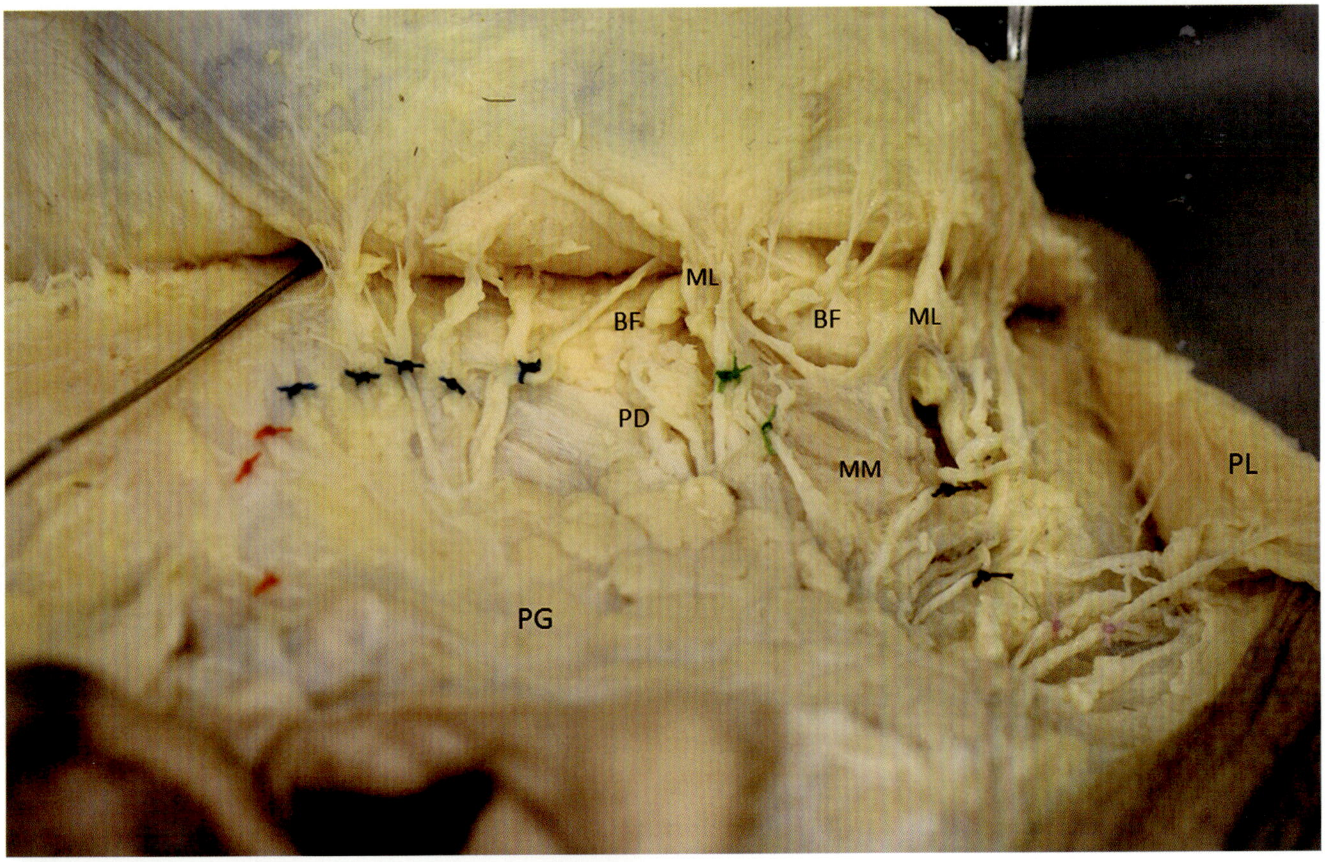

a

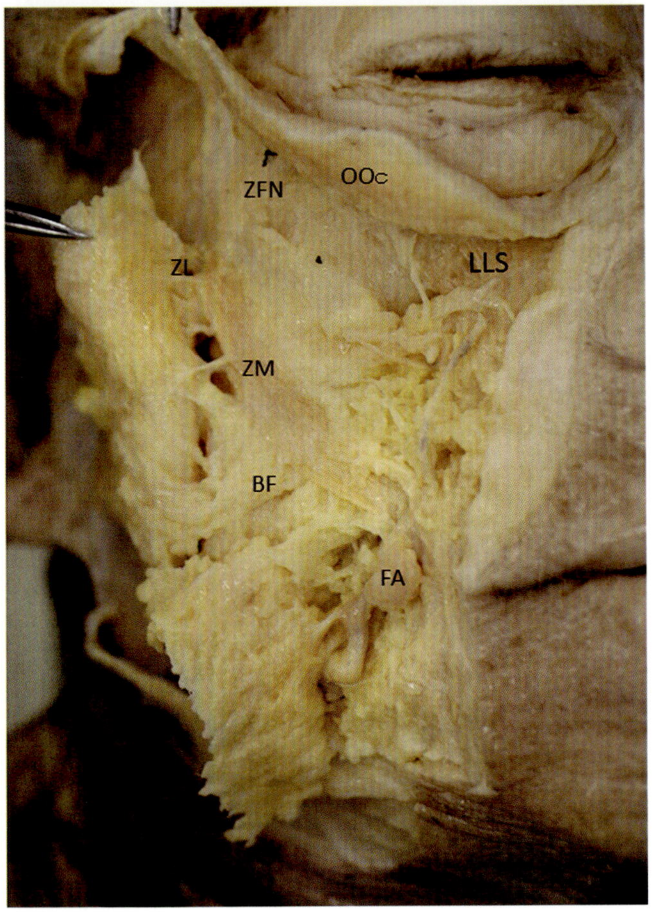

b

Fig. 11.5 Sub-superficial musculoaponeurotic system (SMAS) plane dissection. **(a)** Lateral part. Right lateral view of the right side of the face. The left side of the picture is the cranial aspect, and the right side is the caudal aspect. The area superior to the zygomatic arch was dissected from the more superficial layer to keep the temporal branch on the basal floor. The platysma was cut along the mandibular border. The branches of the facial nerve were marked as follows: temporal branches, orange string knot; zygomatic branches, dark blue; buccal branches, green; marginal mandibular branches, dark brown; and cervical branches, purple. A bar was inserted into the prezygomatic space. **(b)** Medial part. Frontal view of the right side of the face. BF, Buccal fat pad; FA, facial artery; LLS, levator labii superioris muscle; ML, masseteric ligament; MM, masseteric muscle; OOc, orbicularis oculi muscle; PD, parotid duct; PL, platysma; ZFN, zygomaticofacial nerve; ZL, zygomatic ligament; ZM, zygomaticus major muscle.

ligaments. These four ligaments can be classified into two types based on the tissues from which the ligaments arise. The zygomatic ligament and the mandibular ligament arise from the facial skeleton and insert into the dermis, whereas the platysma–auricular ligament and anterior platysma ligament connect the platysma and dermis. Stuzin et al[7] also described two types of retaining ligaments, depending on whether they originate from the bone or from other structures. The ligament arising from the bone, which is compatible with the zygomatic and mandibular ligaments described by Furnas,[15] was classified as a true osteocutaneous ligament. Other ligaments provide coalescence between the deep fascia and superficial fascia. The parotid cutaneous and masseteric cutaneous ligaments are also categorized in this group. Moreover, Moss et al[16] described three type of retaining ligaments: true ligaments, adhesions, and septa. True ligaments are almost identical to the so-called true osteocutaneous ligament described by Stuzin,[7] which arises from either the deep fascia or the periosteum, pierces the SMAS, and distributes the attachment of the ligament to the dermis by spreading like a branching tree. It is located mainly on the medial midface and lower face, and the zygomatic ligament and masseteric ligament are included in this category. Septa are fibrous walls passing between the deep fascia and the SMAS (superficial fascia) and do not adhere to the dermis. This category includes the inferior temporal septum, the superior temporal septum, and the periorbital septum. Finally, adhesions are low-density areas of fibrous or fibrofatty connections between the deep fascia (or pericranium) and the superficial fascia. They also connect the basal tissue and SMAS and do not adhere to the dermis. Adhesions are usually observed in the temporal and forehead regions, excluding the preauricular and parotid regions. Temporal and supraorbital ligamentous adhesions are included in this category.

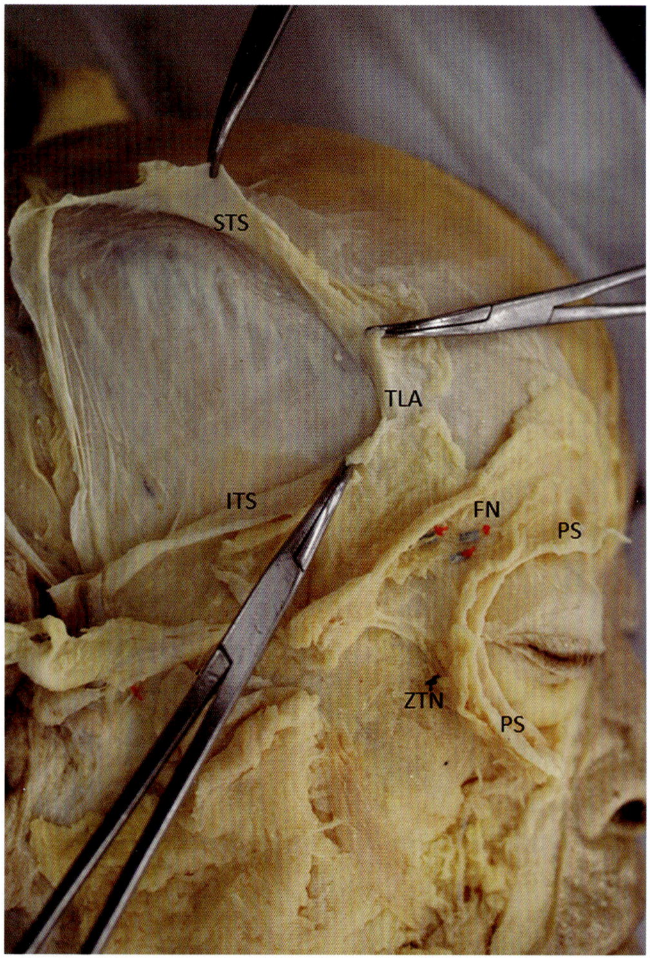

Fig. 11.6 Temporal region. Lateral view of the right side of the face. FN, temporal branches of the facial nerve; ITS, inferior temporal septum; PS, periorbital septum; STS, superior temporal septum; TLA, temporal ligamentous adhesion; ZTN, zygomaticotemporal nerve.

Forehead and Temporal Region

A retaining ligament in the forehead and temporal region was first reported in detail by Moss et al (**Fig. 11.6, Table 11.1**).[16] It includes one adhesion and two septa extending radially in the lateral direction. As previously mentioned, all these structures connect the basal tissue and the SMAS.

Temporal Ligamentous Adhesion

The temporal ligamentous adhesion is located at the lateral part of the supraorbital rim, medial to the anterior end of the temporal line. It is triangular shaped; the base of the triangle lies on a parallel line approximately 10 mm from the supraorbital rim and is approximately 15 mm in length, and the apex lies on the temporal line and is 20 mm in height. Three other ligaments in the forehead and the temporal region converge at this point: the superior temporal septum, inferior temporal septum, and supraorbital adhesion.[16] The superior temporal septum continues to the superior apex of the triangular adhesion, and the inferior temporal septum continues to the lateral apex of the base. The supraorbital adhesion is located along the supraorbital rim medial to the temporal ligamentous adhesion and continues to the medial apex of the triangle.

Superior Temporal Septum

This superior temporal septum starts from the temporal ligamentous adhesion and runs superiorly and laterally along the superior temporal line. It forms the connection between the periosteum and the transitional zone between the superficial temporal fascia and the galea aponeurotica.[16]

Inferior Temporal Septum

The inferior temporal septum starts from the lateral point of the base of the temporal ligamentous adhesion and runs inferiorly and laterally. It is located on an oblique line connecting the temporal ligamentous adhesion and external acoustic meatus. In the vertical section, it arises from the deep temporal fascia

Table 11.1 Retaining ligaments of the forehead and temporal region

Retaining ligament	Location	Type
Temporal ligamentous adhesion	Lateral part of supraorbital rim, medial to the anterior end of the temporal line	Adhesion between the pericranium and the superficial fascia
Supraorbital ligamentous adhesion	Supraorbital rim, medial to the temporal ligamentous adhesion	Adhesion between the pericranium and the superficial fascia
Superior temporal septum	On the superior temporal line	Septum, connecting between the periosteum and superficial fascia (superficial temporal fascia and galea aponeurotica)
Inferior temporal septum	On the line connecting between the temporal ligamentous adhesion and external acoustic meatus	Septum connecting between the deep temporal fascia and superficial temporal fascia

and inserts into the deepest layers of the superficial temporal fascia over the line. The temporal branches of the facial nerve run below the septum.[16]

Supraorbital Ligamentous Adhesion

The supraorbital ligamentous adhesion arises from the frontal bone above the orbital rim and extends in two directions to the corrugator supercilii muscle and temporal ligament.[16]

Periorbital Region (Tear Trough and Orbicularis Retaining Ligament, Periorbital Septum)

The ligaments in the periorbital region course along the orbital rim, covering almost the entire circumference of the orbit (**Table 11.2**). This ligamentous complex is the first reported true osteocutaneous ligament in the lower eyelid and was described by Wong in 2012.[17] The tear trough–orbicularis retaining ligaments comprise the tear trough ligament, which is located medially, and the orbicularis ligament, which is located laterally. The tear trough ligament arises from the inferior orbital rim of the maxilla and connects the boundary of the palpebral and orbital parts of the orbicularis oculi. The medial part of this ligament is located at the level of the medial canthal tendon, immediately inferior to the anterior lacrimal crest. It ends around the medial pupil line and continues laterally to the two orbicularis retaining ligaments. The orbicularis retaining ligament continues to the lateral orbital thickening at the level of the lateral canthus and the lateral brow thickening at the superior lateral angle of the orbital rim, finally ending at the origin of the corrugator supercilii at the superior medial part of the orbital rim.

Middle and Lower Facial Region

Beginning with McGregor's description of the zygomatic ligament, the retaining ligaments in the middle and lower facial regions have been reported in detail by many researchers (**Fig. 11.7, Table 11.3**). In this region, the zygomatic ligament and mandibular ligament are so-called true osteocutaneous ligaments that arise from the periosteum and insert into the dermis. With respect to other ligaments, the masseteric cutaneous ligament forms the coalescence between the deep fascia and the superficial fascia; the fibers of this ligament do not reach the dermis. The platysma auricular ligament is an adhesion only located in the superficial layer, and it connects the platysma and the dermis. In this area, many branches of the facial nerve run

Table 11.2 Retaining ligaments of the periorbital region

Retaining ligament	Location	Type
Tear-trough Ligament	Inferior orbital rim from the medial canthal tendon to medial pupil line	Osteocutaneous ligament
Orbicularis retaining ligament	Continuing to the tear-trough ligament Two ligaments run parallel on the inferior orbital rim and end at the lateral canthus	Osteocutaneous ligament
Lateral orbital thickening	Lateral canthus	Osteocutaneous ligament
Lateral brow thickening	Superior lateral angle of the orbital rim and inferior to the temporal ligamentous adhesion The ligament continues to the medial part of the orbital rim along the superior orbital rim	Osteocutaneous ligament

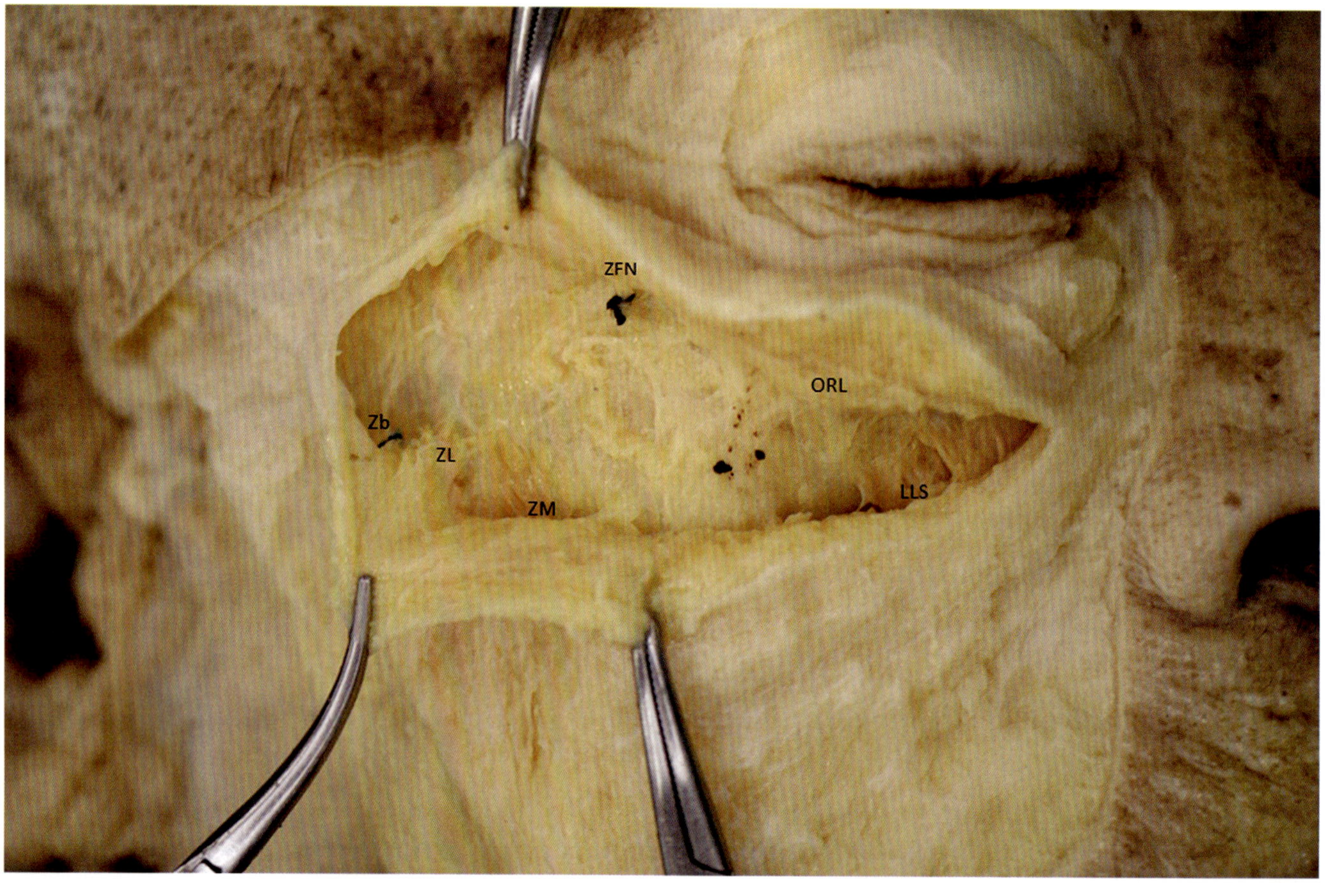

Fig. 11.7 Prezygomatic space. LLS, levator labii superioris; ORN, orbicularis retaining ligament; Zb, zygomatic branch of the facial nerve; ZFN, zygomaticofacial nerve; ZL, zygomatic ligament; ZM, zygomatic major muscle.

Table 11.3 Retaining ligaments of the middle and lower facial region

Retaining ligament	Location	Type
Zygomatic ligament (McGregor's patch)	Usually two bundles About 4.5 cm from the tragus Inferior border of the anterior end of zygomatic arch and behind the insertion of the zygomatic minor	Osteocutaneous ligament
Mandibular ligament	Mandibular bone along a line that is 1cm above the mandibular border and which extends along the anterior third of the mandibular body Immediately in front of the masseter muscle's anterior border.	Osteocutaneous ligament
Masseteric cutaneous ligament	Serious of fibers arising along the anterior border of the masseter muscle	Coalescence between the deep fascia and the SMAS
Platysma cutaneous ligament	Middle and anterior cheek	Aponeurotic connection between the platysma and the dermis
Platysma auricular ligament	Inferior auricular region	Connection between the posterior border of the platysma and the dermis of the inferior auricular region

along the basal floor of the sub-SMAS plane, and some branches run in the vicinity of the ligaments.

Perforating vessels and cutaneous nerves also run with the ligament. Accurate intraoperative identification of these accompanying structures is very important to prevent complications.

Zygomatic Ligament

The zygomatic ligament is a representative true osteocutaneous ligament. It arises from the bone or periosteum and inserts into the dermis, exhibiting treelike spreading. The origin of this ligament is located around the inferior border of the anterior end of the zygomatic arch, behind the insertion of the zygomaticus minor muscle, and about 4.5 cm anteriorly from the tragus.

Two ligamentous bundles are usually present; both are similar in size, measuring approximately 3.0 mm wide, 0.5 mm thick, and 6.0 to 8.0 mm long.[15] One of the upper rami of the zygomatic branch of the facial nerve and a branch of the transverse facial artery usually lie directly beneath this ligament.[15,18] The zygomatic ligament pierces the malar fat pad as it courses toward the overlying dermis and plays a role in supporting the fat pad. As the ligament loosens with aging, the malar fat pad descends and the nasolabial crease deepens. The space on the zygoma anterior to the zygomatic ligament is termed the prezygomatic space. The superior boundary of this space is the orbicularis retaining ligament, and the roof of the space is the orbicularis oculi muscle. The prezygomatic space is filled with the suborbicularis oculi fat pad and provides mobility to the orbicularis oculi muscle during facial expression. The zygomaticotemporal nerve, which is a cutaneous nerve of the face, runs upward toward the dermis, and part of the zygomatic branch of the facial nerve to the orbicularis oculi muscle runs along the roof side of the space.

Mandibular Ligament

Like the zygomatic ligament, the mandibular ligament is also categorized as a true osteocutaneous ligament (**Fig. 11.8**). Furnas[15] reported that the mandibular ligament originates from the mandibular bone along a line that lies approximately 1 cm above the mandibular border and extends along the anterior third of the mandibular body. The mandibular ligament usually appears as a linear series of parallel fibers. A sensory nerve and cutaneous artery usually accompany and run with the ligaments. Mendelson et al[19] reported that the mandibular ligament is located immediately in front of the anterior border of the masseter muscle; this border is curved and extends anteriorly toward the lower edge of the mandible. The mandibular ligament

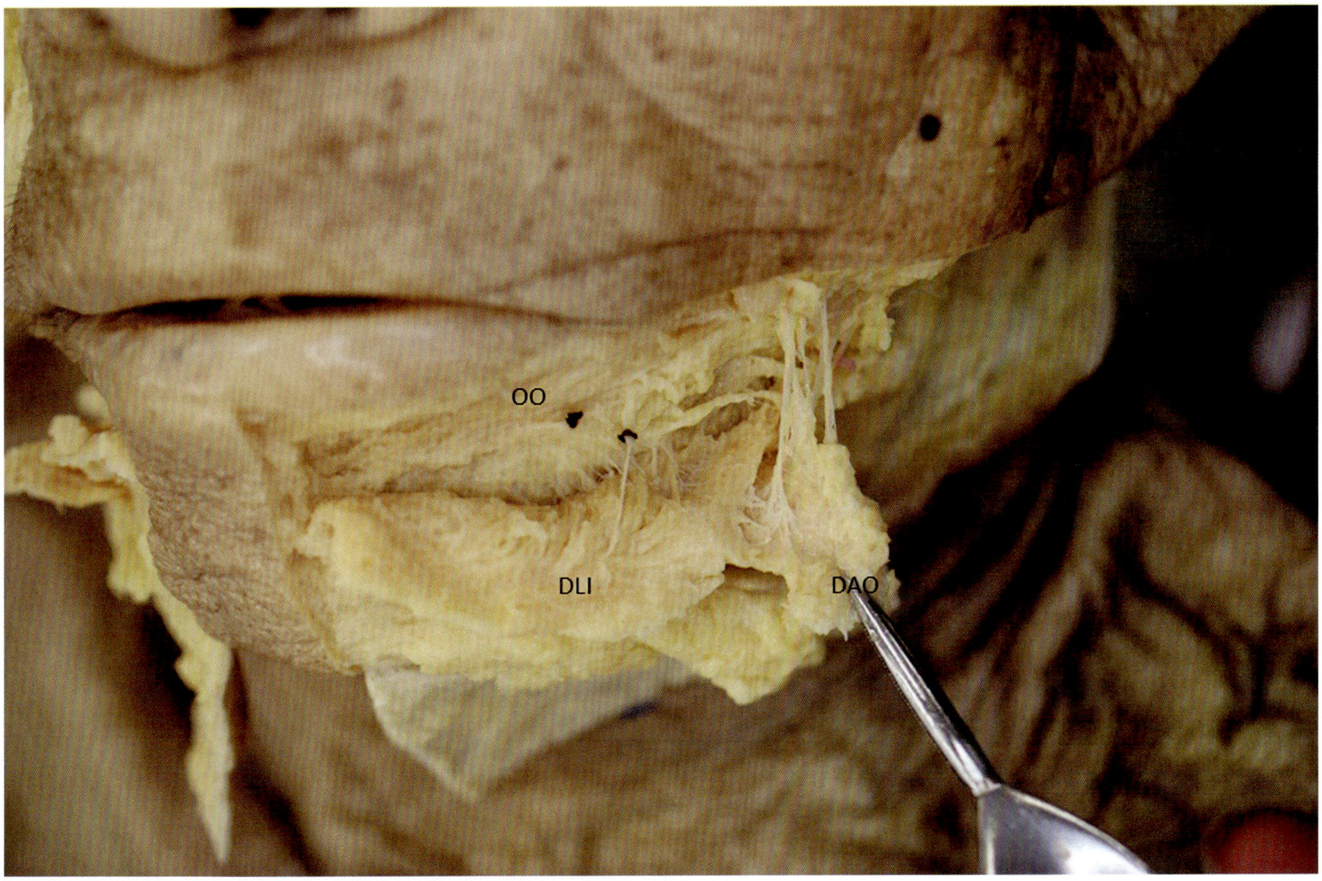

Fig. 11.8 Mandibular area. Frontal view of the left mandibular area. The depressor anguli oris muscle and depressor labii inferioris are elevated. Linear adhesions parallel to the mandibular border are observed. DAO, depressor anguli oris muscle; DLI, depressor labii inferioris, OO, orbicularis oris muscle.

maintains the lateral facial fat in the correct position. Loosening of the ligament with aging causes the fat tissue to droop, forming the facial jowl.

Masseteric Cutaneous Ligament

Stuzin et al[7] stated that a series of fibers arises along the entire anterior border of the masseter muscle superiorly from the malar region and courses inferiorly to the mandibular border. These fibers play a role in supporting the soft tissues of the medial cheek region. This ligament is categorized as *Stuzin's second type* (coalescence between the deep fascia and the SMAS). The zygomatic branch of the facial nerve runs in close proximity to the masseteric cutaneous ligament.[18] The space located posterior to the masseteric cutaneous ligament is termed the *premasseter space*. This space is located between the masseter and platysma and is delineated posteriorly by the posterior border of the masseter and inferiorly by the mandibular border. With age, the fat tissue in this space bulges onto the mandibular ligament and forms the jowls.[19]

Platysma Cutaneous Ligament

Furnas[15] also reported that an aponeurotic connection between the anterior platysma and skin of the middle and anterior cheek is sometimes seen. The incidence of this ligament may not be constant. Ozdemir et al[18] observed this ligament in only a few cases.

Platysma Auricular Ligament

Furnas[15] described the platysma auricular ligament as follows. The posterior border of the platysma recedes into an intricate fascial condensation that often attaches intimately to the overlying skin. This structure provides firm anchorage between the platysma and the dermis of the inferior auricular region.

References

1. Nakajima H, Imanishi N, Minabe T, Kishi K, Aiso S. Anatomical study of subcutaneous adipofascial tissue: a concept of the protective adipofascial system (PAFS) and lubricant adipofascial system (LAFS). Scand J Plast Reconstr Surg Hand Surg 2004;38(5):261–266
2. Mitz V, Peyronie M. The superficial musculo-aponeurotic system (SMAS) in the parotid and cheek area. Plast Reconstr Surg 1976; 58(1):80–88
3. Gosain AK, Yousif NJ, Madiedo G, Larson DL, Matloub HS, Sanger JR. Surgical anatomy of the SMAS: a reinvestigation. Plast Reconstr Surg 1993;92(7):1254–1265
4. Gardetto A, Dabernig J, Rainer C, Piegger J, Piza-Katzer H, Fritsch H. Does a superficial musculoaponeurotic system exist in the face and neck? An anatomical study by the tissue plastination technique. Plast Reconstr Surg 2003;111(2):664–672, discussion 673–675
5. Jost G, Levet Y. Parotid fascia and face lifting: a critical evaluation of the SMAS concept. Plast Reconstr Surg 1984;74(1):42–51
6. Ghassemi A, Prescher A, Riediger D, Axer H. Anatomy of the SMAS revisited. Aesthetic Plast Surg 2003;27(4):258–264
7. Stuzin JM, Baker TJ, Gordon HL. The relationship of the superficial and deep facial fascias: relevance to rhytidectomy and aging. Plast Reconstr Surg 1992;89(3):441–451
8. Freilinger G, Gruber H, Happak W, Pechmann U. Surgical anatomy of the mimic muscle system and the facial nerve: importance for reconstructive and aesthetic surgery. Plast Reconstr Surg 1987; 80(5):686–690
9. Ferreira LM, Hochman B, Locali RF, Rosa-Oliveira LM. A stratigraphic approach to the superficial musculoaponeurotic system and its anatomic correlation with the superficial fascia. Aesthetic Plast Surg 2006;30(5):549–552
10. Thaller SR, Kim S, Patterson H, Wildman M, Daniller A. The submuscular aponeurotic system (SMAS): a histologic and comparative anatomy evaluation. Plast Reconstr Surg 1990;86(4):690–696
11. Fodor PB. From the panniculus carnosum (PC) to the superficial fascia system (SFS). Aesthetic Plast Surg 1993;17(3):179–181
12. Bergman RA, Thompson SA, Afifi AK, Saadeh FA. Compendium of human anatomic variation: text, atlas, and world literature. Baltimore: Urban & Schwarzenberg; 1988:30.
13. Wilhelmi BJ, Mowlavi A, Neumeister MW. The safe face lift with bony anatomic landmarks to elevate the SMAS. Plast Reconstr Surg 2003;111(5):1723–1726
14. Lei T, Cui L, Zhang YZ, et al. Anatomy of the transversus nuchae muscle and its relationship with the superficial musculoaponeurotic system. Plast Reconstr Surg 2010;126(3):1058–1062
15. Furnas DW. The retaining ligaments of the cheek. Plast Reconstr Surg 1989;83(1):11–16
16. Moss CJ, Mendelson BC, Taylor GI. Surgical anatomy of the ligamentous attachments in the temple and periorbital regions. Plast Reconstr Surg 2000;105(4):1475–1490, discussion 1491–1498
17. Wong CH, Hsieh MKH, Mendelson B. The tear trough ligament: anatomical basis for the tear trough deformity. Plast Reconstr Surg 2012;129(6):1392–1402
18. Ozdemir R, Kilinç H, Unlü RE, Uysal AC, Sensöz O, Baran CN. Anatomicohistologic study of the retaining ligaments of the face and use in face lift: retaining ligament correction and SMAS plication. Plast Reconstr Surg 2002;110(4):1134–1149
19. Mendelson BC, Freeman ME, Wu W, Huggins RJ. Surgical anatomy of the lower face: the premasseter space, the jowl, and the labiomandibular fold. Aesthetic Plast Surg 2008;32(2):185–195

12 Mimetic Muscles

Hee-Jin Kim

Layers of the Face

Basic facial soft tissues are composed of five layers: (1) skin, (2) subcutaneous layer, (3) superficial musculoaponeurotic system (SMAS), (4) retaining ligaments and spaces, and (5) periosteum and deep fascia (**Fig. 12.1**). Except for the auricles and nose alae supported by the cartilage under the skin, facial skin glides over the loose areolar connective tissue layer. Facial skin contains numerous sweat and sebaceous glands.

Superficial fascia or subcutaneous connective tissue contains unequal amounts of fat tissue, and these fat tissues make the facial contour smooth between the skin and underlying facial musculatures. In some areas, the fat tissues are broadly distributed. The buccal fat pad forms the bulge over the cheek and continues to the scalp behind the orbit. Facial vessels, trigeminal nerve branches, facial nerve branches, and the muscles of facial expression are contained within the subcutaneous tissue.

The superficial musculoaponeurotic system (SMAS) is the superficial fascial structure composed of muscle fibers and superficial facial fascia. This musculofascial unit is manipulated during facial cosmetic surgery, especially rhytidectomy, and the SMAS extends from the platysma to the galea aponeurotica and is continuous with the temporoparietal fascia and galea. It connects to the dermis through vertical septa.

Facial Expression Muscles and their Actions

Facial muscles are attached to the facial skeleton or membranous superficial fascia beneath the skin (**Fig. 12.2**). The topography of the facial muscles varies between males and females, as well as between individuals of the same sex. It is important to define muscle shapes, their associations with the skin, and their relative functionality to explain the unique expressions people can make. The face is divided into several distinct areas: (1) forehead and temporal region, (2) periorbital region covered by the eyelid, (3) external nose, (4) anterior cheek region (upper lip elevators), (5) perioral region, and (6) chin region and superficial neck.

Generally, the facial muscles are found within the superficial fascia or subcutaneous tissue layer of the face. These muscles are involved in two different roles: (1) control of the opening of the orifices as dilators or sphincters and (2) in the formation of various facial expressions by moving the overlying facial skin. Most of the facial expression muscles originate from the bones of the face or fascia and are inserted into the facial skin. Therefore, facial skin by the contraction of the facial muscle produces the various expressions, such as sadness, anger, joy, fear, disgust, and surprise.

Forehead and Temporal Region

The occipitofrontalis muscle (OFM) is the widest and largest constituent of the complex of muscles underlying the upper face and occipital area, covering from the highest nuchal line to the eyebrows, but the intensity of contractions along that width can differ substantially from person to person. The frontal belly of the OFM is the frontal portion of this muscle, and it arises from the galea aponeurotica and is inserted into the frontal skin above the eyebrow. During anxiety or surprise, this muscle contracts and produces the transverse wrinkles of the forehead.

The OFM is roughly rectangular and has bilateral symmetry; its muscle fibers are approximately vertically oriented and attached to the superficial fascia of the skin in the region where it meets the muscles above the glabella and brow ridges. Its attachment is broader and has longer fibers than the occipitalis. The OFM lies at a uniform depth beneath the skin of the forehead (3–5 mm on average), although that depth can differ considerably (2–7 mm) between individuals and is 1 mm greater on average in men than in women. The OFM does not attach to

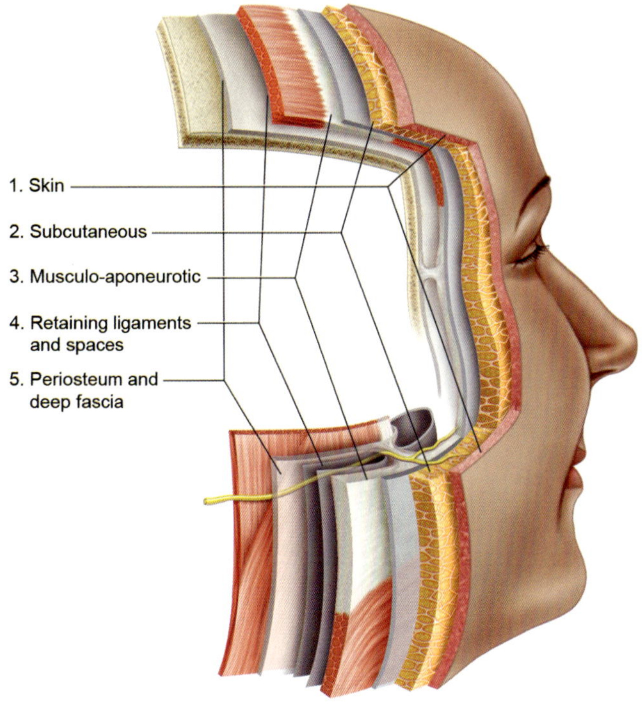

Fig. 12.1 Layers of the face. Facial soft tissues are composed of five layers: (1) skin, (2) subcutaneous layer, (3) superficial musculoaponeurotic system (SMAS), (4) retaining ligaments and spaces, and (5) periosteum and deep fascia.

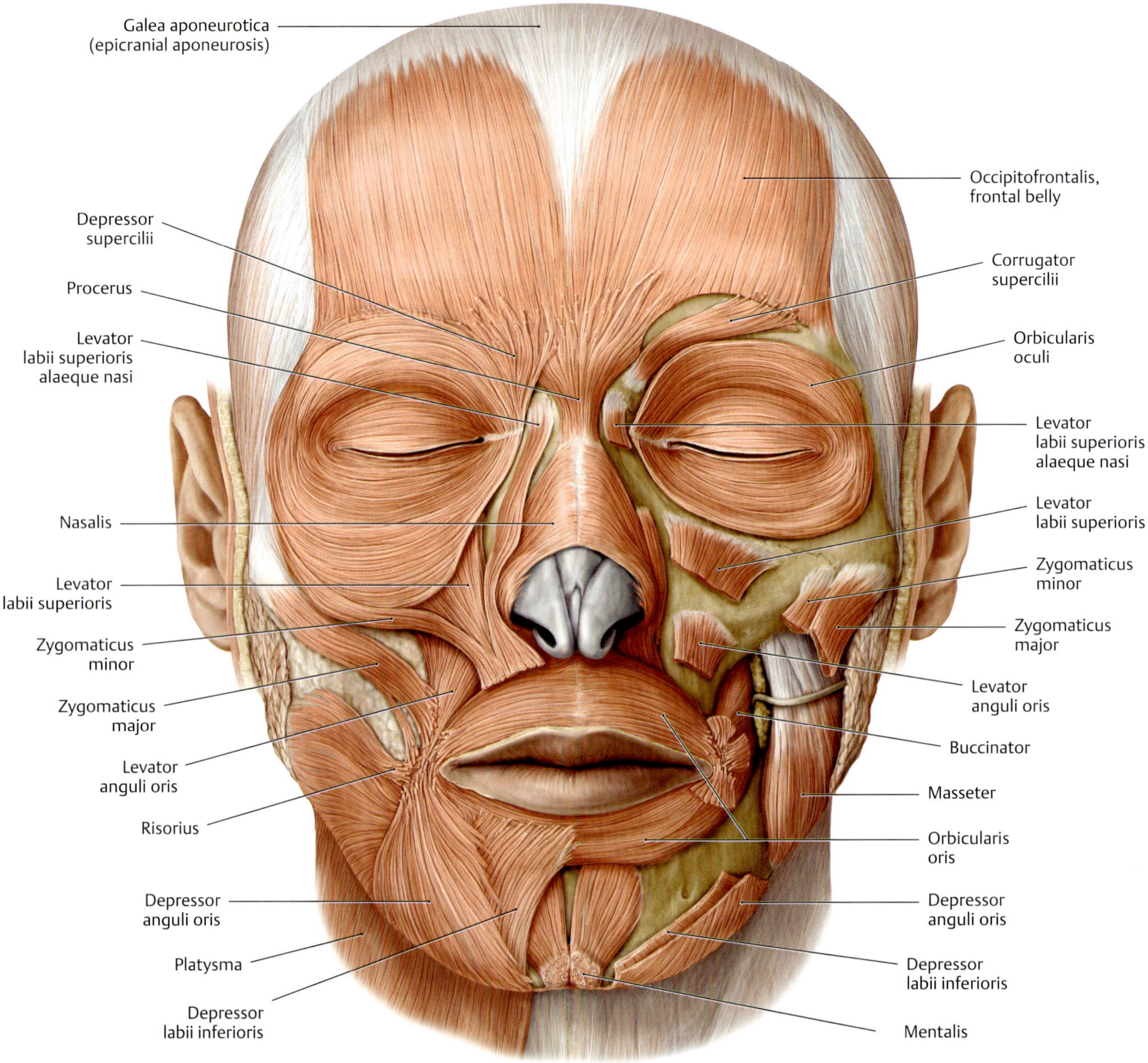

Fig. 12.2 Facial muscles. **(a)** Anterior view. The superficial layer of the muscle is shown on the right half of the face, and the deep layer is shown on the left half.

a bony structure. Instead, its medial fibers continue along procerus, intermediate fibers along the corrugator supercilii (CS) and orbicularis oculi (OOc), and lateral fibers along the OOc over the zygomatic process (**Fig. 12.3**). The temporoparietalis is located between OFM and the anterior and superior auricular muscles, and its development and shape vary.

Periorbital Region

The shape of the eye is clearly framed by the moving muscles surrounding it, which thus determine the basic facial expression. The OOc muscle is located around the orbit and into the eyelids, anterior temporal region, infraorbital cheek, and superciliary region. The OOc is a broad, flat, elliptical muscle composed of three portions: (1) an orbital portion that concentrically encircles the orbit, including the depressor supercilii; (2) a palpebral portion, with finer and paler muscle fibers than the orbital part, that sweeps across the eyelids anterior to the orbital septum and arises from the medial palpebral ligament; and (3) a lacrimal portion that arises from the upper part of the lacrimal crest and passes laterally behind the nasolacrimal sac (**Fig. 12.4**).

The main function of the OOc is to mediate eye closure. The OOc has many neighboring muscles: the corrugator supercilii muscle (CSM), procerus, frontal belly of the OFM, zygomaticus major (ZMj), and zygomaticus minor (ZMi) muscles) and various

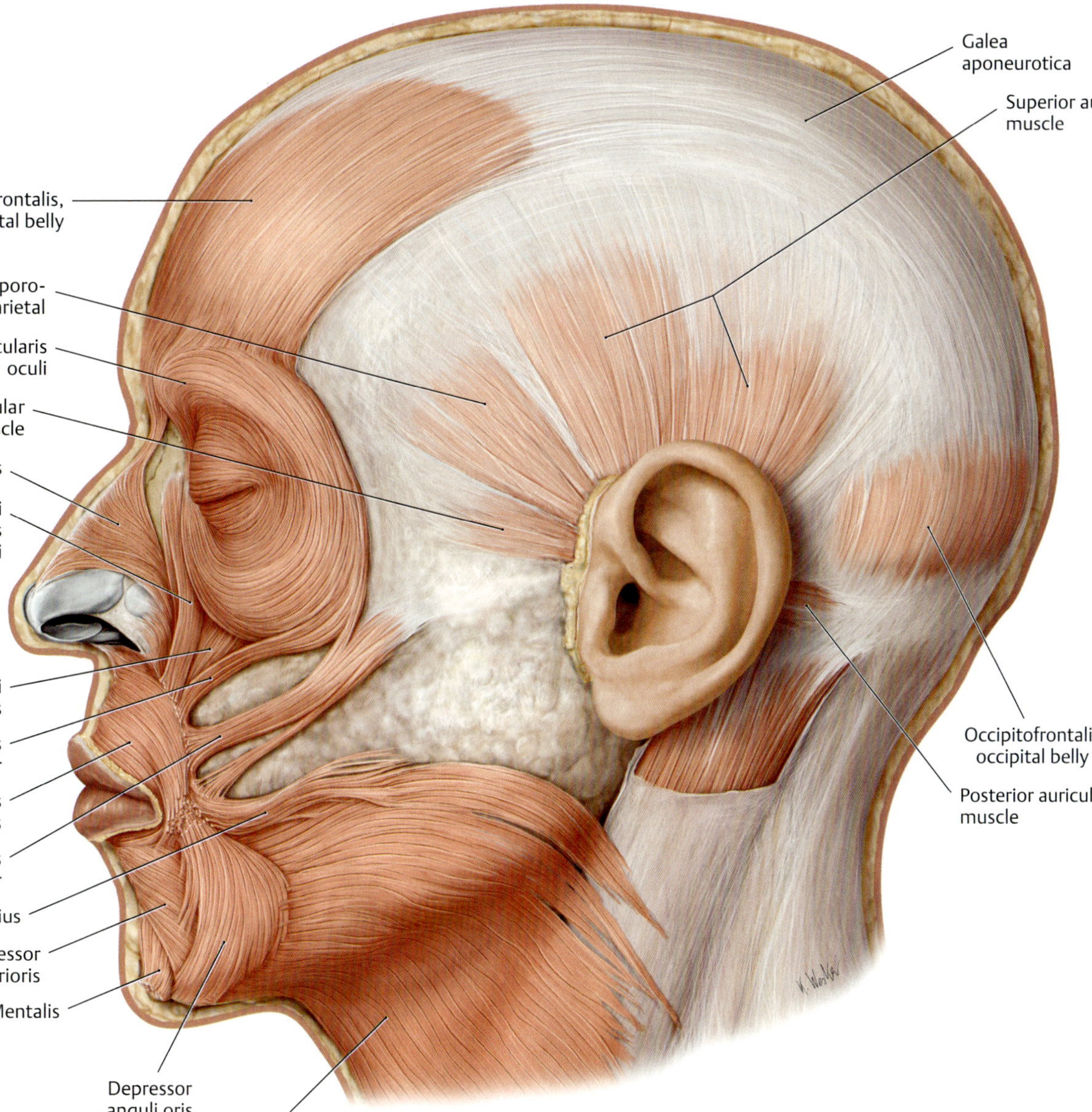

Fig. 12.2 (*continued*) **(b)** Left lateral view. (Reproduced from THIEME Atlas of Anatomy, Head and Neuroanatomy. © Thieme 2010, Illustrations by Karl Wesker.)

direct and indirect muscular connections between the OOc and the surrounding musculature; these may participate in the formation of various facial expressions. A lateral muscular band (malaris muscle) can be observed in 54.1% of Asians. It originates from the superficial temporal fascia and terminates in three different regions: at the zygomatic arch (27.9%), at the cheek region (18%), and at the angle of the mouth (8.2%). It plays a role in facial animation and dimple formation. Medial muscular bands of the orbital portion of OOc are found in 65.6% of Asians. This muscular band helps to prevent further drooping of the OOc. On the other hand, there are many muscular connections between the OOc and ZMi in 88.5% of the cases; this particular anatomical feature may play a specific role in facial expression.

The CSM originates from the periosteum on the frontal bone and merges into the frontal belly of the occipitofrontalis muscle (Fb). The CSM consists of distinct two bellies: transverse and oblique. The origin of the transverse belly of the CSM is more superior and lateral than the origin of the oblique belly, and most are attached into the Fb and the superolateral orbital part of the OOc. The transverse belly is located more deeply and is more horizontal than the oblique belly. The transverse belly is more or less triangular in shape with its inferomedial part as the apex. The oblique belly is classified into two different types: narrow vertical or broad triangular types.[1] The CSM with the OFM cause wrinkling of the skin at the glabella (**Fig. 12.5**).

The depressor supercilii (DS) is a fan or triangular shaped muscle that originates from the frontal process of the maxilla

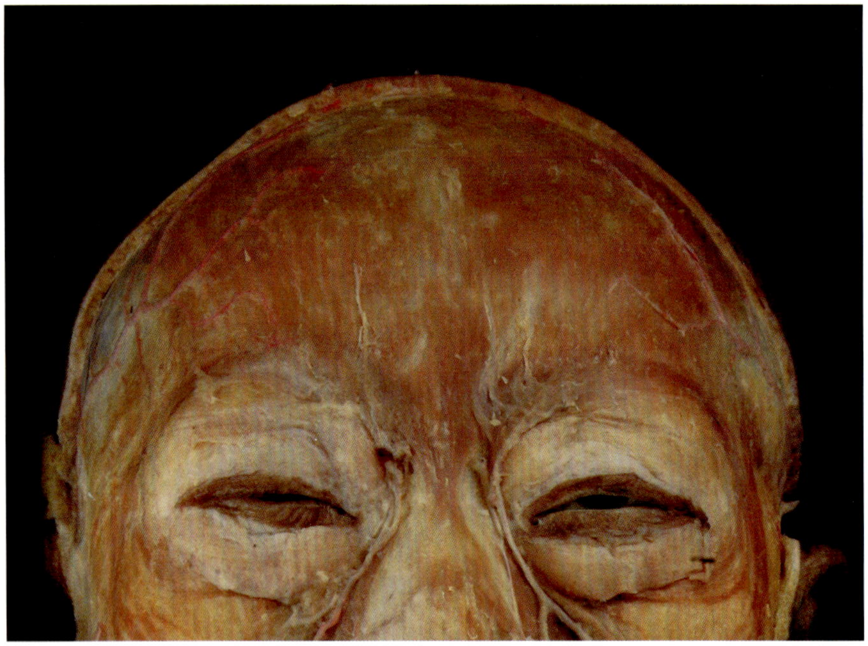

Fig. 12.3 Frontalis. The frontal belly of the occipitofrontalis muscle is the anterior portion of this muscle, and it arises from the galea aponeurotica and is inserted into the frontal skin above the eyebrow.

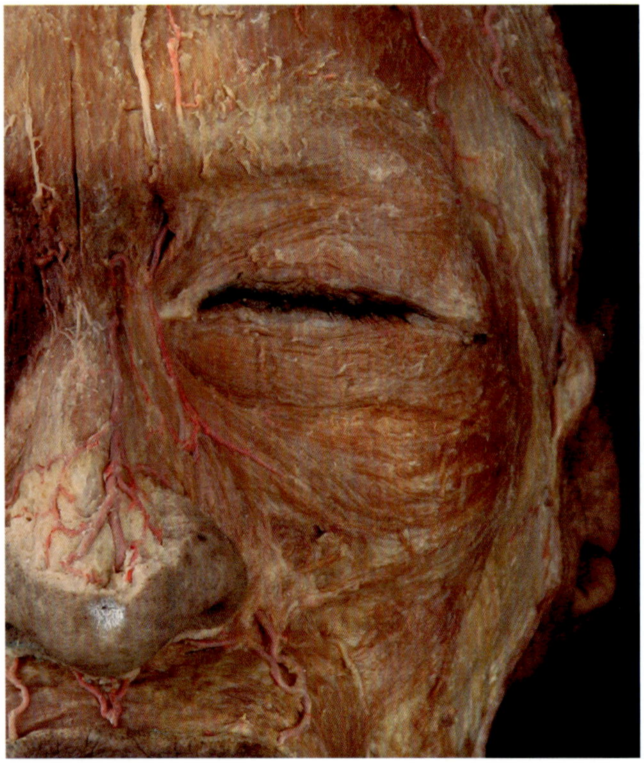

Fig. 12.4 Orbicularis oculi muscle (left side of the face). The orbicularis oculi muscle is located around the orbit and into the eyelids, anterior temporal region, infraorbital cheek and superciliary region.

and the nasal portion of the frontal bone 1 cm above the medial palpebral ligament. At the glabella, DS mixes with fibers of the CS is intermingled with the medial fibers of the OOc. Some muscular fibers of the DS originate from the lacrimal sac, and it plays a role in movement of the eyebrow.

External Nose Region

The nose is a dynamic structure; nasal musculature moves the nasal cartilages and plays an important role in nasal physiology. The transverse part of the nasalis, originating from the maxilla, is thin, flat, and has a triangular shape. It is located deep in the alar part and ascends to the dorsum of the nose. The transverse part of the nasalis, which is C-shaped, surrounds the posterior nasal aperture and ascends anteriorly toward the dorsum of the nose (**Fig. 12.6**). This transverse part lies between the lateral nasal cartilage and the greater alar cartilage and receives some muscle fibers from the superficial layer of levator labii superioris alaquae nasi muscle (LLSAN).

The procerus muscle originates from the fascia covering the dorsum of the nose and inserts superiorly into the skin of the glabella. The contraction of procerus makes the transverse wrinkles on the radix of the nose.

The alar part of nasalis originates with the transverse part of the nasalis from the maxilla and inserts into the alar facial crease and the adjacent deep surface of the external skin of the alar lobule.

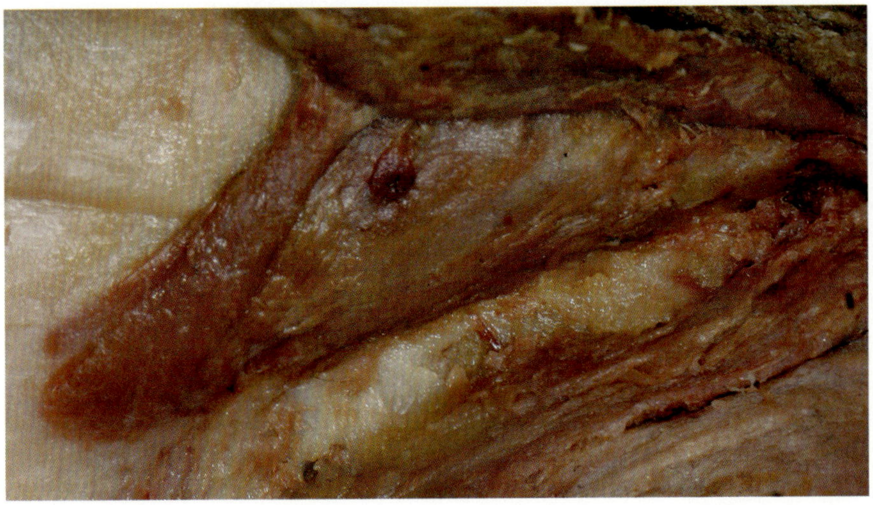

Fig. 12.5 Corrugator supercilii muscle. The corrugator supercilli muscle originates from the periosteum on the frontal bone and merges into the frontal belly of the occipito-frontalis muscle.

The dilator naris vestibularis muscle is located between the external and vestibular skin of the alar lobule.[2] Its muscle fibers radiate along the dome-shaped nasal vestibule. The dilator naris anterior muscle originates from the frontal surfaces of the lateral half of the lateral crus and the accessory alar cartilage adjacent to the lateral crus.

The depressor septi muscle is located in the deep aspect of the lip, continues to the maxillary incisive fossa, and inserts to the mobile portion of the nasal septum. It participates in enlarging the naris by pulling down the tip of the nose.

Anterior Cheek Region (Upper Lip Elevators)

The appearance of the lip framework is determined by the activity of various facial muscles, such as the levator labii superioris (LLS), the LLSAN, and the ZMi/ZMj (**Fig. 12.7**). Among these, the LLS, the LLSAN, and the ZMi determine the amount of lip elevation that occurs during smiling or sadness.

The LLS originates from the orbital rim of the maxilla and zygomatic bone above the infraorbital foramen and inserts into the upper lip area. The LLS is rectangular in 83% and trapezoid in 7%.[3] Its medial fibers are attached to the deep surface of the alar facial crease between the lateral slip of LLSAN and ZMi and are mainly intermingled with the alar part of the nasalis. Some of the deeper muscle fibers of the LLS extend to the vestibular skin of the nasal lobule.

The LLSAN originates from the frontal process of the maxilla and inserts into the upper lip and the ala of the nose. The LLSAN is divided into medial and lateral slips and then is divided into two layers, which are superficial and deep to the levator labii superioris muscle (LLS), respectively. The medial slip is inserted into the alar cartilage, and the lateral slip continues to the lateral part of the upper lip, then to the LLS and the orbicularis oris (OOr). The superficial layer of LLSAN descends on the LLS, and the deep layer is located deep to the LLS. The deep layer of

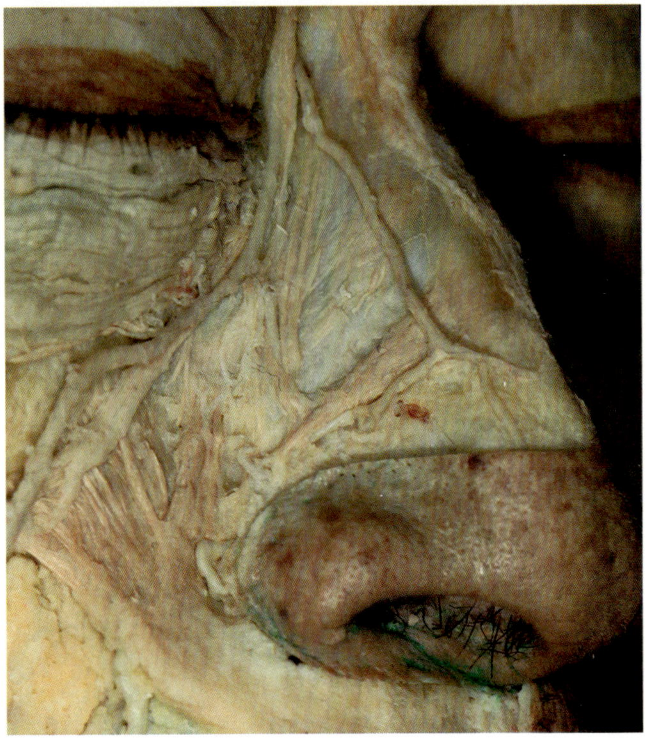

Fig. 12.6 Nasalis (right side of the face).

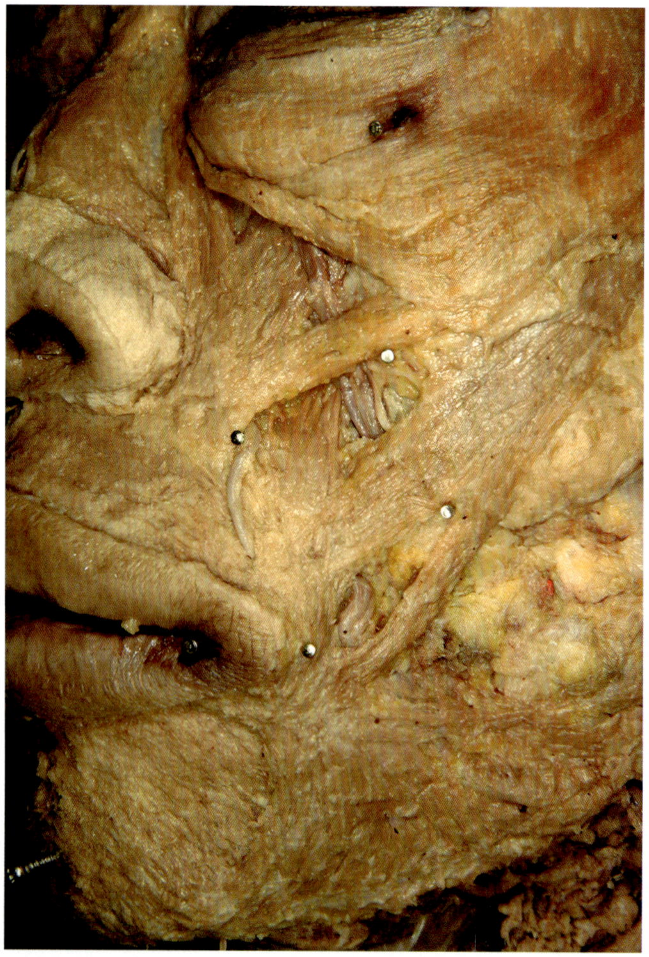

Fig. 12.7 Upper lip elevators (left side). The levator labii superioris (LLS), the levator labii superioris alaeque nasi (LLSAN), and the zygomaticus minor (ZMi) have a role in lip elevation that occurs during smiling or sadness.

LLSAN originates from the superficial layer of LLSAN and the frontal process of the maxilla. It inserts between the levator anguli oris and the OOr muscles. The transverse part of the nasalis originates from the maxilla and ascends passing posterior to the superficial layer of LLSAN (65%), or it originates as two muscle bellies from the maxilla and the upper half of the alar facial crease (35%).[4]

The ZMi originates from the zygomatic bone behind the zygomaticomaxillary suture and inserts into the skin and the upper lip. It is separated superiorly by a narrow triangle-shaped space from the LLS, and it blends with the muscle inferiorly. Besides the bony origin of the ZMi, the lateral belly of the orbital part of the OOc blends with the ZMi in 88.5% of cases. In addition, ZMi attaches into both the upper lip and the ala of the nose in 28% of cases.

The LLSAN and ZMi cover the insertion of the LLS partially or entirely, and these three muscles converge on the area lateral to the ala of the nose. The levator muscles of the upper lip pass through the OOr and participate in the formation of the nasolabial fold.

Perioral Region

In the perioral region, the muscles for facial expression are arranged in four layers based on their origins (**Fig. 12.8**). The individual muscles are arranged in the superficial (first, second, and third) layer and the deepest (fourth) layer, and it has been documented that the ZMj is located in the superficial layer. The deepest, fourth layer is composed of the levator anguli oris, mentalis, and buccinator muscles.

As a constrictor of the mouth, the OOr encircles the mouth and is located within the upper and lower lips. Most muscle fibers originate from the other facial muscles converging to the mouth. A part of intrinsic muscle fibers arise from the labial alveolar bone covering the upper and lower incisors. This muscle acts in closing the mouth and protrusion of the lips in the manner of a sphincter. The OOr divides into four quadrants, which further divide into a pars peripheralis and a pars marginalis. Pars peripheralis is a lateral stem attached to the labial side. Most originate from the modiolus itself, but some continue from the other modiolar muscles. Pars marginalis is narrow and is connected to the red-lip margin. It is involved with speech and production of musical tones. Its medial fibers interface with the contralateral pars marginalis and attaches to the dermis of the lip.

The levator anguli oris muscle (LAO) originates from the canine fossa below the infraorbital foramen and inserts into the modiolus. This muscle intermingles with the OOr, ZMj, and DAO and inserts to the modiolus, thereby raising the corner of the mouth. Infraorbital vessels and a nervous plexus lie between the LAO and LLS.

The depressor anguli oris muscle (DAO) is a triangular muscle on the most superficial layer of the perioral muscles originating from the external oblique line of the mandible. Its continuation forms an oblique line below and lateral to the depressor labii inferioris muscle, and it converges into a narrow fasciculus that blends at the modiolus with the OOr and risorius muscles. Some of its fibers continue below the mental tubercle and cross the midline. Consequently, it interlaces with its contralateral mate creating the transversus menti muscle. The medial border of the DAO overlaps with DLI and its lateral border is adjacent to the risorius, ZMj, and platysma muscles.

The depressor labii inferioris (DLI) originates from the lower part of the oblique line of the mandible between the symphysis menti and the mental foramen and inserts into the lower lip with the paired muscle from the opposite site and with OOr. DLI passes upwards and medially into the skin and mucosa of the lower lip.

The ZMj originates from the facial surface of the zygomatic bone. This muscle descends inferomediall, blends with the OOr, and terminates at the modiolus. The insertion patterns of the zygomaticus major are variable, and the existence of distinct muscle fibers of the ZMj passing deep to the LAO is not always observed. A bifid ZMj, one type of ZMj, separates into two portions, and the LAO passes between the two heads. The ZMa inserts around the modiolar region, and the muscle fibers are interlaced with the buccinator, LAO, and OOr. Even though all these muscles converge and are interdigitated in the modiolar

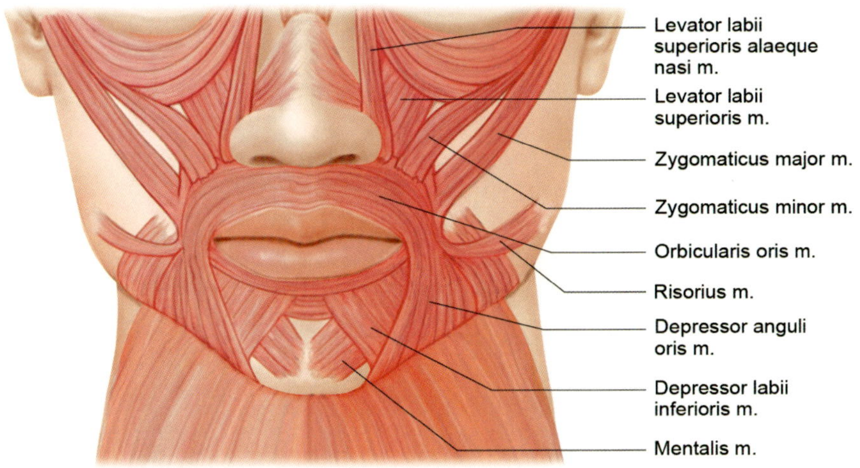

Fig. 12.8 Perioral region.

region, knowledge of the relationship between the deep muscle band of the ZMj and the buccinator is crucial in the understanding of facial animation. In every case, the main insertion of the deep muscle band of the ZMj is at the anterior margin of the buccinator and its fascia. This anatomical relationship provides the synchronous pulling of the anterior region of the buccinator with the corresponding buccal mucosa outward and upward to create a smile. The outward movement of the anterior margin of the buccinator and the contraction of the lip elevators naturally compress the cheek fat mass above the nasolabial fold, and this cheek mass becomes quite prominent. These muscle actions also widen the nasal width because of the expansion of the midface contour, followed by the muscle pulling upward and laterally.

The risorius is a thin and slender muscle and is usually located 20 to 50 mm lateral to the cheilion and 0 to 15 mm below the intercheilion horizontal line. Most risorius muscle fibers originate from the SMAS and some fibers from the parotid fascia or masseteric fascia. In some cases, this muscle receives the upper muscle fibers of platysma. It terminates in the modiolus region and acts by pulling the corner of the mouth when smiling. Risorius can be categorized into three common types: zygomaticus risorius, platysma risorius, and triangularis risorius.[5] It also inserts into the modiolus in three distinct layers in relation to the DAO: superficial, flush, and deep (**Fig. 12.9**).

The buccinator originates from three regions: pterygomandibular raphe, maxillary, and mandibular alveolar processes. It is located between the maxilla and the mandible. The buccinator is rectangular and has four bands: (1) a band originating from the maxilla, (2) a band from the anterior margin of the pterygomandibular raphe, (3) a band extending from the mandible, and (4) an additional inferior band also extending from the mandible. The buccinator is reinforced by the incisivus labii inferioris (ILI).[6] A few fibers spring from a fine tendinous band that bridges between the maxilla and the pterygoid hamulus (**Fig. 12.10**).

Chin Region and Superficial Neck

The mentalis muscle (MT) is the only elevator of the lower lip and the chin, and it provides the major vertical support for the lower lip. The absence of this muscular function would result in the lower central incisors being visible at rest. Resection of the MT may cause the patient to drool and may affect denture stability. MT is cone-shaped; the apex of this muscle originates from the incisive fossa of the mandible. The medial fibers of both

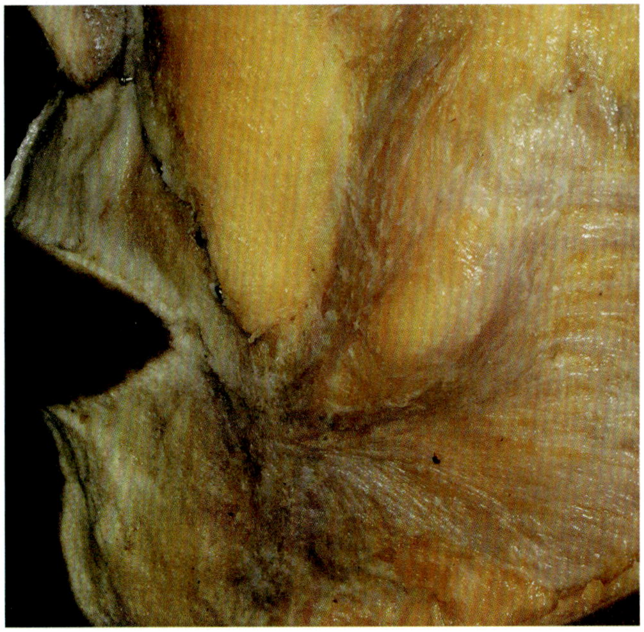

Fig. 12.9 Risorius (left side).

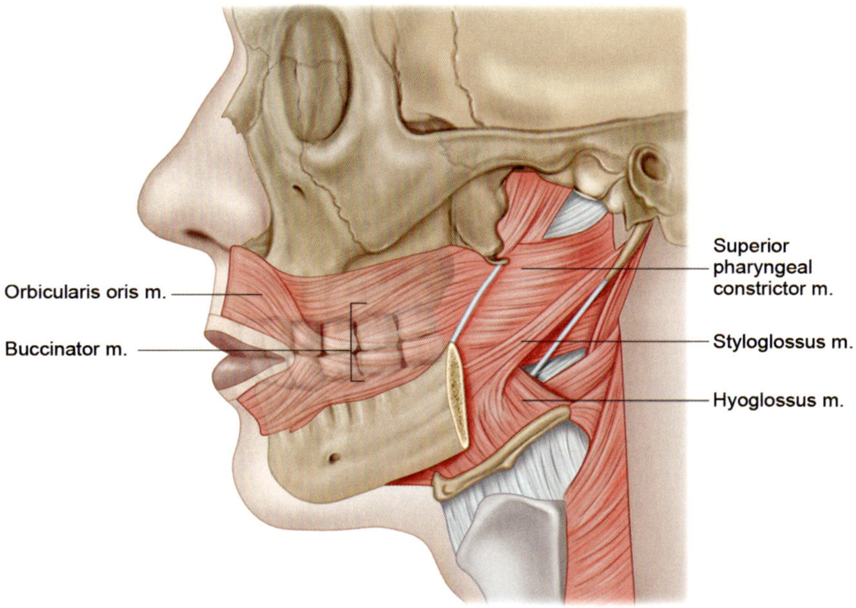

Fig. 12.10 Buccinator.

MTs descend anteromedially and cross over together, forming a dome-shaped chin prominence. The lateral fibers of the MT descend mostly inferomedially. The upper fibers are short and horizontal, whereas the lower fibers are long and descend inferomedially or vertically.[7] MT contraction causes the skin over the mentum to wrinkle. The upper fibers of the MT intermingle with the inferior margin of the OOr. In addition, the originating muscle fibers of the ILI intermingle with the upper lateral MT (**Fig. 12.11**).

The platysma attaches to the lower border of the mandible and consists of two types of fibers. A flattened bundle passes superomedially to the lateral border of the DAO, and others continue deep into DAO and reappear at its medial border. Lack of decussation creates a cervical defect, resulting in a reduction in elasticity of the cervical skin and platysma with ageing, which gives rise to the so-called turkey gobbler neck. Platysmal fibers do not merely decussate and interlace from each side, but sometimes one side of the muscle overlaps and covers the other side.[8]

Modiolus

The modiolus is a fibromuscular structure that decussates between the OOr muscle and the labial retractors, ending at the lateral border of the cheilion (**Fig. 12.12**).[9] It extends 20 mm above and below a horizontal line through the buccal angle. It is strongly associated with facial expression, beauty, aging, and formation of the nasolabial fold. The modiolus is a dense, compact, and mobile muscular mass located at the lateral border of the corner of the mouth and is formed by a convergence of muscle fibers from the zygomaticus major, levator labii superioris, depressor labii inferioris, DAO, risorius, OOr, buccinators, and LAO muscles. The formation of subtle and detailed facial ex-

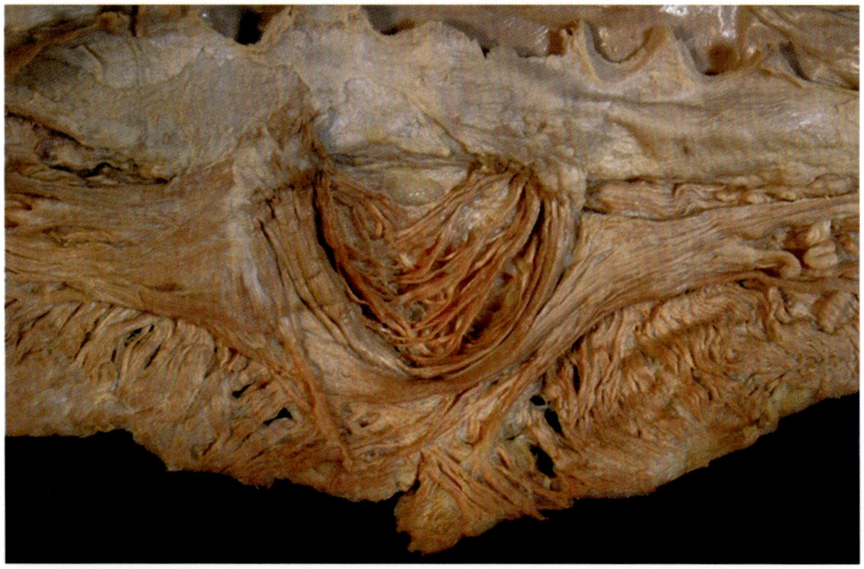

Fig. 12.11 Mentalis muscle.

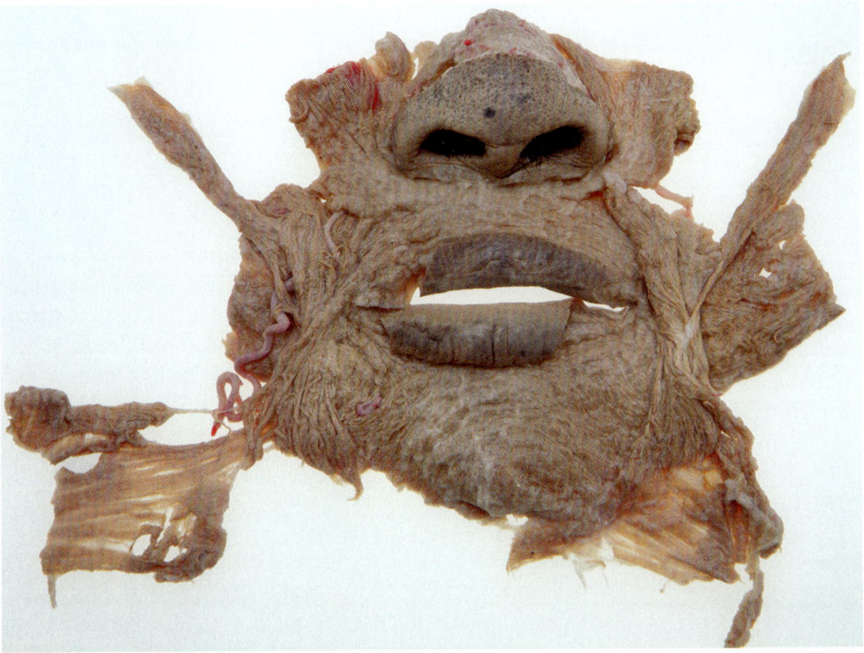

Fig. 12.12 Modiolus (left side). The modiolus is a fibromuscular structure that decussates between the orbicularis oris muscle and the labial retractors ending at the lateral border of the cheilion.

pressions of the inferior face, such as those reflecting determination, satisfaction, smiling, purposeful action, and sadness, are possible by contracting these muscles, which terminate at the modiolus. A tendinous tissue nodule in the modiolus is found in about 20% of cases. The facial artery passes approximately 1 mm lateral to the lateral border of the modiolus.

References

1. Yang HM, Kim HJ. Anatomical study of the corrugator supercilii muscle and its clinical implication with botulinum toxin A injection. Surg Radiol Anat 2013;35(9):817–821
2. Hur MS, Hu KS, Youn KH, Song WC, Abe S, Kim HJ. New anatomical profile of the nasal musculature: dilator naris vestibularis, dilator naris anterior, and alar part of the nasalis. Clin Anat 2011;24(2): 162–167
3. Hur MS, Youn KH, Hu KS, et al. New anatomic considerations on the levator labii superioris related with the nasal ala. J Craniofac Surg 2010;21(1):258–260
4. Hur MS, Hu KS, Park JT, Youn KH, Kim HJ. New anatomical insight of the levator labii superioris alaeque nasi and the transverse part of the nasalis. Surg Radiol Anat 2010;32(8):753–756
5. Kim HS, Pae C, Bae KS, et al. An anatomical study of the risorius in Asians and its insertion at the modiolus. Surg Radiol Anat 2015; 37:147–151
6. Hur MS, Hu KS, Kwak HH, Lee KS, Kim HJ. Inferior bundle (fourth band) of the buccinator and the incisivus labii inferioris muscle. J Craniofac Surg 2011;22(1):289–292
7. Hur MS, Kim HJ, Choi BY, Hu KS, Kim HJ, Lee KS. Morphology of the mentalis muscle and its relationship with the orbicularis oris and incisivus labii inferioris muscles. J Craniofac Surg 2013;24(2): 602–604
8. Kim HJ, Hu KS, Kang MK, Hwang K, Chung IH. Decussation patterns of the platysma in Koreans. Br J Plast Surg 2001;54(5):400–402
9. Yu SK, Lee MH, Kim HS, Park JT, Kim HJ, Kim HJ. Histomorphologic approach for the modiolus with reference to reconstructive and aesthetic surgery. J Craniofac Surg 2013;24(4):1414–1417

13 Orbital Anatomy

Swapna Vemuri and Jeremiah P. Tao

Clinical Anatomy

The orbit is conical and has a volume of about 30 cm^3. The anterior orbital rim has horizontal and vertical diameters of 4.0 cm and 3.5 cm, respectively; however, the orbital dimension widens posteriorly, with a maximum diameter 1 cm posterior to the rim. The distance from the anterior orbital rim to the apex is approximately 4.5 to 5 cm along the medial orbital wall, whereas the distance from the lateral orbital rim to the superior orbital fissure is about 4 cm.[1,2]

The medial orbital walls are parallel to each other and approximately 2.5 cm apart. The lateral wall forms a 45-degree angle with the ipsilateral medial wall. The two lateral walls form a 90-degree angle (**Fig. 13.1**).

Orbital Bones

Orbital Rim

The orbital rim is composed of the frontal, zygomatic, and maxillary bones that adjoin at suture lines (frontozygomatic, zygomaticomaxillary, and frontomaxillary, respectively). The lateral and superior rims are the strongest. The orbital rim creates the anterior lacrimal crest and then spirals posteriorly to end at the posterior lacrimal crest. The lacrimal sac fossa is found between the two crests (**Fig. 13.2a**).

Orbital Walls

Seven orbital bones compose the four walls of the orbit (**Fig. 13.2a**).

Orbital Roof

The orbital roof, which is the floor of the anterior cranial fossa, consists of the frontal and lesser wing of sphenoid bones. The supraorbital notch or foramen, through which the supraorbital nerve (CN V_1) and vessels travel, divides the medial one-third and lateral two-thirds of the superior orbital rim. The lacrimal gland is found laterally in the lacrimal gland fossa.

Lateral Orbital Wall

The lateral orbital wall, separated from the roof by the superior orbital fissure, consists of the zygomatic and greater wing of the sphenoid bones (**Fig. 13.2b**). The zygomaticofacial and zygomaticotemporal canals transmit vessels and zygomatic nerve branches. Occasionally, a meningo-orbital foramen is identified lateral to the superior orbital fissure and transmits a branch of the middle meningeal artery.[3,4] Whitnall's tubercle is a protuberance on the inner aspect of the lateral orbital rim approximately 4 mm posterior to the rim and 10 mm inferior to the frontozygomatic suture. The lateral canthal tendon, lateral horn of the levator aponeurosis, Lockwood's ligament, and check ligament of the lateral rectus muscle attach to the tubercle.

Orbital Floor

The orbital floor, separated from the lateral wall by the inferior orbital fissure, consists of the zygomatic, maxillary, and palatine bones. The floor forms the roof of the maxillary sinus. The infraorbital groove or canal, through which the infraorbital nerve (CN V_2 branch) and artery travel, divides the floor. The infraorbital nerve and artery then exit through the infraorbital foramen, which is approximately 1 cm inferior to the orbital rim on the anterior maxillary bone face (**Fig. 13.2c**).

Medial Orbital Wall

The medial orbital wall consists of the maxillary, lacrimal, ethmoid, and sphenoid bones. The anterior and posterior ethmoidal foramina, with ethmoidal vessels passing through, are found on the medial wall along the frontoethmoidal suture. Along the medial wall, the distance between the anterior lacrimal crest, anterior ethmoidal foramen, posterior ethmoidal foramen, and orbital apex is approximately 24 mm, 12 mm, 6 mm, respectively (**Fig. 13.2d**).

Additional Fissures, Canals, and Foramina and Contents

The superior orbital fissure (SOF) is located between the greater and lesser wings of sphenoid. The annulus of Zinn, a tendinous ring at the orbital apex formed by the extraocular rectus muscles, divides the SOF. The annulus also encircles the optic foramen, which is medial to the SOF. Above the annulus, the lacrimal and frontal nerves (CN V_1 branches), trochlear nerve (CN IV), and superior ophthalmic vein pass through the SOF. The superior and inferior branches of the oculomotor nerve (CN III), abducens nerve (CN VI), and nasociliary nerve (CN V_1) pass through the annulus. The inferior ophthalmic vein may pass below the annulus (**Fig. 13.3**).

The optic foramen is located medial to the SOF in the lesser wing of the sphenoid and separated by a bony optic strut. It extends posteriorly as the optic canal that has an approximate diameter of 6 mm and a length of 10 mm. The optic nerve and ophthalmic artery pass through the optic canal.

The inferior orbital fissure (IOF) is located inferior to the SOF between the greater wing of sphenoid (lateral orbital wall) and

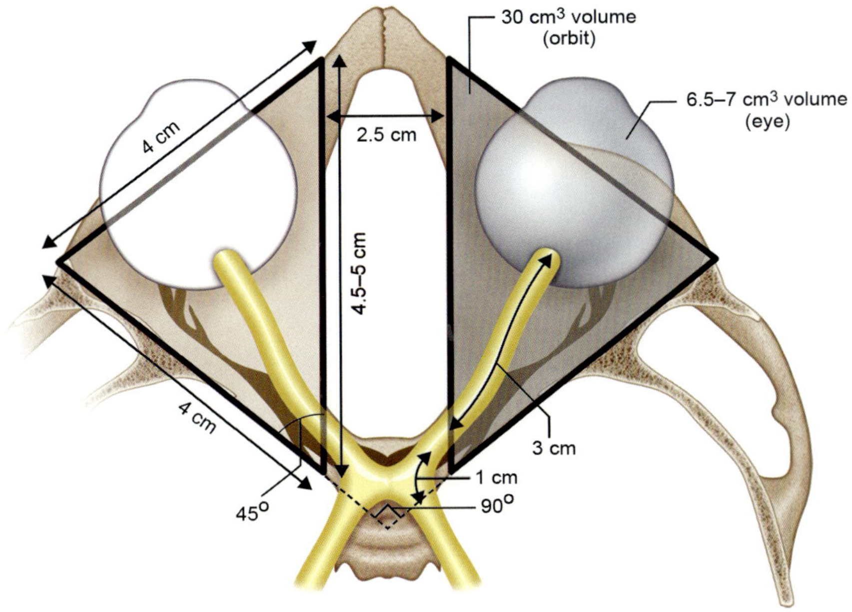

Fig. 13.1 Orbital dimensions and volumes.

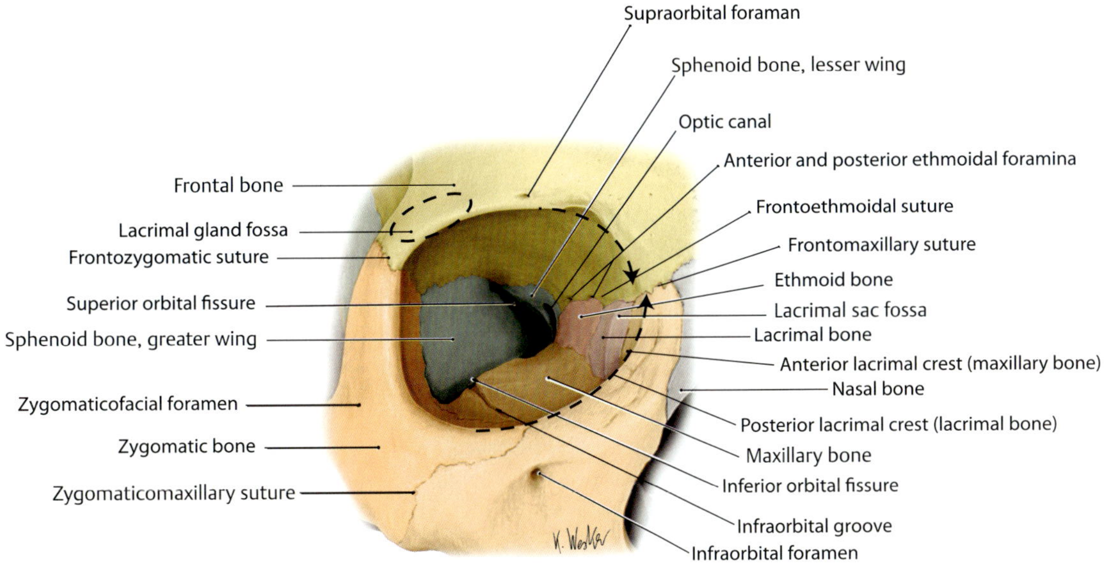

a

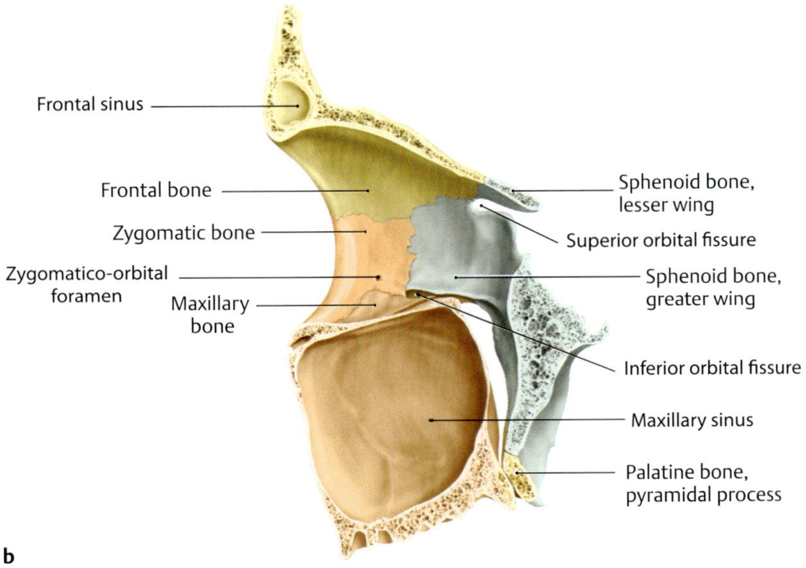

b

Fig. 13.2 **(a)** Orbital bones, sutures, foramina, and fissures. Anterior view. The orbital rim is composed of the frontal, zygomatic, and maxillary bones that adjoin at suture lines (frontozygomatic, zygomaticomaxillary, and frontomaxillary, respectively). **(b)** Lateral wall, right orbit. The lateral orbital wall, separated from the roof by the superior orbital fissure, consists of the zygomatic and greater wing of sphenoid bones. (*continued on page 122*)

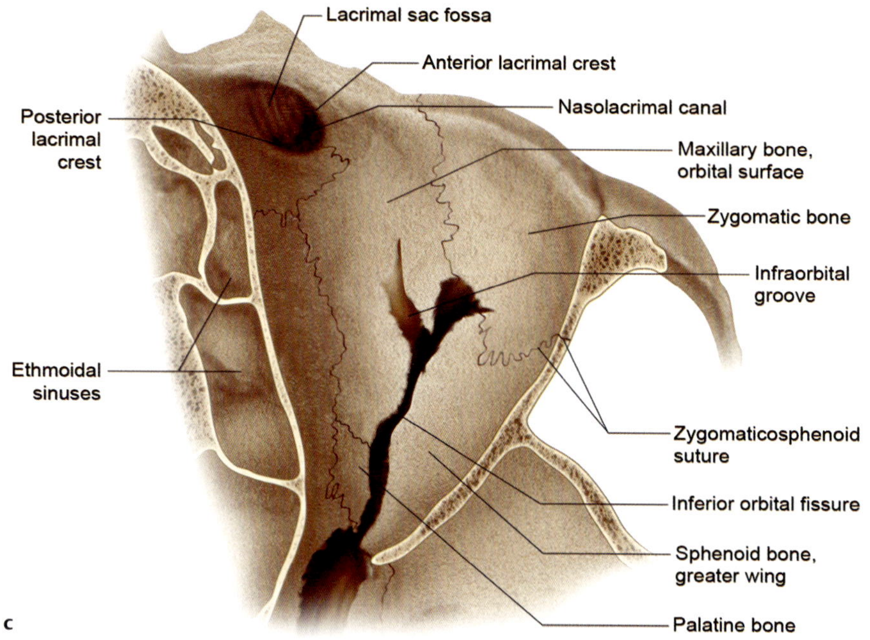

c

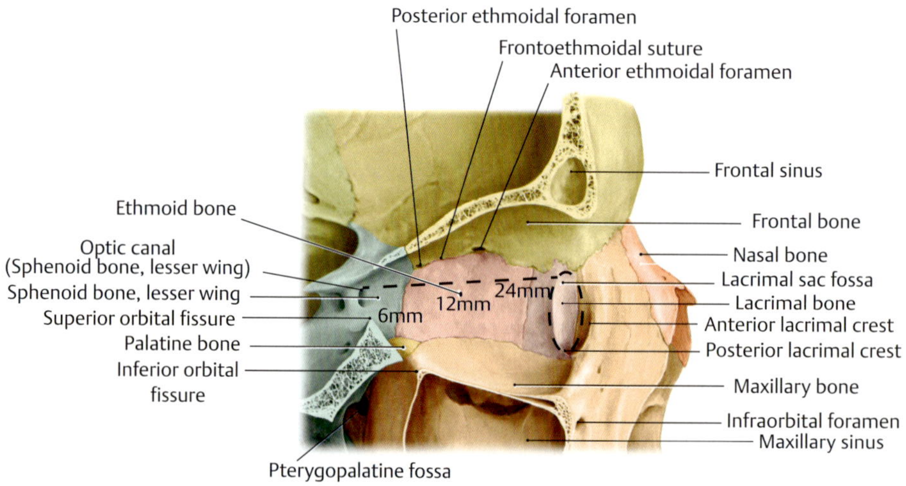

d

Fig. 13.2 (*continued*) **(c)** Orbital floor, right orbit. The orbital floor, separated from the lateral wall by the inferior orbital fissure, consists of the zygomatic, maxillary, and palatine bones. **(d)** Medial wall, right orbit. The medial orbital wall consists of the maxillary, lacrimal, ethmoid, and sphenoid bones. (Modified from THIEME Atlas of Anatomy, Head and Neuroanatomy. © Thieme 2010, Illustrations by Karl Wesker.)

palatine and maxillary bones (orbital floor). The infraorbital and zygomatic nerves (CN V_2), infraorbital artery, inferior ophthalmic vein, and pterygopalatine ganglion autonomic branches pass through the IOF.

Periorbita and Fascial Tissues

Periosteum covers the orbital bones and is known as periorbita along the orbital walls (**Fig. 13.4**). It is loosely adherent over the walls but tightly adherent at suture lines, the orbital rim where it forms the arcus marginalis, foramina, and fissures. The orbital septum originates from the arcus marginalis. At the optic canal, periorbita is continuous with the dural sheath of the optic nerve.

Orbital fascia is complexly organized.[5] Tenon's capsule, a fibrous membrane, extends from the posterior globe and fuses with conjunctiva anteriorly at the limbus. Fibrous septa extend from Tenon's to divide lobules of orbital fat. Extraocular muscles pass through Tenon's fascia to insert onto the globe. Muscular fascial sheaths are found surrounding each extraocular muscle with projections to the orbital walls, known as check ligaments. The fascial sheath in the anterior orbit is also found in between each muscle to create the intermuscular septum.

Surgical Annotation

Orbital Surgical Spaces and Approaches

The organization of orbital fascia and structures compartmentalizes the orbit. From deep to superficial, the surgical spaces of the orbit include the following: intraconal, sub-Tenon's, extraocular muscles, extraconal, subperiosteal, and extraorbital (**Fig. 13.5**). The appropriate orbital surgical approach is determined

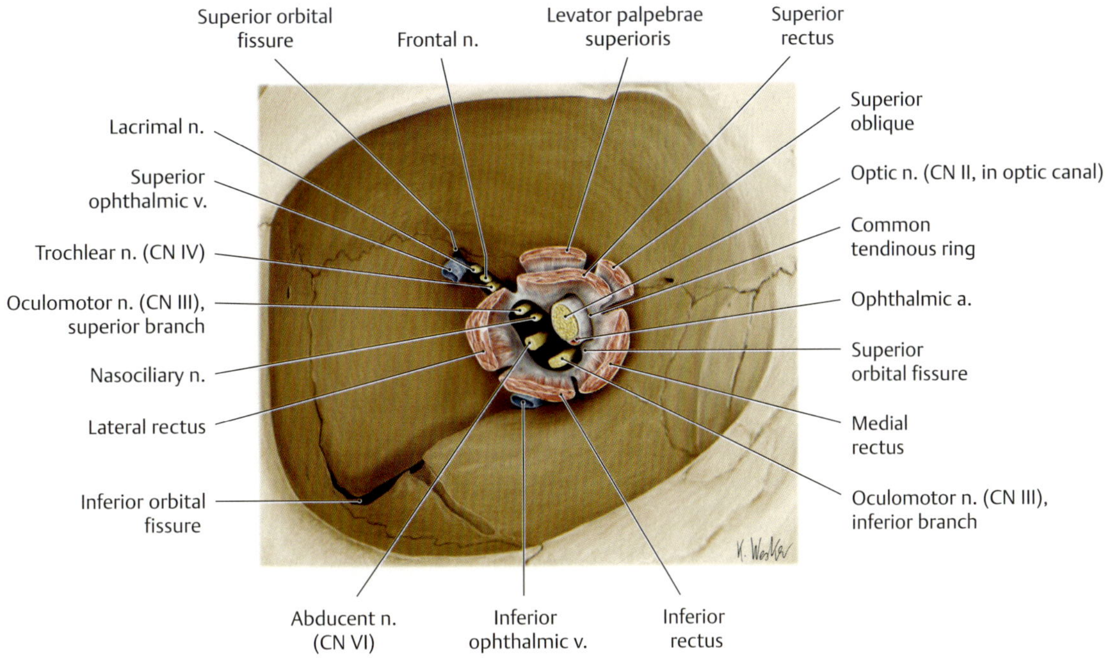

Fig. 13.3 Structures of the orbital apex including muscle origin, annulus of Zinn, fissures, and contents. Right orbit, anterior view, with most of the orbital contents removed. (Reproduced from THIEME Atlas of Anatomy, Head and Neuroanatomy. © Thieme 2010, Illustration by Karl Wesker.)

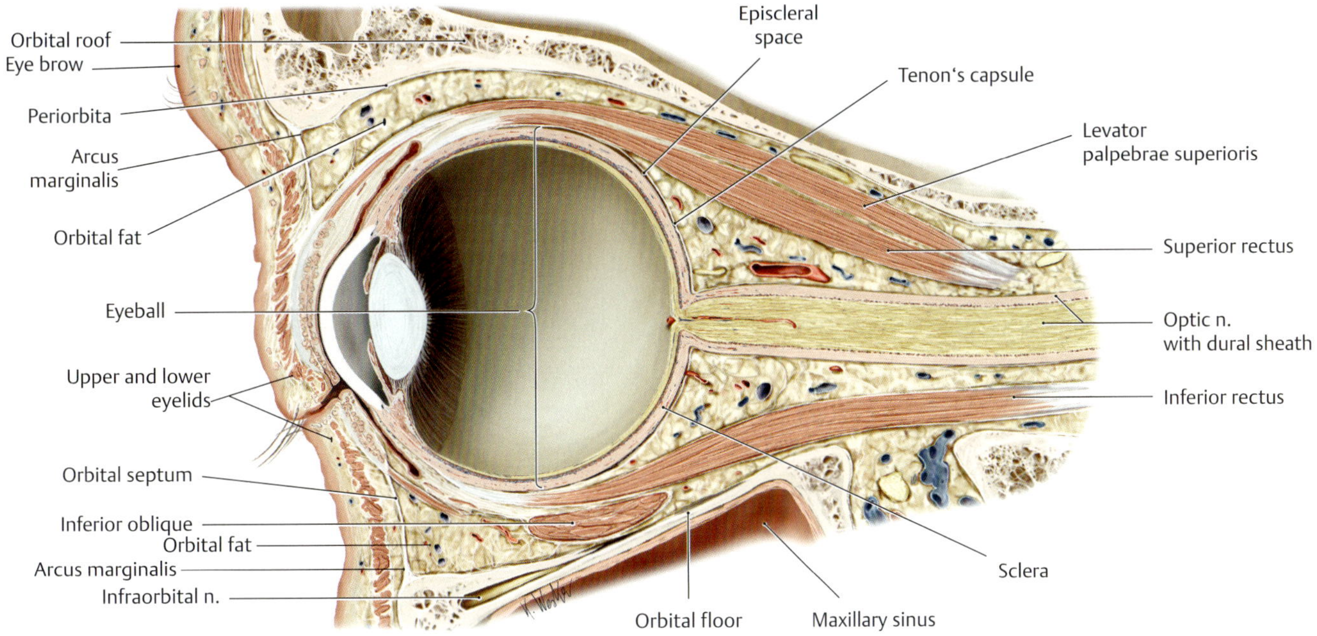

Fig. 13.4 Sagittal view of right orbit demonstrating periorbita, fascia, and relationship of extraorbital and intraorbital structures. Periorbita covers the orbital bones. It is loosely adherent over the walls but tightly adherent at suture lines. (Modified from THIEME Atlas of Anatomy, Head and Neuroanatomy. © Thieme 2010, Illustration by Karl Wesker.)

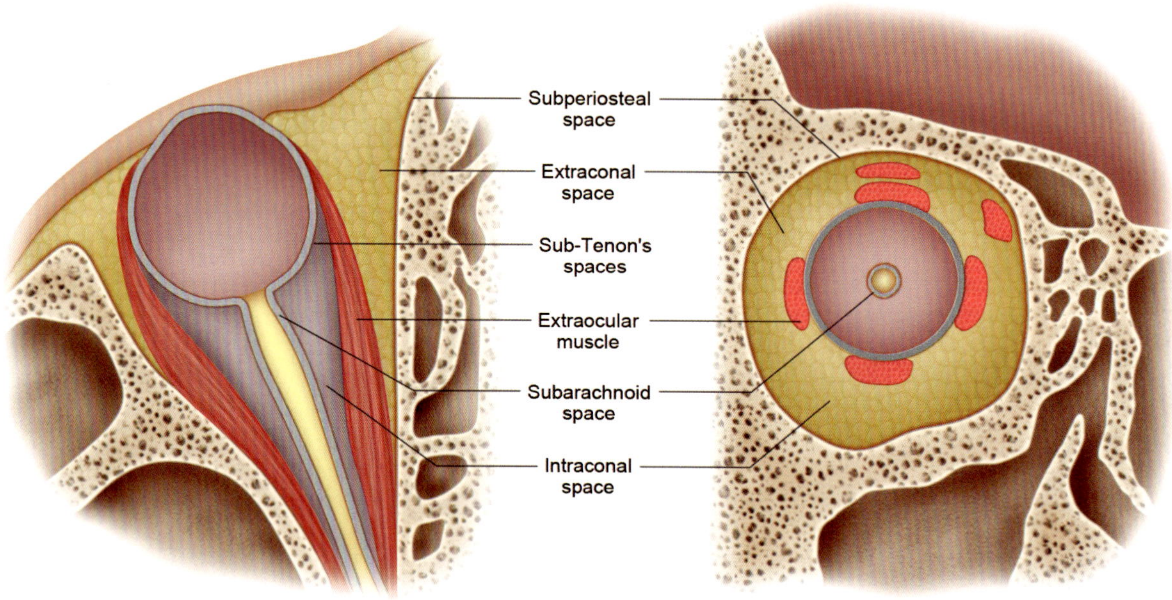

Fig. 13.5 Axial and coronal views of right orbit demonstrating surgical spaces. From deep to superficial, the surgical spaces of the orbit include the following: intraconal, sub-Tenon's, extraocular muscles, extraconal, subperiosteal, and extraorbital.

by the location of pathology with regards to surgical space, depth in orbit relative to the globe equator, and location relative to optic nerve.

Anatomical Considerations during Orbital Surgery

Orbital Wall Surgery

Due to the tight space and numerous vital structures in this region, orbital surgery poses significant risks. A thorough understanding of orbital anatomy is essential for safe surgery.

Orbital Floor

The most commonly fractured orbital wall is the floor. The inferomedial wall (medial to the infraorbital canal) is particularly susceptible. During orbital floor surgery (i.e., fracture repair or bone decompression), the safest dissection plane is subperiosteal. The authors prefer a tranconjunctival approach combined with lateral canthotomy and inferior cantholysis, however, transcutaneous approaches are alternative options. The following are important considerations, once in the orbit:

- Anteromedially, the inferior oblique muscle originates on the maxillary bone just behind the inferior orbital rim and lateral to the lacrimal sac fossa. Dissection near the anteromedial floor can result in its unintentional disruption along with damage to the lacrimal sac.
- The infraorbital nerve travels in the infraorbital groove along the central floor and should be visualized and preserved. Damage to the nerve results in bother some infraorbital hypoesthesia. Elevation of periosteum over the canal may induce small to medium size arterial bleeding. Electrocautery to these vessels should be performed cautiously and with a minimal energy technique.
- Lateral to the infraorbital groove, along the posterior floor, the contents of the infraorbital fissure can be found entering the fissure and should not be confused with entrapped orbital soft tissues.
- The postero-medial floor has a relatively steep supero-medial incline. This can result in difficulty visualizing the posteromedial ledge of a floor fracture from the head-of-bed surgeon perspective. Entering the maxillary sinus and following its roof anteriorly may aid in the identification of the posterior ledge.
- The posterior wall of the maxillary sinus is an excellent landmark for the orbit apex. Intraorbital dissection posterior to this depth is risky and is usually not necessary.

Medial Orbital Wall

The following are important considerations for orbit medial wall surgery (fracture repair or decompression):

- The medial canthal tendon inserts onto the anterior and posterior lacrimal crest with the lacrimal sac located in the lacrimal sac fossa. The cutaneous approach to the medial orbit offers a panoramic view of the medial orbit, however medial canthal tendon disinsertion is necessary and a canthopexy suture is placed to forestall telecanthus.[6,7]
- The transcaruncular approach avoids a cutaneous incision with preservation of the medial canthal tendon while offering good access to the medial wall.[8] The leading periosteal edge for subperiosteal dissection must begin at the posterior lacrimal crest with care not to violate the lacrimal sac. Herniation of surrounding orbital fat and a tighter surgical space

are disadvantages of this approach compared to the transcutaneous approach.

- Periosteal elevation should begin on the thicker frontal bone maxillary process. A subperiosteal plane is more difficult to achieve on the thin ethmoid bone that fractures easily with manipulation.
- The anterior and posterior ethmoidal foramina mark the level of the fovea ethmoidalis, the roof of the ethmoid sinus. This is the superior extent of medial orbital decompression as there is risk of disrupting the cribriform plate and entering the anterior cranial fossa with a resultant cerebrospinal fluid (CSF) leak or intracranial hemorrhage.
- The anterior and posterior ethmoidal arteries pose a risk of orbital hemorrhage if lacerated.
- Dissection greater than a 4 cm depth from the orbital rim along the medial wall risks damage to the optic nerve.

Lateral Orbital Wall

The anterior lateral orbital wall is strong; however, the posterior border of the deep lateral orbital wall is thin.[2,9] When performing lateral wall surgery (i.e., zygomaticomaxillary complex fracture repair or decompression) the following should be considered:

- The distance along the lateral wall from the orbital rim to the SOF is about 4 cm.
- During deep lateral wall decompression, the diploic trigone of the greater wing of sphenoid (found lateral to the SOF), lacrimal sac fossa, and body of the zygoma may be sculpted to allow for globe retropulsion.[10] Because these areas of bone can vary in thickness, computed tomography helps determine the volume when planning for surgery. These areas lie adjacent to intracranial cavities, which may result in a CSF leak during decompression. Care must be taken to avoid dural penetration.
- The meningo-orbital foramen with a branch of the middle meningeal artery may be encountered lateral to SOF during deep lateral wall dissection. This is an additional potential intracranial extension that must be avoided.
- Zygomaticomalar complex (ZMC), or tripod, fractures consist of fractures at the frontozygomatic, zygomaticomaxillary, and zygomaticosphenoid sutures and the zygomatic arch. Often in a ZMC fracture, the zygomatic bone telescopes around the frontal bone at the suture in addition to a medial rotation of the fractured zygomatic bone segment. Adequate realignment during fracture repair requires torqueing the fragmented segment and relieving the telescoping to restore more normal orbital anatomy. Realignment of the zygomaticosphenoid suture is essential. The intraorbital view of the lateral wall offers the best vantage point to ensure proper ZMC fracture reduction.

References

1. Lemke BN, Lucarelli MJ. Anatomy of ocular adnexa and orbit. In: Smith BC, editor. Ophthalmic Plastic and Reconstructive Surgery. 2nd ed. St. Louis, MO: CV Mosby; 1997:3–78
2. Whitnall SE. The Anatomy of the Human Orbit and Accessory Organs of Vision. New York: Oxford University Press; 1932:1–252
3. Mysorekar VR, Nandedkar AN. The groove in the lateral wall of the human orbit. J Anat 1987;151:255–257
4. Kwiatkowski J, Wysocki J, Nitek S. The morphology and morphometry of the so-called "meningo-orbital foramen" in humans. Folia Morphol (Warsz) 2003;62(4):323–325
5. Koornneef L. Details of the orbital connective tissue system in the adult. In: Koornneef L, ed. Spatial Aspects of Orbital Musculo-Fibrous Tissue in Man: A new anatomical and histological approach. Amsterdam: Swets and Zeitlinger; 1977
6. Nunery WR, Tao JP, Johl S. Nylon foil "wraparound" repair of combined orbital floor and medial wall fractures. Ophthal Plast Reconstr Surg 2008;24(4):271–275
7. Timoney PJ, Sokol JA, Hauck MJ, Lee HB, Nunery WR. Transcutaneous medial canthal tendon incision to the medial orbit. Ophthal Plast Reconstr Surg 2012;28(2):140–144
8. Shorr N, Baylis HI, Goldberg RA, Perry JD. Transcaruncular approach to the medial orbit and orbital apex. Ophthalmology 2000; 107(8):1459–1463
9. Kakizaki H, Nakano T, Asamoto K, Iwaki M. Posterior border of the deep lateral orbital wall—appearance, width, and distance from the orbital rim. Ophthal Plast Reconstr Surg 2008;24(4):262–265
10. Goldberg RA, Kim AJ, Kerivan KM. The lacrimal keyhole, orbital door jamb, and basin of the inferior orbital fissure. Three areas of deep bone in the lateral orbit. Arch Ophthalmol 1998;116(12): 1618–1624

14 Orbital Soft Tissues

Swapna Vemuri and Jeremiah P. Tao

Extraocular Muscles and Innervation

The six extraocular muscles (medial, lateral, superior and inferior recti, and superior and inferior oblique muscles) move the globe. With the exception of the inferior oblique muscle, which originates on the anteromedial orbital floor, all the extraocular muscles originate at the orbital apex (**Fig. 14.1a**). The rectus muscles originate at the fibrous annulus of Zinn. These muscles course anteriorly, penetrate Tenon's capsule, and insert onto the anterior aspect of the globe, forming the spiral of Tillaux (**Fig. 14.1b**). The rectus muscles form the muscle cone and delineate the intraconal and extraconal spaces.

The levator palpebrae superioris muscle originates on the lesser wing of sphenoid superior to the annulus. The superior oblique muscle also originates on the lesser wing of sphenoid medial to the levator muscle origin, continues anteriorly through the trochlea, then courses posterolaterally under the superior rectus muscle to insert onto the globe. The inferior oblique originates on the maxillary bone lateral to the lacrimal sac fossa, continues posterolaterally under the inferior rectus, and inserts onto the globe posterior to the macula.

The extraocular muscles are innervated by cranial nerves (CN) III (oculomotor), IV (trochlear), and VI (abducens). CN III divides into superior and inferior branches in the cavernous sinus before entering the orbit. The superior branch innervates the levator and superior rectus muscles. The inferior branch innervates the medial rectus, inferior rectus, and inferior oblique muscles. CN IV innervates the superior oblique muscle. CN VI innervates the lateral rectus muscle. Cranial nerves III and VI enter the orbit through the superior orbital fissure, travel through the intraconal space, and innervate the rectus muscles at the posterior one-third and anterior two-thirds junction. The blood supply for the rectus muscles arises from muscular anterior ciliary artery branches of the ophthalmic artery, lacrimal artery, and infraorbital artery. The inferior division of CN III to the inferior oblique travels lateral to the inferior rectus to innervate the muscle on the posterior surface. A parasympathetic branch to the ciliary ganglion travels with this inferior oblique muscle branch. CN IV travels extraconally to innervate the superior oblique on the superior surface at the posterior third of the muscle.

Optic Nerve

The optic nerve (CN II) can be divided into intraocular, intraorbital, intracanalicular, and intracranial segments measuring approximately 1 mm, 25 to 30 mm, 10 mm, and 10 mm long, respectively. The intraorbital optic nerve exits the posterior aspect of the globe and increases in diameter as it extends posteriorly through the orbit. Its intraorbital length is greater than the distance from the posterior globe to the optic canal (18 mm), allowing for eye movement and a safety margin in the event of proptosis. The optic nerve, with a 4-mm diameter and surrounded by the meninges (pia, arachnoid, and dura mater), then enters the optic foramen, which is 6.5 mm in diameter. Dura fuses with the annulus of Zinn and the optic canal periosteum, resulting in immobilization of the optic nerve. The optic nerve courses through the optic canal, which is about 10 mm long, and continues intracranially until it reaches the optic chiasm. Surgical management of intraconal pathology requires a keen understanding of the optic nerve course.

Orbital Nerves

In addition to the cranial nerves previously described, sensory, motor, and autonomic nerves supply the orbit.

Sensory Innervation

The ophthalmic (V_1) and maxillary (V_2) divisions of the trigeminal nerve (CN V) provide sensory innervation to the orbital and periorbital regions (**Fig. 14.2**).

Ophthalmic Nerve

The ophthalmic nerve (CN V_1) divides into the frontal and lacrimal nerves, which enter the orbit above the annulus of Zinn, and the nasociliary nerve, which enters through the annulus. The frontal nerve divides further; the supratrochlear nerve innervates the medial upper lid, glabellar region, and medial conjunctiva, and the supraorbital nerve innervates the medial forehead. The lacrimal nerve innervates the lateral upper lid, lacrimal gland, and lateral conjunctiva. The nasociliary nerve crosses the optic nerve superiorly from lateral to medial and courses between the superior oblique and medial rectus muscles before further dividing. Anterior and posterior ethmoidal nerves innervate the middle and inferior turbinates, nasal septum, lateral nasal wall, and tip of the nose (terminal infratrochlear nerve). Ciliary nerves provide sensory innervation to the ciliary body, iris, and cornea along with sympathetic innervation to the dilator pupillae muscle.

Ciliary Ganglion

The ciliary ganglion, which is located lateral to the optic nerve and medial to the lateral rectus muscle, is about 1.5 cm posterior

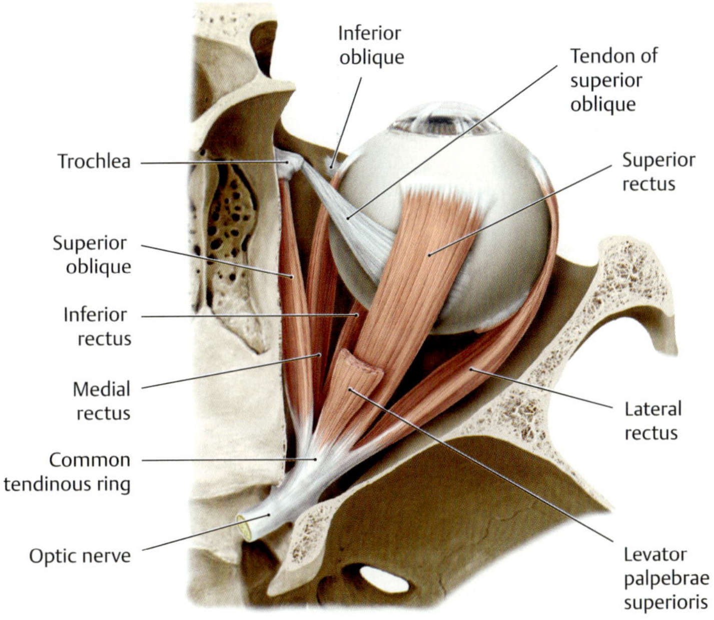

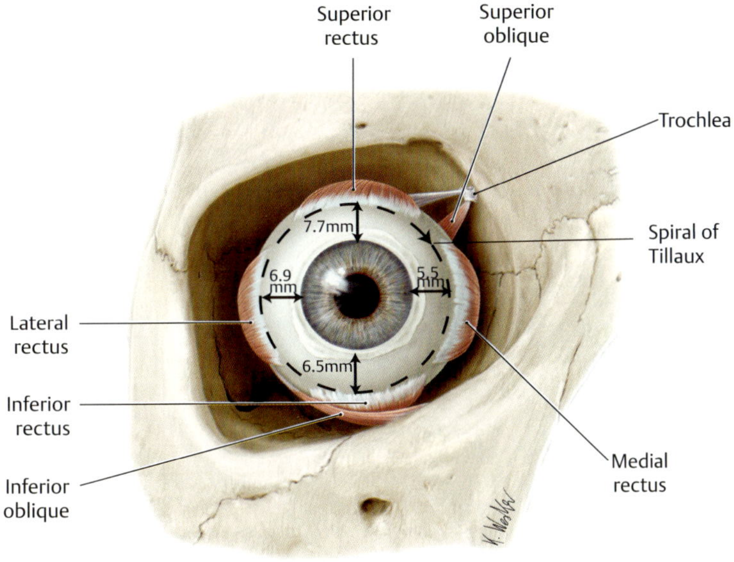

Fig. 14.1 Extraocular muscles, right eye. **(a)** Superior view. **(b)** Anterior view. Muscle insertions onto the anterior aspect of the globe beginning with the medial rectus and ending with the superior rectus create the spiral of Tillaux. The distance between the muscle insertion and limbus are indicated. (Modified from THIEME Atlas of Anatomy, Head and Neuroanatomy. © Thieme 2010, Illustrations by Karl Wesker.)

to the globe. Sensory (V_1) and sympathetic fibers pass through without synapsing, whereas parasympathetic fibers synapse in the ganglion. The ganglion can be encountered during lateral orbital intraconal surgery.

Maxillary Nerve

The maxillary nerve (CN V_2) divides into the infraorbital, zygomatic, nasal branches, palatine, superior alveolar, and pharyngeal nerves. After leaving the trigeminal ganglion, the maxillary nerve enters the foramen rotundum into the pterygopalatine fossa. The nerve enters the inferior orbital fissure to continue through the infraorbital groove and canal to exit anteriorly through the infraorbital foramen as the infraorbital nerve. The infraorbital nerve divides into the inferior palpebral branch, nasal branch, and superior labial branch to supply the inferior eyelid, lateral nose, and upper lip, respectively. The zygomatic nerve divides in the inferior orbital fissure into the zygomaticofacial and zygomaticotemporal nerves to exit through the respective foramina and innervate the cheek and lateral forehead, respectively.

The infraorbital, zygomaticofacial, and zygomaticotemporal may be encountered during surgery of the midface. Care should be taken to preserve these sensory nerves; however, compromise to the zygomaticofacial and zygomaticotemporal nerves may be less consequential than infraorbital nerve damage that may result in symptomatic hypoesthesia.

Motor Innervation

Motor innervation to the facial muscles is supplied by the facial nerve (CN VII), which is described in further detail along with facial anatomy in other chapters. In the periorbital region, the

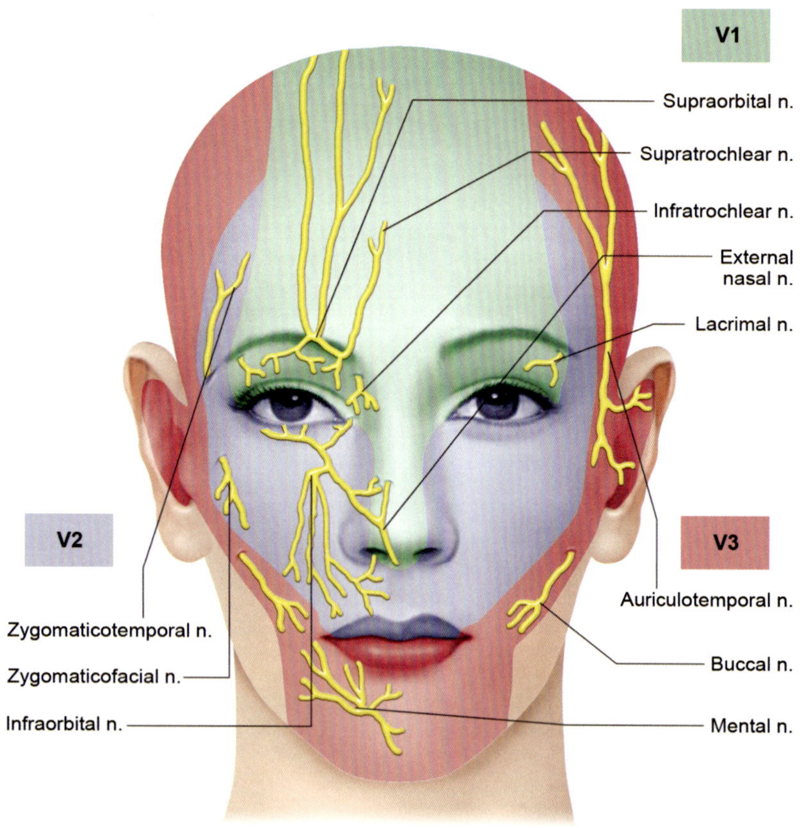

Fig. 14.2 Trigeminal nerve (CN V) cutaneous distribution. The ophthalmic (V1) and maxillary (V2) divisions of the trigeminal nerve (CN V) provide cutaneous innervation to the orbital and periorbital regions.

facial nerve lies in a deep plane as it emerges from the parotid gland (**Fig. 14.3**). The temporal branch courses superiorly and crosses over the zygomatic arch about midway between the lateral canthus and tragus. Dissection in the subperiosteal plane is safe in this region. Superior to the arch, the facial nerve lies beneath the superficial temporalis fascia, which is an extension of the superficial musculoaponeurotic system (SMAS). To avoid damaging the facial nerve in this region, dissection should be performed deep to SMAS, just anterior to the deep temporalis fascia. In addition, a branch can be found along a line from approximately 1 cm inferior to the tragus to 1.5 cm superior to the lateral brow. Inferior to the arch, dissection superficial to SMAS and the parotid gland avoids the facial nerve.

Autonomic Innervation

The sympathetic nerves from the superior cervical ganglion enter the carotid canal as a plexus around the internal carotid artery (ICA). Sympathetics to the lacrimal gland leave the ICA to exit the petrous bone and eventually parallel the parasympathetic fibers to the lacrimal gland. The fibers to the dilator pupillae muscle leave the ICA in the cavernous sinus and travel with CN VI and then the nasociliary branch of V_1 before leaving the cavernous sinus. These fibers pass through the ciliary ganglion without synapsing, travel with the long ciliary nerves, and result in pupil dilation. The fibers to Müller muscle travel along ophthalmic artery branches to stimulate upper lid elevation. Sympathetic innervation results in lower lid retraction via the inferior tarsal muscle and causes hidrosis.

Parasympathetic fibers from the Edinger-Westphal nucleus travel with the inferior division of the oculomotor nerve, synapse in the ciliary ganglion, and continue with the branch to the inferior oblique muscle. They enter the globe as posterior ciliary nerves and cause accommodation through ciliary muscle contraction and pupil constriction through the pupillary sphincter muscle. Parasympathetic fibers from the pterygopalatine ganglion travel through the inferior orbital fissure then with the lacrimal nerve to innervate the lacrimal gland.

Orbital Vessels

The periorbital and facial region receives blood supply from both the ICA and external carotid arteries, resulting in rich anastomoses and vascular supply (**Fig. 14.4**). In the cavernous sinus, the ICA gives off the ophthalmic artery, which then travels inferior to the optic nerve through the optic canal. The pial branch of the ophthalmic artery supplies the intracanalicular optic nerve. The central retinal artery branches off about 10 mm posterior to the globe. Additional branches include the lacrimal, supraorbital, ethmoidal, and extraocular muscle branches; long posterior ciliary arteries; and terminal branches (supratrochlear, medial palpebral, and dorsal nasal). The external carotid artery branches include the maxillary and facial artery. The an-

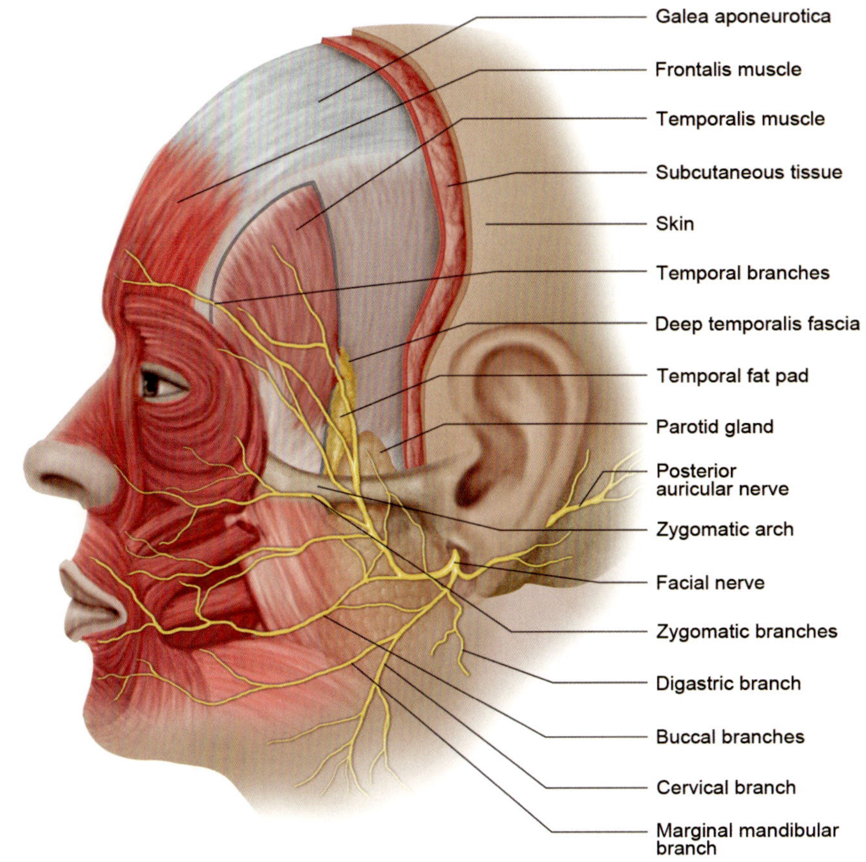

Fig. 14.3 Facial nerve (CN VII) distribution. Left lateral view of the face. Motor innervation to the facial muscles is supplied by the facial nerve (CN VII). In the periorbital region, the facial nerve lies in a deep plane as it emerges from the parotid gland.

gular artery, a branch of the facial artery, courses about 5 mm anterior to the medial canthal tendon (MCT) insertion and may be encountered along with the angular vein during dissection in this area. The superior ophthalmic vein provides orbital venous drainage. It courses from superomedially to laterally in the orbit as it enters the cavernous sinus.

Orbital Lymphatics

Lymphatics were previously thought to be absent in the orbit; however, recent studies challenge this notion.[1,2]

Orbital Fat

Orbital fat surrounds the globe and orbital structures. Anteriorly, extraconal orbital fat is found in the postseptal plane in the upper and lower lids. The superior orbital fat is divided by the trochlea into the medial and central fat pads (**Fig. 14.5**).

The inferior orbital fat is divided into the medial, central, and lateral fat pads (**Fig. 14.5**). The inferior oblique muscle courses between the medial and central fat pads. The lateral and central fat pads are separated by the fascial arcuate expansion of the inferior oblique muscle.

Surgical Annotation: Precautions during Orbital Fat Pad Manipulation

During upper or lower lid blepharoplasty, debulking of the fat pads can result in insidious bleeding into the fat and subsequently retrobulbar. If hemostasis is not ensured before wound closure, an orbital compartment syndrome may result in vision compromise. Aggressive orbital fat pad removal in the upper and lower lids was once thought to improve cosmetic outcomes. Conservative excision and fat preservation, especially laterally, may be associated with improved aesthetic results and avoid hollowing.

Upper Eyelid

The orbital lobe of the lacrimal gland is found in the postseptal, or preaponeurotic, plane lateral to the orbital fat pads, and may be easily confused for orbital fat; therefore, careful dissection is required if the central fat pad is debulked during an upper lid blepharoplasty. The lacrimal gland appears more pink and lobulated and is more firm compared with the orbital fat.

Lower Eyelid

The inferior oblique muscle is encountered between the central and medial fat pads of the lower eyelid. During lower lid

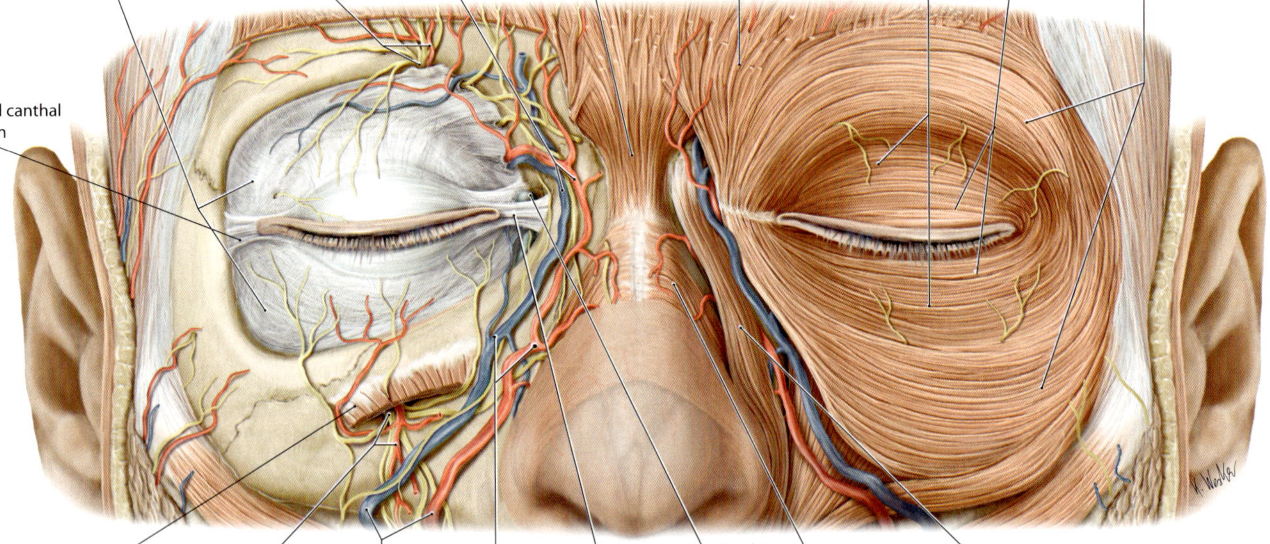

Fig. 14.4 Periorbital neurovascular structures. Right orbit: Orbicularis oculi muscle removed. The periorbital and facial region receives blood supply from both the internal and external carotid arteries resulting in rich anastomoses and vascular supply. (Modified from THIEME Atlas of Anatomy, Head and Neuroanatomy. © Thieme 2010, Illustration by Karl Wesker.)

blepharoplasty and fat redistribution, the fat pads must be gently separated from their connective tissue attachments to the inferior oblique before translocation. A restrictive strabismus may otherwise result. Some surgical techniques involve direct visualization of the inferior oblique muscle and release from surrounding soft tissues.[3]

Lacrimal System

Lacrimal Gland

The lacrimal gland and accessory glands of Wolfring and Kraus produce the aqueous layer of the tear film. The lacrimal gland is thought to produce chiefly reflex tears and to contribute to basal tear secretion provided by the glands of Wolfring and Kraus located in the superior or inferior tarsal border and fornix, respectively. The lacrimal gland is located in the lacrimal gland fossa in the lateral aspect of the frontal bone. It consists of an orbital lobe, which is visible during an upper eyelid dissection, and a palpebral lobe, which can be visualized in the superolateral fornix by manually elevating the eyelid. The lateral horn of the levator aponeurosis separates the two lobes, with secretory ductules connecting them. To avoid damage to these ductules, an incisional lacrimal gland biopsy should be performed on the orbital lobe.

The lacrimal gland has been found to receive both sympathetic and parasympathetic innervation, and innervation from CN V and VII. The lacrimal nerve of CN V_1 carries sensory information from the gland and upper lid.

Nasolacrimal System and Lacrimal Pump

The eyelids help pump tears produced by the lacrimal apparatus across the ocular surface to drain medially through the upper and lower lid 0.3 mm diameter puncta. The puncta are positioned opposed to the globe. With punctual eversion, tears are unable to drain appropriately, resulting in epiphora. Lateralization of the puncta suggests medial canthal tendon laxity or disruption.

After entering the puncta, tears travel 2 mm vertically to the ampulla of the canaliculi, then 8 mm horizontally through the canaliculi. In more than 90 percent of individuals, the superior and inferior canaliculi merge into a common canaliculus before draining into the nasolacrimal sac.[4,5]

The lacrimal sac measures about 12 mm vertically, extending about 3 to 5 mm superior to the MCT. It is located in the lacrimal sac fossa, which is created by the maxillary bone anteriorly and lacrimal bone posteriorly.

The lacrimal sac then opens into a nasolacrimal duct, which courses posteriorly, laterally, and inferiorly for 18 mm in an os-

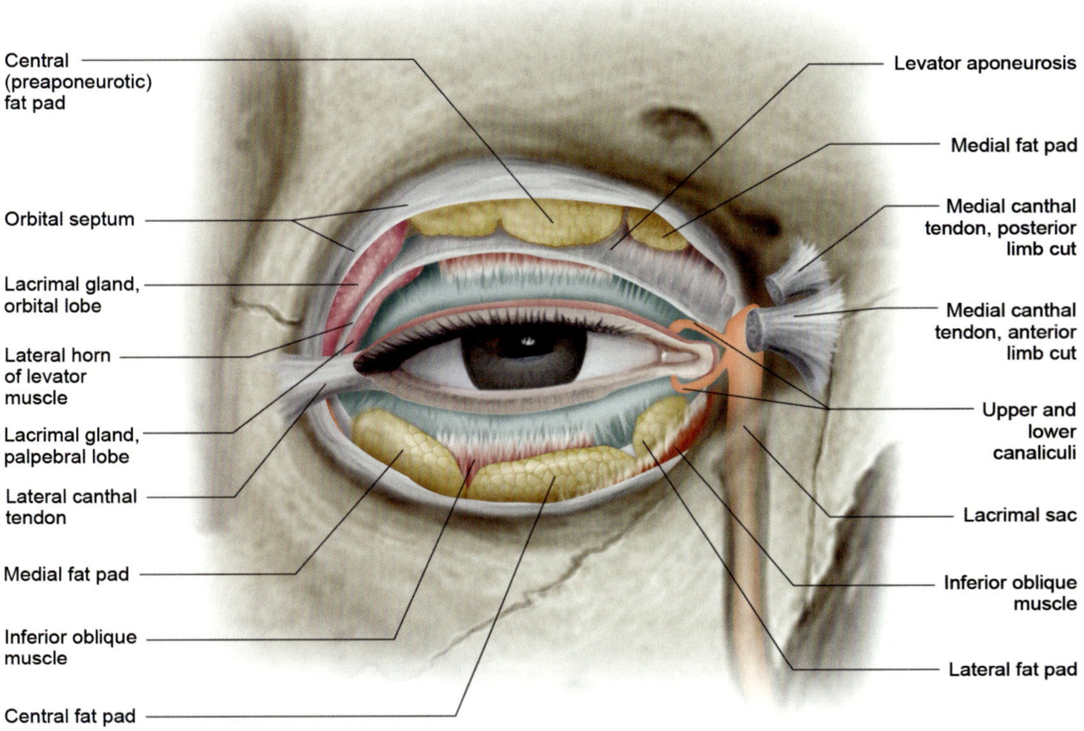

Fig. 14.5 Orbital fat pad distribution in relation to surrounding structures, right orbit. Orbital fat surrounds the globe and orbital structures. Anteriorly, extraconal orbital fat is found in the postseptal plane in the upper and lower lids. The superior orbital fat is divided by the trochlea into the medial and central fat pads. The inferior orbital fat is divided into the medial, central, and lateral fat pads.

seous nasolacrimal canal. The duct opens beneath the inferior turbinate into the inferior meatus. The duct opening is about 25 mm posterior to the anterior naris (**Fig. 14.6**).

Various valves have also been described in the nasolacrimal system. The valve of Rosenmüller at the opening of the common canaliculus to the lacrimal sac prevents reflux of tears. The valve of Krause is found between the sac and duct. The valve of Hasner is located at the duct opening into the inferior meatus (**Fig. 14.6**).

Lid position and tone are important to allow for adequate lacrimal pump function. In addition, the organization of the structures around the nasolacrimal system contributes to appropriate tear drainage.

The pretarsal orbicularis muscle surrounds the canaliculi. Periorbital fascia and the thick anterior and thin posterior limbs of the MCT encircle the lacrimal sac. The anterior limb inserts onto the anterior lacrimal crest and the posterior limb inserts onto the posterior lacrimal crest (**Fig. 14.4**). The deep pretarsal orbicularis muscle, also called the Horner muscle, courses posterior to the lacrimal sac and posterior limb of the MCT to insert onto the posterior lacrimal crest.

During a transcaruncular approach to the medial orbit, blunt dissection along Horner's muscle allows identification of the posterior lacrimal crest. A periosteal incision and elevation gives access to the subperiosteal plane along the medial orbit.

Surgical Annotation: Anatomical Considerations during Nasolacrimal Surgery

Nasolacrimal Intubation

During canalicular intubation, gentle introduction of a stent after the previously described anatomy prevents creation of false passageways. When retrieving a canalicular intubation stent through the nose, a retrieving instrument introduced parallel to the floor of the nasal cavity, along the lateral nasal wall, and in a posterolateral direction helps locate the stent. Occasionally, the inferior turbinate may need to be fractured if it is too close to the lateral nasal wall.

Dacryocystorhinostomy

A dacryocystorhinostomy (DCR), whether external or endoscopic, involves fistulization of the lacrimal sac into the nasal cavity for management of nasolacrimal duct obstruction. The lacrimal sac is located in a fossa between the anterior lacrimal crest of the maxillary bone and the posterior lacrimal crest of the lacrimal bone. For an external DCR, after making a transcutaneous incision along the medial canthus, dissection

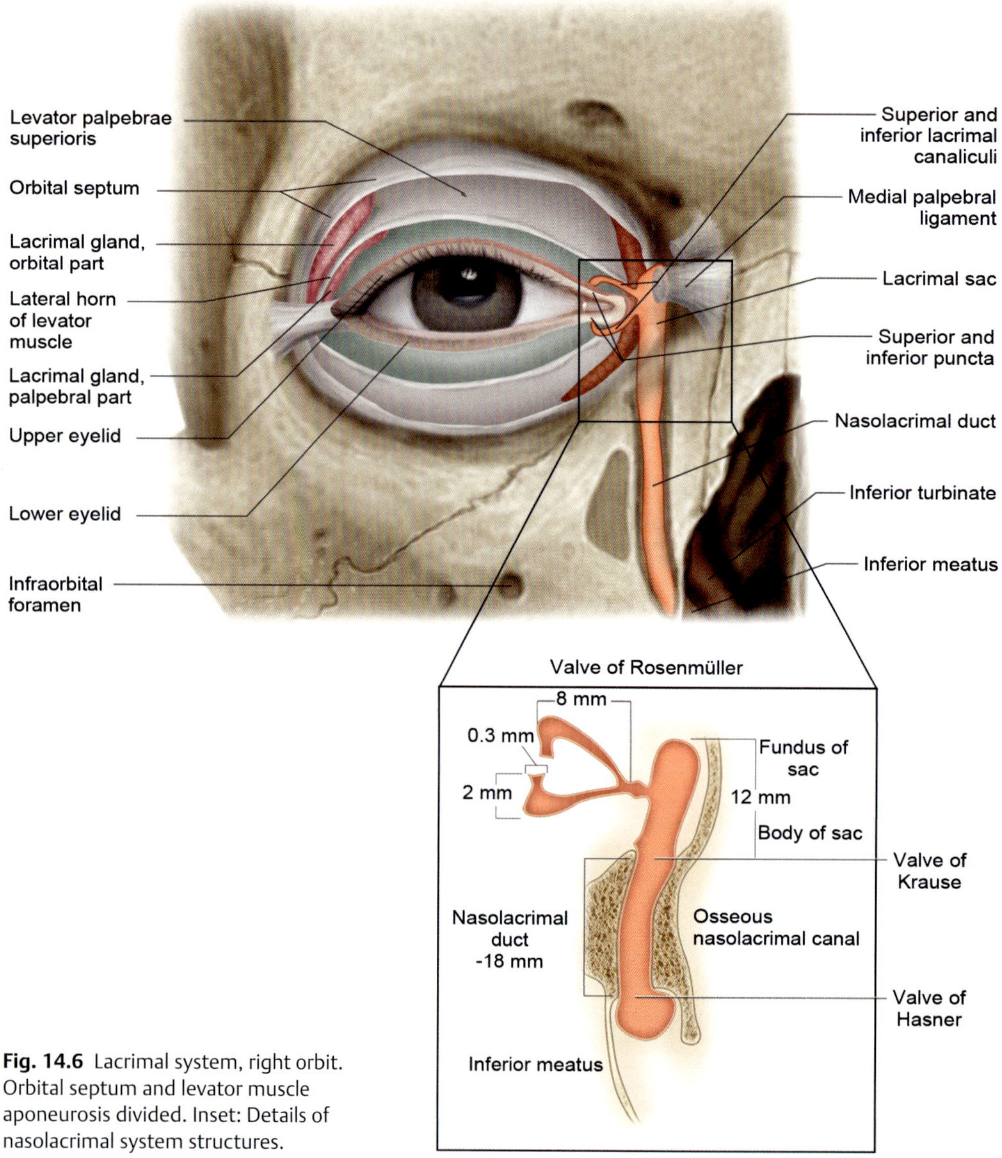

Fig. 14.6 Lacrimal system, right orbit. Orbital septum and levator muscle aponeurosis divided. Inset: Details of nasolacrimal system structures.

continues down to periosteum. The anterior lacrimal crest is exposed, the sac is elevated out of the fossa, and the posterior lacrimal crest is visualized. Although the anterior limb of the MCT may be intentionally disinserted, too posterior of a dissection may result in disinsertion of the posterior limb of the MCT at the posterior lacrimal crest and loss of lid apposition to the globe.

An osteotomy is created anterior to the middle meatus to enter the nasal cavity. In many individuals, ethmoidal air cells are present medial to the lacrimal sac fossa or at least extend anterior to the posterior lacrimal crest.[6,7] The ethmoidal air cells may have to be removed for the new osteotomy to communicate with the nasal cavity and not with the ethmoid sinus. A larger osteotomy and the absence of obstruction of the common internal ostium may increase the chance of a successful DCR.[8] A distance of at least 5 mm has been suggested between the common internal ostium and osteotomy margin.[9]

If a patient has persistent epiphora despite a patent DCR, lacrimal sump syndrome should be considered.[10] Inadequate drainage of tears that accumulate in an intact inferior lacrimal sac with possible bone remaining medially may result in this finding. This can be avoided by ensuring that the osteotomy and lacrimal sac marsupialization extend inferior to the proximal nasolacrimal duct.

References

1. Sherman DD, Gonnering RS, Wallow IHL, et al. Identification of orbital lymphatics: enzyme histochemical light microscopic and electron microscopic studies. Ophthal Plast Reconstr Surg 1993; 9(3):153–169
2. Gausas RE, Gonnering RS, Lemke BN, Dortzbach RK, Sherman DD. Identification of human orbital lymphatics. Ophthal Plast Reconstr Surg 1999;15(4):252–259
3. Massry G. "The inverse shoe shine sign" in transconjunctival lower blepharoplasty with fat repositioning. Ophthal Plast Reconstr Surg 2012;28(3):234–235
4. Jones LT. An anatomical approach to problems of the eyelids and lacrimal apparatus. Arch Ophthalmol 1961;66:111–124
5. Lemke BN. Lacrimal anatomy. Adv Ophthalmic Plast Reconstr Surg 1984;3:11–23
6. Whitnall SE. The relations of the lacrimal sac fossa to the ethmoidal cells. Ophthalmic Res 1911;30:321–325
7. Blaylock WK, Moore CA, Linberg JV. Anterior ethmoid anatomy facilitates dacryocystorhinostomy. Arch Ophthalmol 1990;108(12): 1774–1777
8. Linberg JV, Anderson RL, Bumsted RM, Barreras R. Study of intranasal ostium external dacryocystorhinostomy. Arch Ophthalmol 1982;100(11):1758–1762
9. Jones LT. The cure of epiphora due to canalicular disorders, trauma and surgical failures on the lacrimal passages. Trans Am Acad Ophthalmol Otolaryngol 1962;66:506–524
10. Jordan DR, McDonald H. Failed dacryocystorhinostomy: the sump syndrome. Ophthalmic Surg 1993;24(10):692–693

15 Eyelid Anatomy

Catherine Y. Liu, Swapna Vemuri, and Jeremiah P. Tao

Surface Anatomy

The eyelids provide globe protection, contribute to tear production, and distribute tears. The adjacent forehead and midface influence correct eyelid positioning. Understanding these relationships is essential in eyelid surgery.

The upper and lower eyelids, along with the upper and lower puncta, oppose the globe. The upper lid naturally rests 1 to 2 mm below the superior limbus and peaks 1 mm medial to the center of the pupil. The lower lid rests at the inferior limbus and peaks 1 mm lateral to the center of the pupil. Horizontal and vertical interpalpebral fissures are about 30 mm and 10 mm, respectively. The lateral canthal angle is about 2 mm higher than the medial canthal angle. The medial canthal angle is slightly rounded compared with the sharply peaked lateral canthal angle (**Fig. 15.1**).

The eyebrows set above the superior orbital rim but slightly lower at the rim in males. The brow usually peaks at the lateral limbus. The forehead extends from the hairline to the glabella and superior orbital rim. The midface extends from the lower lids tapering medially to the nasolabial folds to encompass a triangular area. Facial mimetic muscles, those contributing to facial expression, influence brow position, and also cause skin furrows, including in the forehead, periorbital region, and midface.

Eyelid Anatomy

Upper Eyelid Layers

The layers of the upper eyelid vary depending on the location in the eyelid (**Fig. 15.2a**). Anterior to the tarsus, the structures from anterior to posterior include skin, orbicularis oculi muscle, tarsus, and conjunctiva. A few millimeters above the tarsus, structures include skin, orbicularis, orbital septum, orbital fat, levator palpebrae superioris muscle, Müller muscle, and conjunctiva. The orbital septum fuses with the levator muscle about 2 to 5 mm superior to the tarsus in non-Asians and anterior to tarsus in Asians. Orbital fat descends inferiorly to fill the space between the septum and levator, which results in a fuller lid appearance.

Lower Eyelid Layers

The layers of the lower lid are similar those of the upper except that the lid retractors consist of the capsulopalpebral fascia, analogous to the levator muscle, and the inferior tarsal muscle, analogous to Müller muscle (**Fig. 15.2a**).

Skin

The eyelid skin is the thinnest in the body. The lid also lacks subcutaneous tissue so the skin attaches directly to the underlying orbicularis muscle. In the upper lid, the levator muscle sends fascial attachments to the overlying orbicularis and skin to create an upper lid crease. The crease is about 10 mm or 8 to 9 mm above the lid margin in females and males, respectively. In Asians, it may be closer to the lid margin or absent. The upper lid skin is continuous with that of the thicker skin of the brow. The superior sulcus is located below the brow and tends to hollow with age.

Protractors

Orbicularis oculi muscle contraction results in eyelid closure. Its fibers are concentric around the eyelids. It is divided into the pretarsal, preseptal, and orbital regions (**Fig. 15.3**). The pretarsal and preseptal orbicularis are involved in involuntary blink, whereas the orbital portion is involved in voluntary lid closure. The orbicularis oculi contributes to the lacrimal pump.

The pretarsal orbicularis oculi divides into a superficial and deep head at the medial canthus. The superficial head fuses with the medial canthal tendon (**Fig. 15.4**). The deep head, also known as Horner's muscle, inserts onto the posterior lacrimal crest. Contraction pulls the lid medially and posteriorly against the globe. Laterally, the fibers from the upper and lower lids fuse into a common tendon and insert onto Whitnall's tubercle.

The preseptal orbicularis also divides into a superficial and deep head that insert onto the medial canthus. The superficial

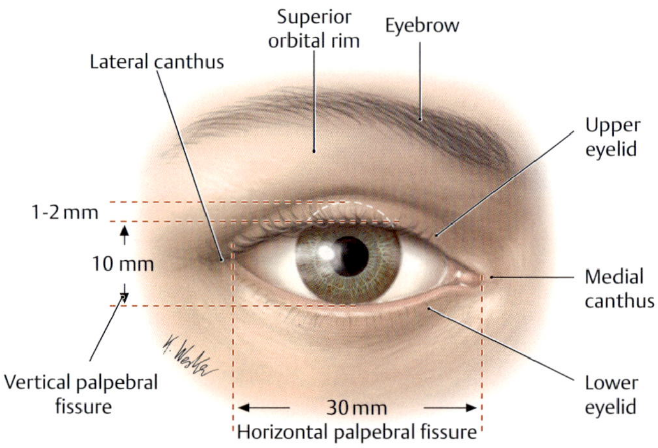

Fig. 15.1 Surface anatomy of periorbital region. Right eye, anterior view. (Modified from THIEME Atlas of Anatomy, Head and Neuroanatomy. © Thieme 2010, Illustrations by Karl Wesker.)

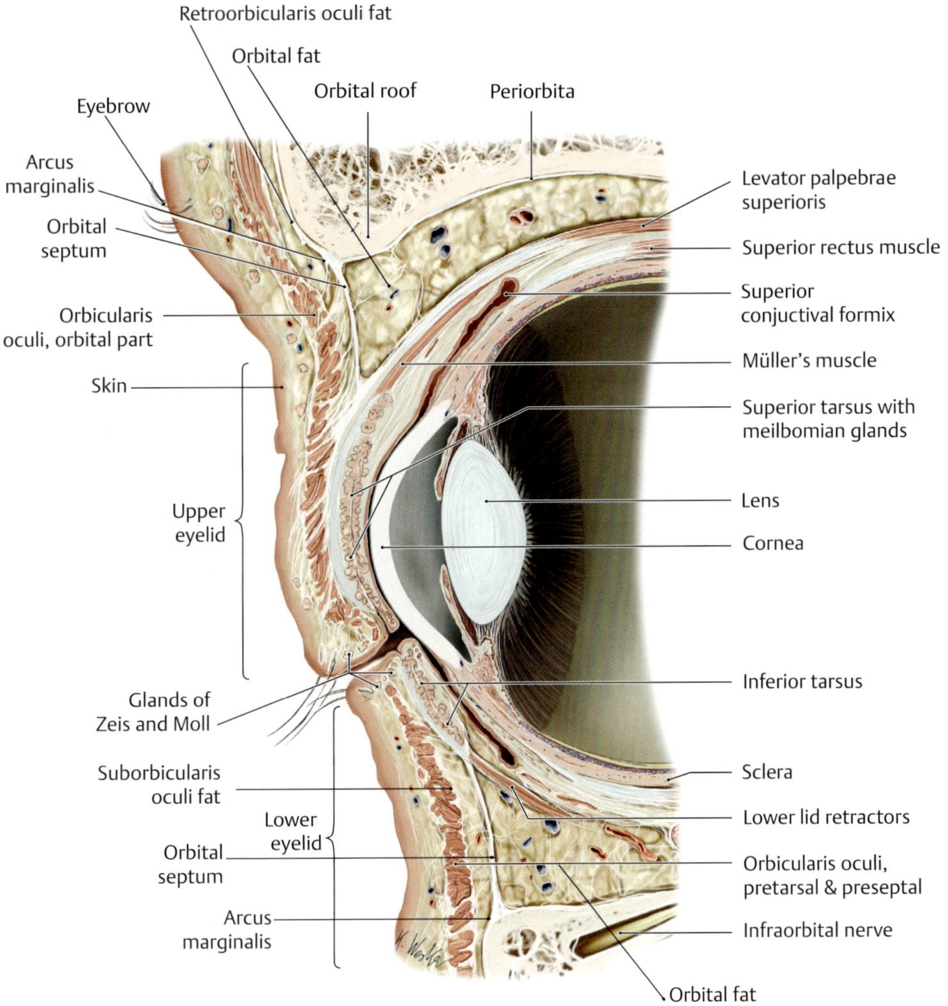

a

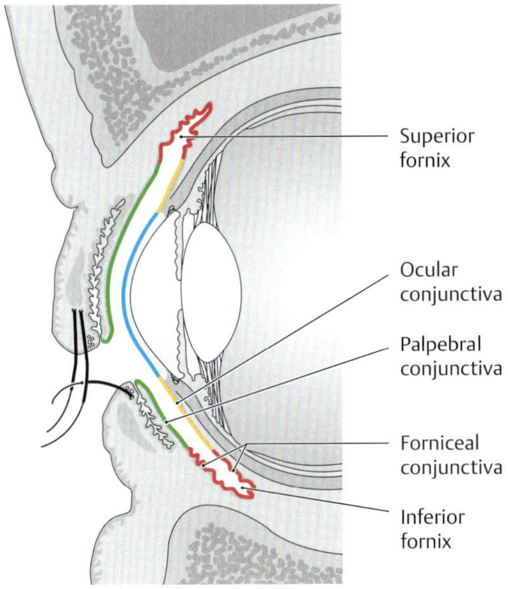

b

Fig. 15.2 Structure of eyelids and conjunctiva. **(a)** Sagittal view of eyelids and surrounding structures. **(b)** Anatomy of conjunctiva. (Modified from THIEME Atlas of Anatomy, Head and Neuroanatomy. © Thieme 2010, Illustrations by Karl Wesker.)

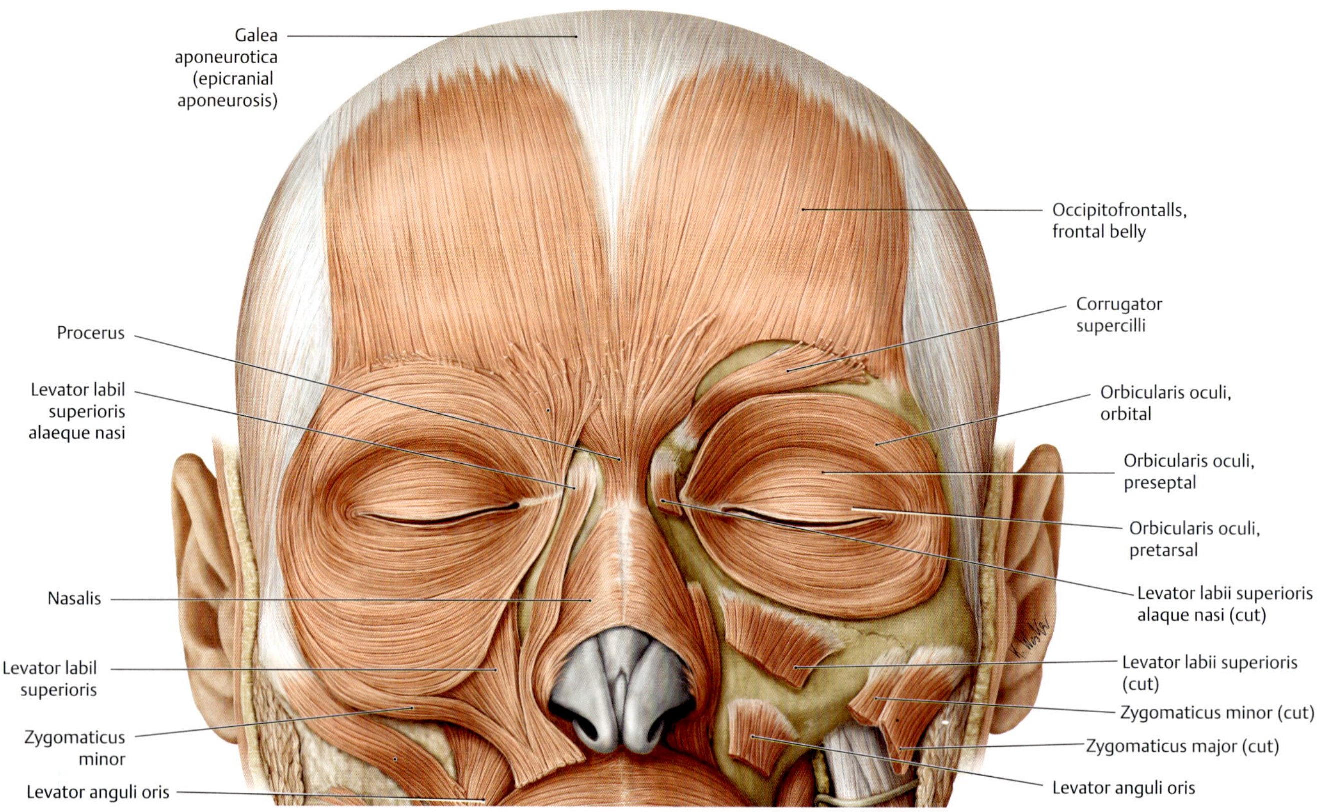

Fig. 15.3 Periorbital facial mimetic muscles. Orbicularis oculi muscle contraction results in eyelid closure. Its fibers are concentric around the eyelids. It is divided into the pretarsal, preseptal, and orbital regions. The pretarsal and preseptal orbicularis are involved in involuntary blink; the orbital portion is involved in voluntary lid closure. (Modified from THIEME Atlas of Anatomy, Head and Neuroanatomy. © Thieme 2010, Illustrations by Karl Wesker.)

head inserts onto the medial canthal tendon and the deep head inserts onto the lacrimal sac fascia. Laterally, the upper and lower fibers join to form the lateral palpebral raphe and connect to the underling lateral canthal tendon.

The orbital orbicularis arises from the medial orbital rim, broadens outward in concentric bands superiorly and inferiorly, and joins at the lateral orbital rim to form a continuous ellipse. It extends beyond the orbital rim.

Lateral and Medial Canthal Tendons

The medial canthal tendon (MCT) splits into anterior and posterior limbs, which attach to the corresponding lacrimal crest encircling the lacrimal sac (**Fig. 15.4**).The anterior limb of the MCT gives the lid structural support whereas the posterior limb keeps the eyelid apposed to the globe. The lateral canthal tendon is formed by superior and inferior limb that fuses to form a common tendon inserting onto Whitnall's tubercle.

Surgical Annotation. Lateral and Medial Canthal Reanchoring

In lateral canthal anchoring (canthoplasty or canthopexy), the lid is sutured to inner aspect of the lateral orbital rim (about 10 mm posterior to the anterior rim) and slightly above the medial canthal angle. Usually the suture is secured to periosteum, but a drill hole may be helpful if the periosteal tissue is inadequate (i.e., scar). In patients with a prominent globe, the lid should be reanchored slightly more anteriorly on the inner aspect of the rim in order to avoid slipping of the lower lid under the globe.

Medial canthal tendon reanchoring or tightening of the anterior limb is to the anterior lacrimal crest. Tightening of the posterior limb presents a greater challenge given the lacrimal sac obscures access to the posterior lacrimal crest.

Orbital Septum

The orbital septum is a connective tissue structure that forms from the periosteum of the orbital rim at the arcus marginalis (**Fig. 15.2a**). It divides the lid into anterior (skin and orbicularis) and posterior (tarsus, conjunctiva, and lid retractors) lamella.

Orbital Fat Pads

Orbital fat, also known as preaponeurotic fat, is sandwiched between the septum and the lid retractors. As discussed in Chapter 14, there is a medial and central fat pad in the upper lid and a medial, central, and lateral fat pad in the lower lid. These fat pads can atrophy with age, creating a hollowed superior or

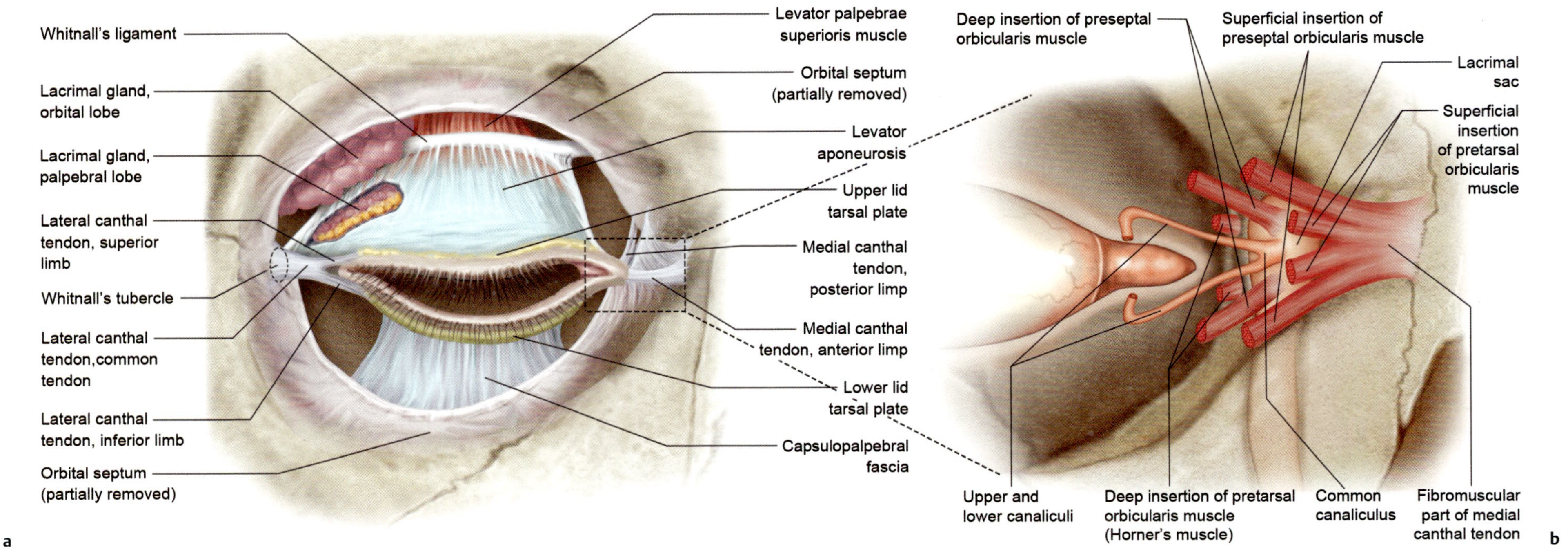

Fig. 15.4 Details of eyelid anatomy. **(a)** Upper and lower tarsal plates and attachments. **(b)** Anatomy of orbicularis oculi muscle at the medial canthus.

inferior sulcus or a bulge behind a weakened septum, causing orbital fat prolapse and bulging.

Retractors

Levator Palpebrae Superioris Muscle

The levator palpebrae muscle arises from the lesser wing of the sphenoid bone above the superior rectus attachment. It projects anteriorly toward the globe (**Fig. 15.2a, Fig. 15.4**). Whitnall's ligament is a band of fibrous tissue derived from the muscle itself that attaches medially to the trochlea and laterally to the capsule of the lacrimal gland and lateral orbital wall (**Fig. 15.4**). Near Whitnall's ligament, the levator muscle changes course from anterior-posterior to superior-inferior and also transitions to an aponeurosis. The aponeurosis sends fascial slips posteriorly to attach to the anterior surface of tarsus and anteriorly to the orbicularis muscle and skin to form the lid crease. The lateral and medial levator horns anchor to periosteum. The lateral horn divides the lacrimal gland orbital and palpebral lobes as described in Chapter14. The levator muscle contributes about 10 to 12 mm of upper lid elevation. It is innervated by cranial nerve (CN) III.

Müller's Muscle

Müller's muscle is found posterior to the levator muscle (**Fig. 15.2a**). It is a smooth muscle that is innervated by sympathetic nerves. It contributes about 2 mm of lid elevation. It arises from behind the levator close to the junction where the muscle fibers transition to an aponeurosis. It inserts onto the superior border of the tarsus. Müller's muscle may serve as a coupling mechanism for transmitting levator aponeurosis forces to the tarsus.

Surgical Annotation

External Levator Advancement Ptosis Surgery

With aponeurotic upper lid ptosis, the levator aponeurosis may elongate or disinsert, resulting in ptosis associated with a high lid crease. During external aponeurotic ptosis repair, the levator muscle is reanchored to the tarsus. The orbital septum should be carefully dissected free from the levator. Suturing the septum may tether the eyelid, impair eyelid excursion, and cause lagophthalmos.

Capsulopalpebral Fascia and Inferior Tarsal Muscle

The lower lid retractors contract to depress the lid in down gaze and also help to maintain tarsal position. The capsulopalpebral fascia arises from the inferior rectus muscle sheath, splits to enwrap the inferior oblique muscle, and fuses to form the Lockwood's suspensory ligament (**Fig. 15.2a**). It continues superiorly to fuse with the orbital septum and insert on the inferior tarsal border. The inferior tarsal muscle is poorly developed but lies along the posterior surface of the capsulopalpebral fascia (**Fig. 15.2a, Fig. 15.4**).

During a transconjunctival surgical approach, conjunctiva and lower lid retractors are incised and reapproximated often without compromising lid stability. With lower lid dissection, the lower lid retractors course posteriorly into the orbit, which helps to distinguish them from the orbital septum that arises from the arcus marginalis along the inferior orbital rim.

Tarsus and Conjunctiva

The tarsus is a dense, connective tissue plate that gives structural support to the eyelid (**Fig. 15.2a, Fig. 15.4**). It is about 1 mm thick, and its vertical height measures about 8 to 10 mm in the upper lid and 4 mm in the lower lid but tapers medially and laterally. The tarsus contains meibomian glands, which secrete the sebaceous layer of the tear film. There are about 25 glands in the upper lid and 20 glands in the lower lid. The lateral and medial canthal tendons anchor tarsus to periosteum. Palpebral conjunctiva lines the posterior surface of tarsus and continues superiorly or inferiorly to the fornix then reflects on the globe as bulbar conjunctiva (**Fig. 15.2b**). The conjunctiva contains goblet cells, which provide the mucus layer of the tear film.

Eyelid Margin

The eyelid margin is a confluence of several eyelid structures (**Fig. 15.5**). Starting posteriorly and in contact with the globe is the mucosal surface of the conjunctiva, creating the mucocutaneous junction. Continuing anteriorly, the meibomian gland openings of tarsus are visible. The muscle of Riolan, representing the pretarsal orbicularis muscle, makes up the gray line. Finally, the skin is the most anterior structure with hair follicles emanating. About 100 eyelashes are found in the upper lid and about 50 in the lower lid organized into two or three irregular rows. Glands of Zeis are oil glands associated with hair follicles. Glands of Moll are eccrine, or sweat, glands that are located at the eyelid margin.

The gray line is an important landmark during surgical realignment of the lid margin such as during a marginal laceration repair or wedge lesion excision repair. Without precise align-

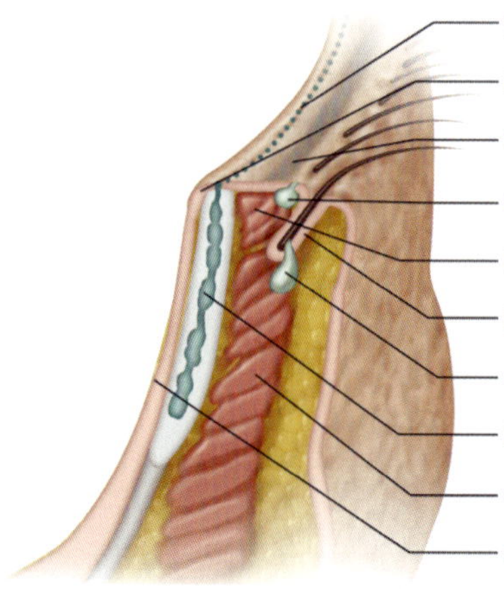

Fig. 15.5 Lower eyelid margin anatomy.

ment, a notch or step-off can result, resulting in ocular surface exposure, poor cosmesis, or both.

Forehead, Temporal, and Midface Anatomy

The facial planes guide surgical dissection. They vary slightly based on the facial region but they include the following: skin, subcutaneous tissue, superficial musculoaponeurotic system (SMAS) and facial mimetic muscles, loose areolar tissue, and deep facial fascia.

Forehead

The forehead represents the upper third of the face. The layers of the forehead include skin, subcutaneous tissue, frontalis muscle (encompassed in the galea aponeurotica and continuous with SMAS), loose areolar tissue, periosteum, and frontal bone (**Fig. 15.6**). Sensory branches from CN V_1 and vessels can be found coursing on the anterior surface of the frontalis muscle.

Temporal Forehead

The temporal region consists of skin, subcutaneous tissue, superficial temporalis or temporoparietal fascia (continuous with SMAS), loose areolar tissue, deep temporal fascia surrounding the superficial temporal fat pad, and temporalis muscle (**Fig. 15.6**). The superficial temporal artery, which is obtained during a temporal artery biopsy, is found in loose areolar tissue between the superficial and deep temporalis fasciae; however, care must be taken to avoid damaging the facial nerve that courses in the superficial temporal fascia.

Eyebrow

The skin of the brow is thicker than that of the eyelid and thinner than that of the forehead. Elevators and depressors influence brow position, which in turn influences upper lid position. Frontalis muscle contraction elevates the upper lid about 2 mm. The orbicularis, corrugator, and procerus muscles depress the brow (**Fig. 15.3**).

The frontalis muscle interdigitates with the orbicularis oculi muscle above the superior orbital rim. Posterior to the muscle is the brow fat pad, also known as the retro-orbicularis oculi fat pad (ROOF). It is separated from the orbital fat pads by the orbital septum (**Fig. 15.2a**). With aging, the brow pad can contribute to sub-brow fullness and subsequent upper lid droop and fullness. ROOF is continuous with the suborbicularis oculi fat (SOOF) of the lower lid.

Midface

The planes of the midface are especially important to understand for effective treatment of lower lid retraction or midfacial rejuvenation. Sub-orbicularis oculi fat (SOOF) is positioned between the orbicularis oculi muscle and periosteum (**Fig. 15.2a**).The SMAS surrounds the facial mimetic muscles. Ligamentous attachments between SMAS and skin dermis as well as SMAS and the underlying bone contribute to facial expression and support respectively. The orbitomalar ligament attaches the orbicularis oculi muscle that is encompassed in the SMAS to the inferior orbital rim.[1] The zygomatic ligament extends from the periosteum of the zygoma and zygomatic arch and through the malar fat pat to the malar skin.

Surgical Annotation

Lower Lid Malposition

In addition to downward vectors of the lower lid, midfacial ptosis and descent can also greatly influence lower lid positioning.[1] When performing surgery of the lower lid or midface, minimal (if any) skin, muscle, or soft tissue should be excised in the zone extending from the lower lid margin to the mouth. The lower lid is susceptible to any inferior vectors such as anterior lamellar shortening (e.g., cicatrix), ligamentous attenuation, or soft tissue debulking. In addition to directing wound closure and tension horizontally or at least obliquely, tissue recruitment and resuspension in the superolateral aspect of the lower lid and lateral canthus increase the likelihood of surgical success and longevity.

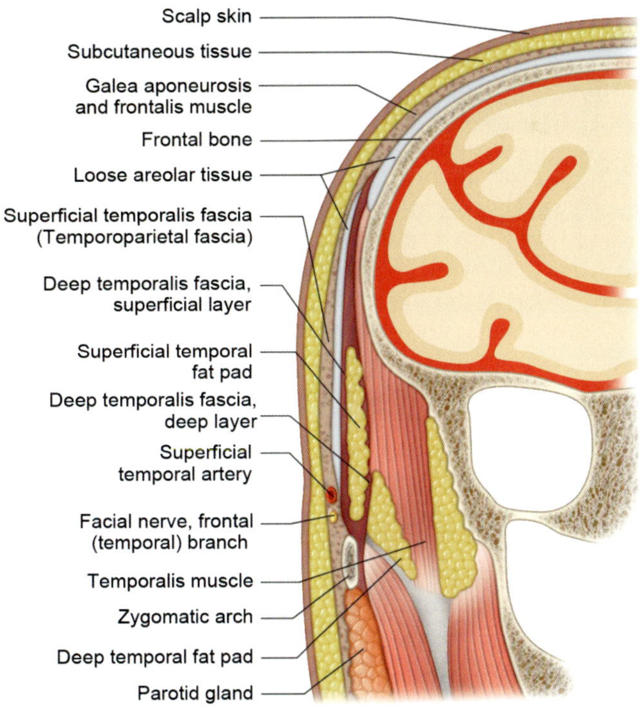

Fig. 15.6 Layers of forehead and temporal forehead regions. The temporal region consists of skin, subcutaneous tissue, superficial temporalis or temporoparietal fascia (continuous with the superficial musculoaponeurotic system [SMAS]), loose areolar tissue, and deep temporal fascia surrounding the superficial temporal fat pad and temporalis muscle.

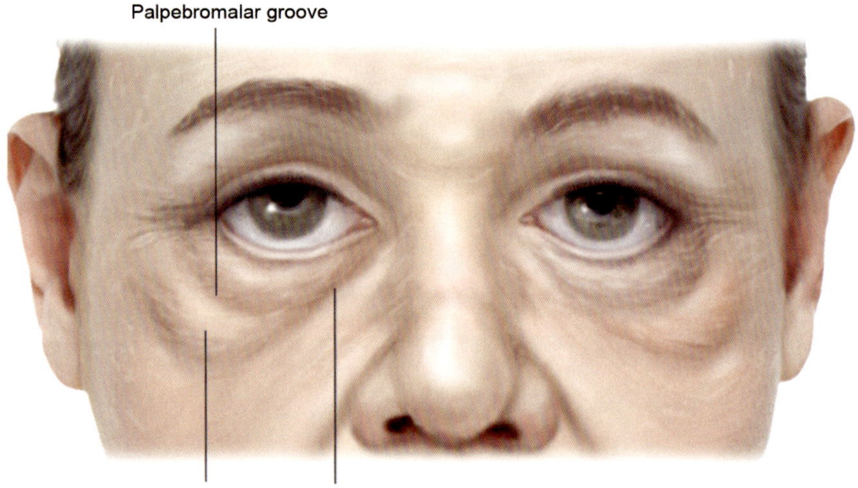

Fig. 15.7 Aging changes of the face. Nasojugal groove (tear trough), palpebromalar groove, and malar mound identified on an aging face.

Addressing the Nasojugal Groove, Palpebromalar Groove, and Malar Region

With age, the midfacial soft tissues descend, ligaments attenuate, and orbital fat herniates. Weakening of the orbital septum and elongation of the orbitomalar ligament results in anterior protrusion of orbital fat with accentuation of the nasojugal groove, or tear trough, and palpebromalar groove (**Fig. 15.7**).[2] Effective surgical management of the tear-trough deformity and palpebromalar grooves requires release of the orbitomalar ligament at the arcus marginalis along with orbital fat pad redistribution and orbicularis muscle tightening.[3]

In the malar region, SOOF descends with age. Zygomatic ligament suspension and SMAS and SOOF dissection, mobilization, and elevation either subperiosteally or preperiosteally improve midface descent.[4,5] Attention to these components addresses the double convexity that occurs with aging. The chief structure that must be preserved with these dissections is the infraorbital nerve that exits the anterior maxilla approximately 1 cm below the rim, centrally. Laterally, the zygomaticofacial and zygomaticotemporal nerves may be encountered. Injury to these smaller sensory nerves may be less consequential than the large infraorbital nerve.

Nerves, Vessels, and Lymphatics

Nerves

In addition to the innervation previously described, the ophthalmic (CN V_1) and maxillary (CN V_2) divisions of the trigeminal nerve carry sensory fibers from the periorbital region. Facial mimetic muscles receive motor innervation from branches of the facial nerve (CN VII). Further details of innervation to periorbital structures are discussed in Chapter 13.

Vessels

The internal and external carotid arteries supply the periorbital region, resulting in rich anastomoses. These anastomoses form two arterial arcades of the upper lid: the marginal and peripheral arcades. The marginal arcade is located about 2 mm away from the lid margin anterior to tarsus. The peripheral arcade is located between the Müller's and levator muscles. During external ptosis repair, the peripheral arcade can be visualized as tortuous vessels on the anterior surface of Müller's muscle and helps distinguish the muscle from levator. Both arcades may significantly bleed during lid surgery. The inferior marginal arcade lies at the inferior tarsal border of the lower lid.

Venous drainage of pretarsal tissues is into the angular and superficial temporal veins. Post-tarsal tissue drains into the deeper veins of the orbit, including the orbital veins, pterygoid plexus, and deep branches of the anterior facial vein. Chapter 13 further describes the vascular supply of the periorbital region.

Lymphatics

The medial and central lower lids have been suggested to drain into the submandibular lymph nodes, the upper lid, medial canthus, and lateral lower lid into the preauricular lymph nodes[6]; however, recent studies show that substantial variability exists. Recent evidence suggests that the preauricular lymph node basin may be responsible for most eyelid lymphatic drainage.[7,8]

References

1. Lucarelli MJ, Khwarg SI, Lemke BN, Kozel JS, Dortzbach RK. The anatomy of midfacial ptosis. Ophthal Plast Reconstr Surg 2000; 16(1):7–22
2. Kikkawa DO, Lemke BN, Dortzbach RK. Relations of the superficial musculoaponeurotic system to the orbit and characterization of the orbitomalar ligament. Ophthal Plast Reconstr Surg 1996; 12(2):77–88
3. Korn BS, Kikkawa DO, Cohen SR. Transcutaneous lower eyelid blepharoplasty with orbitomalar suspension: retrospective review of 212 consecutive cases. Plast Reconstr Surg 2010;125(1):315–323
4. Hoenig JA, Shorr N, Shorr J. The suborbicularis oculi fat in aesthetic and reconstructive surgery. Int Ophthalmol Clin 1997; 37(3):179–191
5. Aiache AE, Ramirez OH. The suborbicularis oculi fat pads: an anatomic and clinical study. Plast Reconstr Surg 1995;95(1):37–42
6. Cook BE Jr, Lucarelli MJ, Lemke BN, et al. Eyelid lymphatics II: a search for drainage patterns in the monkey and correlations with human lymphatics. Ophthal Plast Reconstr Surg 2002;18(2):99–106
7. Nijhawan N, Marriott C, Harvey JT. Lymphatic drainage patterns of the human eyelid: assessed by lymphoscintigraphy. Ophthal Plast Reconstr Surg 2010;26(4):281–285
8. Echegoyen JC, Hirabayashi KE, Lin KY, Tao JP. Imaging of eyelid lymphatic drainage. Saudi J Ophthalmol 2012;26(4):441–443

16 Nasal Cavity and Paranasal Sinuses

Joe Iwanaga, Tsuyoshi Saga, and Koichi Watanabe

Introduction

The nasal cavity is located in the central region of the face and is divided by the nasal septum into a pair of cavities. These two cavities constitute the uppermost portion of the respiratory tract and continue anteriorly to the outer environment via the nares and posteriorly to the nasopharynx via the choanae. The nasal cavity is divided into two regions: the nasal vestibule and the nasal cavity. The nasal vestibule is the initial part of the nasal cavity as entered through the nares; it is lined by epithelium and contains hair (vibrissae) and sebaceous glands. The nasal cavity is the large space following the nasal vestibule and is lined by mucosa. It is divided into four meatuses (the superior, middle, inferior, and common meatus) by three nasal conchae that arise medially from the lateral nasal wall and curve inferiorly. Each meatus with the exception of the common meatus is located inferior to the conchae. The superior meatus is inferior to the superior concha, the middle meatus is inferior to the middle concha, and the inferior meatus is inferior to the inferior concha. The common meatus is the medial portion of the nasal cavity; it is located on both sides of the nasal septum and extends vertically. The nasal cavity is also divided into two regions according to function: the olfactory region and the respiratory region. The olfactory region is located in the upper part of the nasal cavity and is lined by olfactory epithelium, which contains olfactory receptors. The residual part of the nasal cavity has a respiratory function.[1–3]

Roof of the Nasal Cavity

The roof of the nasal cavity comprises the nasal bone, frontal bone, ethmoid bone, and sphenoid bone (**Fig. 16.1**). In the coronal section, it is triangular; the roof is extremely narrow, and the floor is wide. In a sagittal section, its height is greatest in the central region, which contains the cribriform plate of the ethmoid bone; the roof then decreases in height as it progresses in the anterior and posterior directions. The roof is adjacent to three paranasal sinuses: the frontal sinus, sphenoid sinus, and ethmoid sinus.[1–3]

Floor of the Nasal Cavity

The floor of the nasal cavity mainly consists of the superior surface of the maxilla and palatine bone, which together constitute the hard palate (**Fig. 16.2**). The maxilla occupies the anterior two-thirds of the floor, and the palatine bone occupies the posterior one-third. The incisive canal is located in the anterior part of the floor, immediately lateral to the nasal septum. The nasopalatine nerve and terminal end of the greater palatine artery pass through the incisive canal.[1–3]

Medial Wall (Nasal Septum)

The nasal septum forms the medial wall of the nasal cavity and divides the entire nasal cavity into two (**Fig. 16.3**). Histologically, the nasal septum is made up of a cartilaginous part and a bony part. The septal nasal cartilage forms the cartilaginous part and occupies the anterior part of the nasal septum. The posterior part is the bony part and is made up primarily of the vomer in the inferior posterior region and the perpendicular plate of the ethmoid bone in superior region. The most anteroinferior part of the nasal septum, which is positioned more anteroinferior to the edge of the nasal septal cartilage, is called the columella. The nasal septum often curves and shifts to either the right or left and sometimes obstructs the common nasal meatus on one side. The reported frequency of nontraumatic septal deviation is 20% to 58%.[4–6] Guyuron et al[7] classified septonasal deviation into six types: septal tilt, C-shaped deformity (either anteroposterior or cephalocaudal), S-shaped deformity (either anteroposterior or cephalocaudal), and localized deformity. The most common type of deviation is the septal tilt type, in which the septum has no curve but is tilted toward one side in the coronal section. This type is observed in approximately 40% of patients with septonasal deviation. The second most common type is the C-shaped anteroposterior deviation, which occurs in approximately 32% of patients. In this type, the septum exhibits a C-shaped curve in the coronal section. The C-shaped cephalocaudal deviation, in which the septum forms a C shape in the coronal section, is observed in approximately 4% of patients.

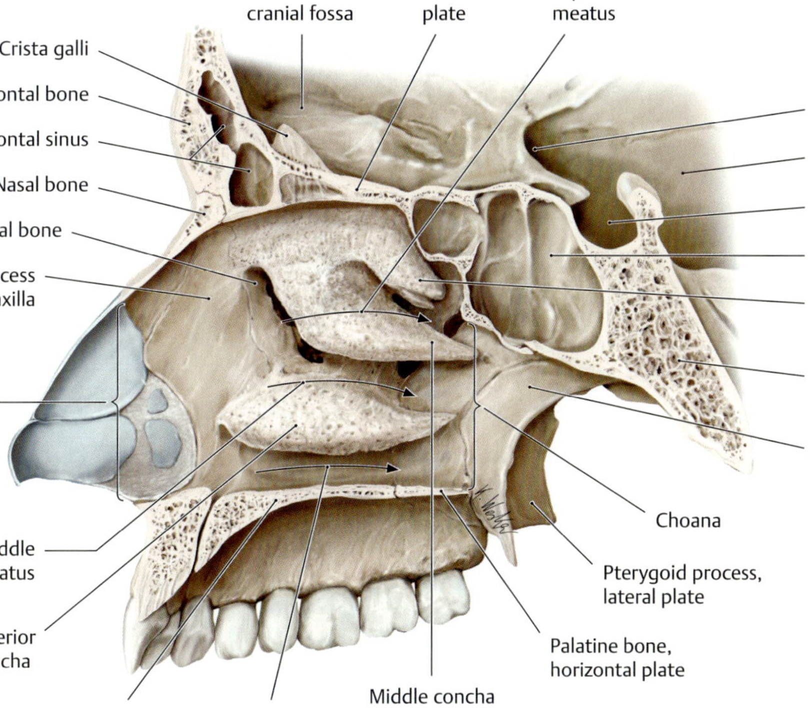

Fig. 16.1 Sagittal section of the nasal cavity (right side). (From THIEME Atlas of Anatomy, Head and Neuroanatomy. © Thieme 2010, Illustration by Karl Wesker.)

Anteroposterior and cephalocaudal S-shaped deviations are observed in 9% and 1% of patients, respectively. Finally, localized deformities are observed in about 14% of patients with septonasal deviation.[7]

An important region of the nasal septum is Kiesselbach's or Little's area, located in the anterior part of the nasal septum. Five arteries supplying the nasal septum anastomose at this point to create an arterial plexus (**Fig. 16.4**). This area is frequently involved in chronic epistaxis, especially in children.

Lateral Wall of the Nasal Cavity

The lateral wall of the nasal cavity is characterized by three conchae that are long in the anteroposterior direction and protrude medially toward the nasal cavity; their free edge rolls inferiorly (**Fig. 16.4**). These conchae are termed the superior nasal concha, middle nasal concha, and inferior nasal concha, and the meatuses below these conchae are called the superior nasal meatus, middle nasal meatus, and inferior nasal meatus, respectively. At the posterior end of these conchae, the three meatuses conflate and meet at the nasopharynx; this point is termed the nasopharyngeal meatus. An atrophic supreme nasal concha is sometimes found above the superior concha.[8] The posterosuperior part of the nasal cavity, which forms the space between the nasal roof and superior concha, is the sphenoethmoidal recess.

Some important structures are located around the middle meatus. The ethmoid bulla, which contains the ethmoid bulla cells of the ethmoid sinus, projects from the medial wall of the orbit. Part of the ethmoid bulla is exposed on the superior part of the lateral wall of the middle nasal meatus. The uncinate process is the thin, bony projection located above the attachment of the inferior nasal concha. The deep groove between the ethmoid bulla and uncinate process is called the semilunar hiatus.

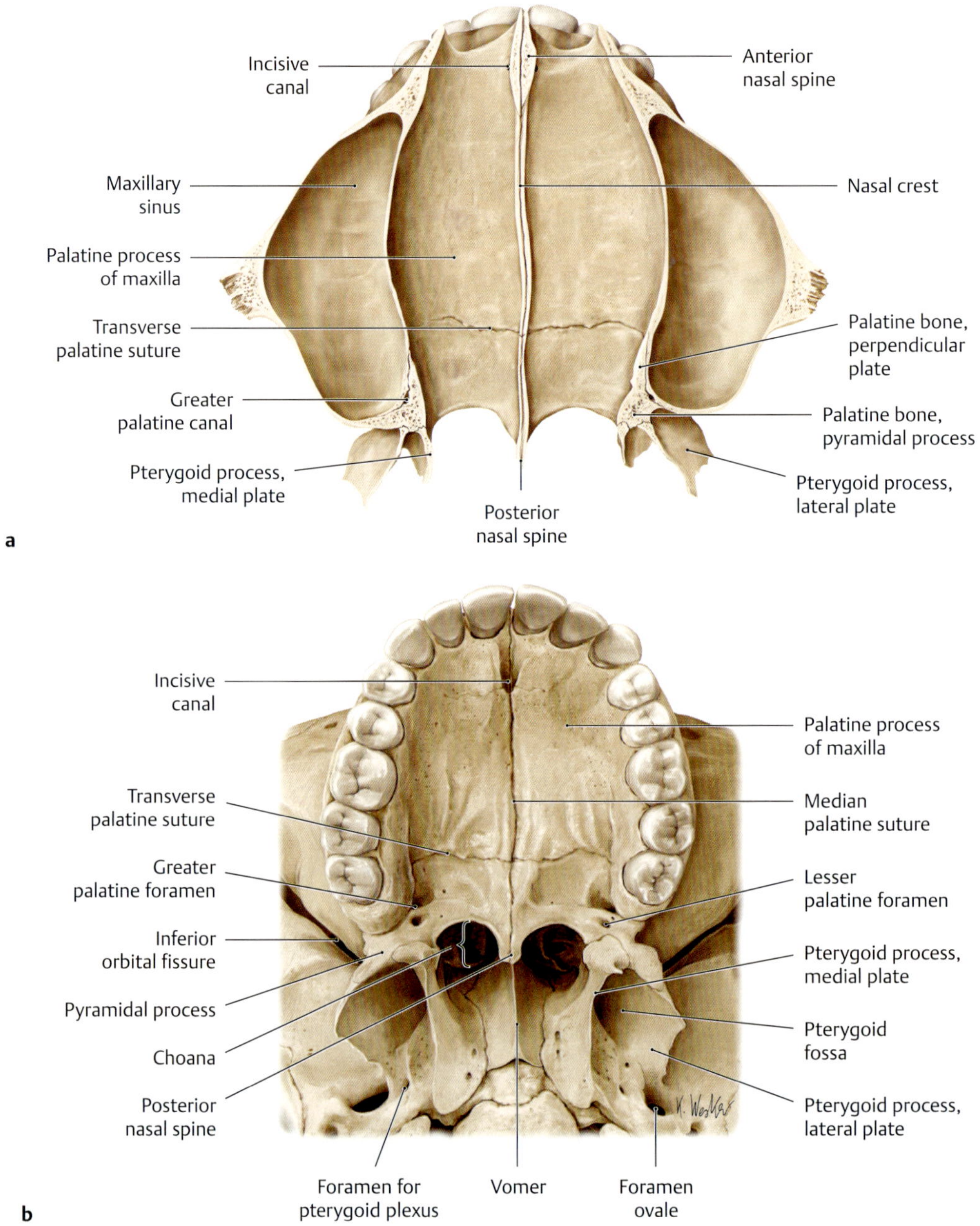

Fig. 16.2 Floor of the nasal cavity. The floor of the nasal cavity comprises mainly the superior surface of the maxilla and palatine bone. In the anterior part of the floor, the incisive canal is observed immediately lateral to the nasal septum. **(a)** Superior view. **(b)** Inferior view. (From THIEME Atlas of Anatomy, Head and Neuroanatomy. © Thieme 2010, Illustrations by Karl Wesker.)

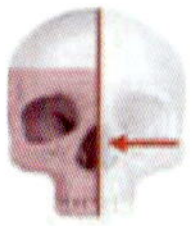

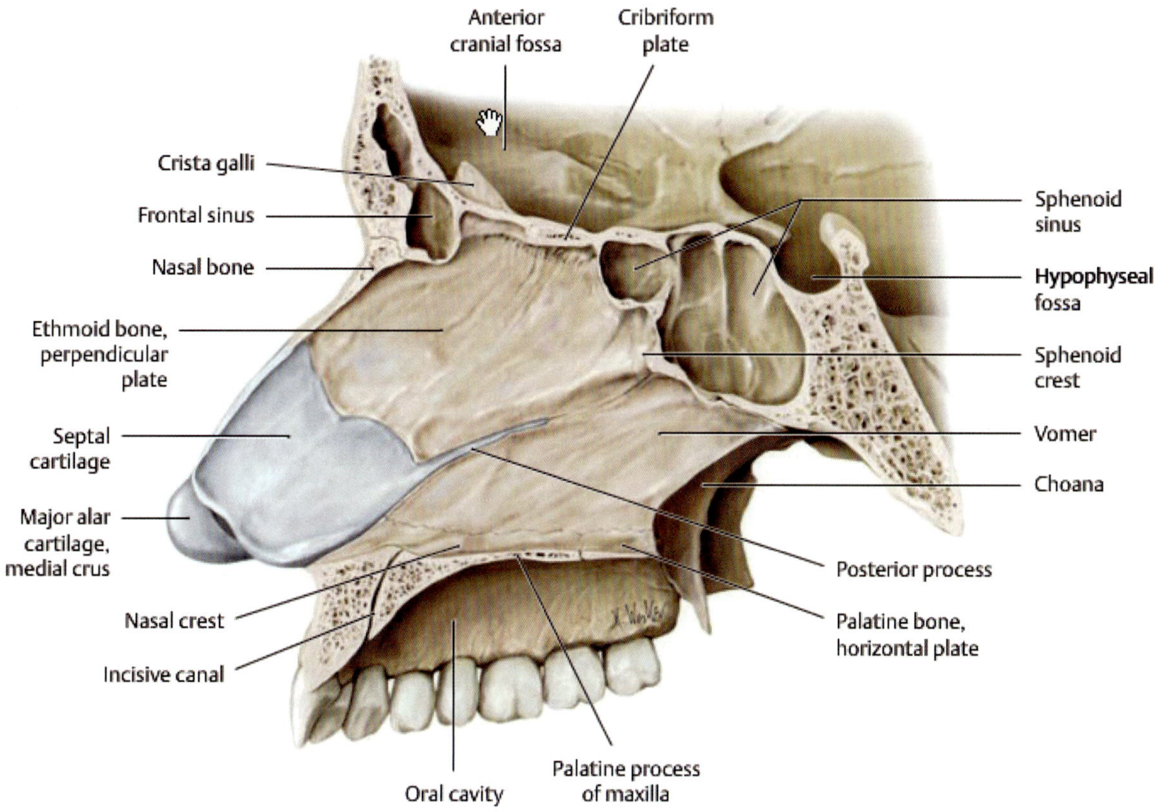

Fig. 16.3 Nasal septum. Parasagittal section viewed from the left side. Histologically, the nasal septum comprises two parts: the cartilaginous part and the bony part. The septal nasal cartilage forms the cartilaginous part and occupies the anterior part of the nasal septum. The posterior part is the bony part and mainly comprises the vomer in the inferior posterior part and the perpendicular plate of the ethmoid bone in the superior part. (From THIEME Atlas of Anatomy, Head and Neuroanatomy. © Thieme 2010, Illustration by Karl Wesker.)

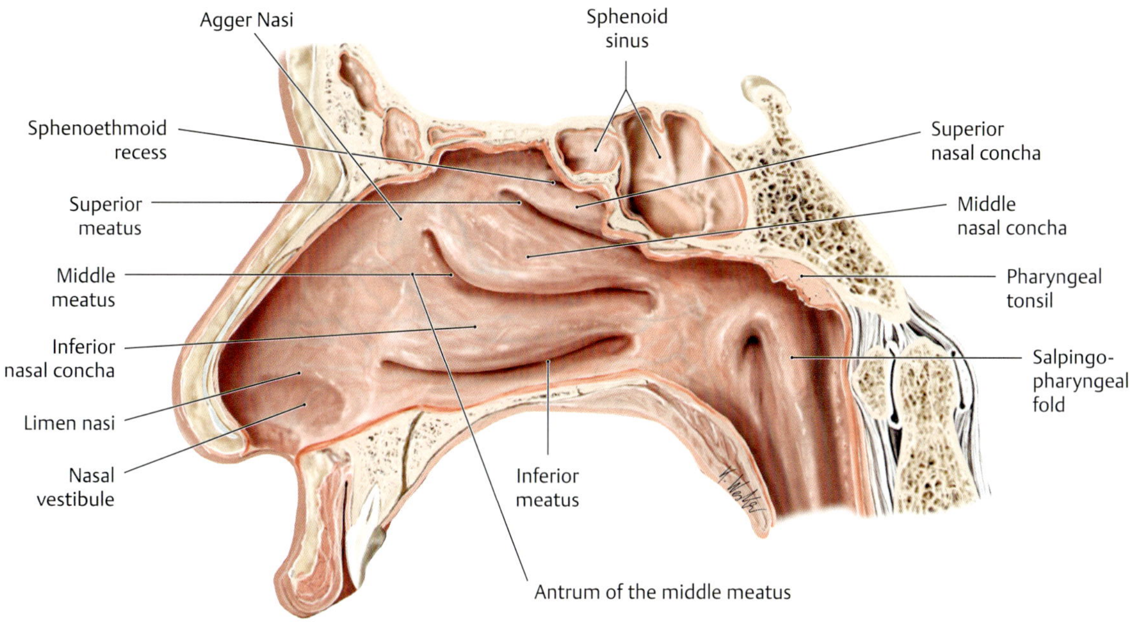

Fig. 16.4 Right lateral wall of the nasal cavity. (Modified from THIEME Atlas of Anatomy, Head and Neuroanatomy. © Thieme, 2010, Illustration by Karl Wesker.)

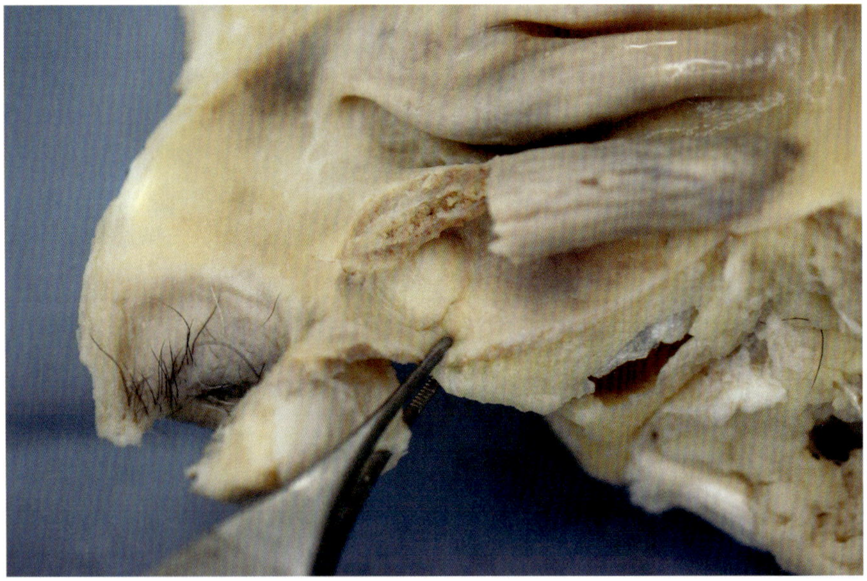

Fig. 16.5 Left inferior nasal meatus (cadaver dissection). Anterior part of the inferior nasal concha was cut. Slitlike opening of the nasolacrimal duct is observed just beneath the attachment of the inferior nasal concha.

The semilunar hiatus is divided into two parts in its anterior region by the projection of the ethmoid bulla: the superior and inferior semilunar hiatus. These structures are involved in connecting the paranasal sinuses. The ethmoidal infundibulum is the funnel-shaped space inside the medial wall of the nasal cavity. It is surrounded by the uncinate process medially and ethmoid bulla laterally and continues to the semilunar hiatus posteriorly. The bony bulge anterior to the anterior end of the middle nasal concha is called the agger nasi. The outward bulge immediately anterior to the middle meatus is called the antrum of the middle meatus.[1–3]

The opening of the nasolacrimal duct is located in the anterosuperior part of the inferior meatus, just below the attachment of the inferior concha (**Fig. 16.5**). The openings of each paranasal sinus and the nasolacrimal duct are described in the section that discusses the paranasal sinuses, nasolacrimal ducts, and their openings into the nasal cavity.

Blood Supply of the Nasal Cavity

The nasal cavity, including both the medial and lateral walls, is supplied by five arteries: the anterior ethmoidal artery, posterior ethmoidal artery, sphenopalatine artery, greater palatine artery, and superior labial artery (**Fig. 16.6**).[2]

Both the anterior ethmoidal artery and posterior ethmoidal artery are branches of the ophthalmic artery. They branch within the orbital cavity, enter the nasal cavity through the ethmoidal bone, and mainly supply the upper region of the cavity. A branch of the anterior ethmoidal artery runs anteriorly,

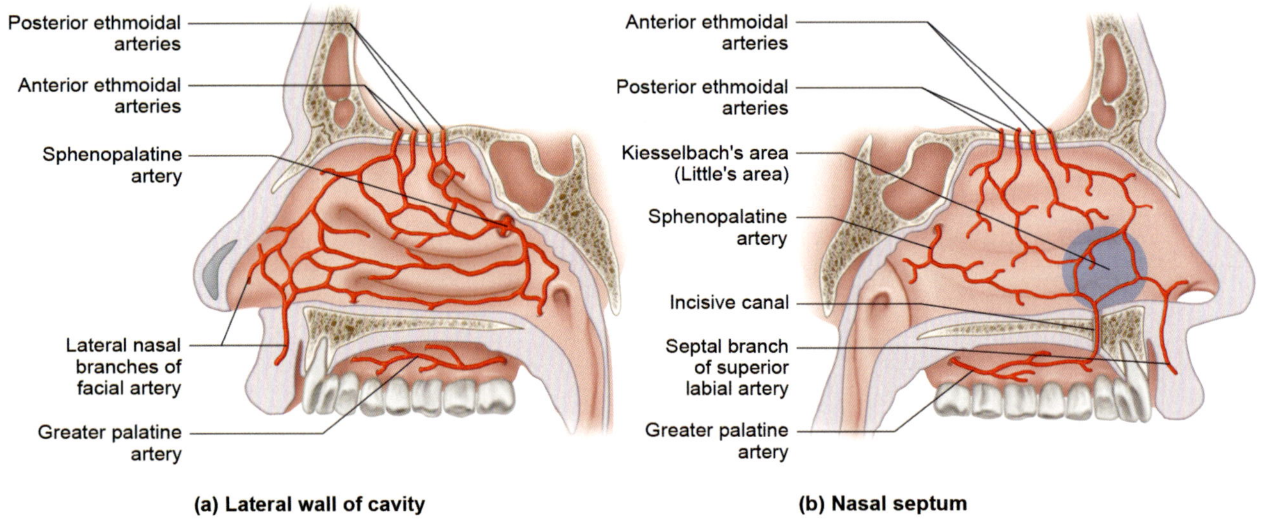

Fig. 16.6 Arterial blood supply of the nasal cavity. **(a)** Arterial blood supply of the nasal septum. Kiesselbach's area is located in the anterior part of the nasal septum. Five arteries supplying the nasal septum anastomose in this region and form the arterial plexus. **(b)** Arterial blood supply of the lateral nasal wall.

pierces the nasal bone, and distributes its blood supply to the nasal epithelium. The main artery supplying the nasal cavity is the sphenopalatine artery. This artery arises from the maxillary artery in the pterygopalatine fossa and enters the nasal cavity through the sphenopalatine foramen, which is located on the lateral wall posterior to the superior nasal meatus. After entering the nasal cavity, the artery gives off various branches. The two main branches course to the posterior part of the nasal septum and posterior part of the lateral nasal wall. The greater palatine artery, which is the terminal branch of the descending palatine artery, enters the nasal cavity through the incisive canal and distributes its blood supply to the lower part of the nasal cavity. The superior labial artery, which is a branch of the facial artery, also enters the nasal cavity through the soft tissue in the upper lip and distributes its blood supply to the anterior and lower parts of the nasal cavity. These arteries anastomose with one another on both the lateral nasal wall and the nasal septum. The region in which these five arteries meet and anastomose at the anterior part of the nasal septum is called Kiesselbach's area (**Fig. 16.6b**).[1–3,9]

Sensory Innervation of the Nasal Cavity

The sensory innervation of the nasal cavity is separated into two areas by the line connecting the anterior nasal spine and the sphenoethmoidal recess (**Fig. 16.7**). The upper area of the nasal cavity contains the anterior ethmoidal nerve, which is a branch of the ophthalmic nerve (first division of the trigeminal nerve). This nerve, accompanied by the anterior ethmoidal artery, enters the nasal cavity through the ethmoid bone and

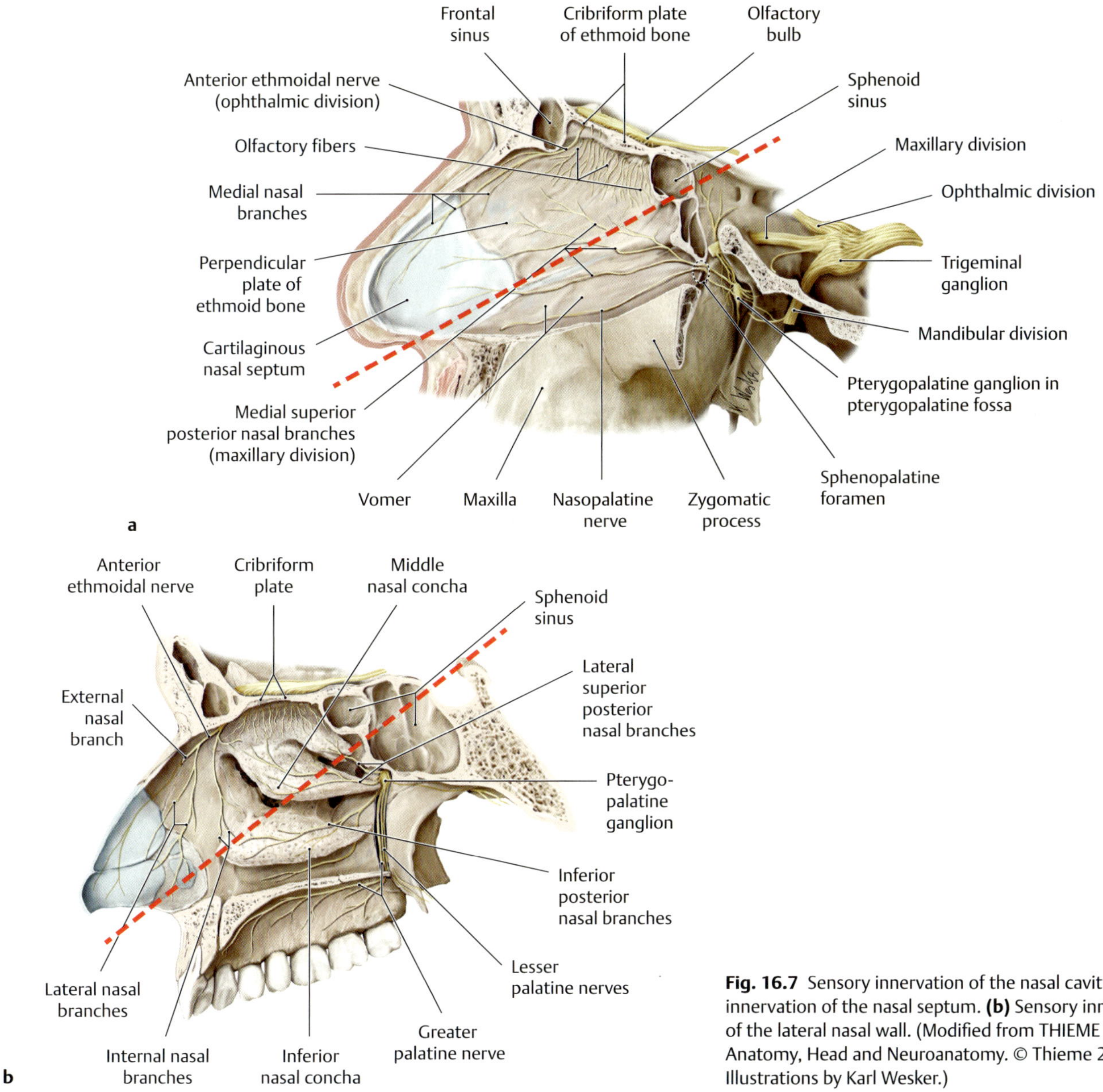

Fig. 16.7 Sensory innervation of the nasal cavity **(a)** Sensory innervation of the nasal septum. **(b)** Sensory innervation of the lateral nasal wall. (Modified from THIEME Atlas of Anatomy, Head and Neuroanatomy. © Thieme 2010, Illustrations by Karl Wesker.)

courses through the anterior and superior parts of the nasal cavity. The lower area of the nasal cavity is innervated by a branch derived from the maxillary nerve (second division of the trigeminal nerve). The nasopalatine nerve and medial superior posterior branch of the greater palatine nerve innervate the nasal septum in this region of the nasal cavity. The medial superior posterior branch innervates the upper half of this area, and the nasopalatine nerve innervates the lower half. The lateral superior posterior nasal branch and inferior posterior nasal branch of the greater palatine nerve innervate the lateral nasal wall in this region of the nasal cavity.

Paranasal Sinuses, Nasolacrimal Ducts, and their Opening to the Nasal Cavity

Frontal Sinus

The frontal sinus is usually divided into two parts around the midline (**Table 16.1, Fig. 16.8**). It is sometimes made up of multiple air cells. The bilateral frontal sinuses extend into the frontal bone and are located posterior to the supraciliary arches of the frontal bone. The sinuses are adjacent to the cranial cavity, orbital cavity, ethmoidal cells, and nasal cavity. The sinuses sometimes extend quite widely, spreading posteriorly and covering the entire orbital roof. Cases of aplasia have also been described. In one report, the sinus was 24.3 mm (range, 5.0–66.0 mm) in height, 29.0 mm (range, 17.0–49.0 mm) wide from the midline coursing in the lateral direction, and 20.5 mm (range, 10.0–46.5 mm) long in the anteroposterior direction.[3] The sinus continues downward and passes through the ethmoid bone on the way to their opening of the nasal cavity. The part of the frontal sinus contained within the ethmoid bone is called the frontal recess, which serves as a drainage pathway of the frontal sinus. The sinuses usually open into the semilunar hiatus or the ethmoidal infundibulum. The drainage pattern depends on the location at which the uncinate process attaches anteriorly. If the uncinate process inserts into the lamina orbitalis (lamina papyracea), the ethmoidal infundibulum ends blindly at the superior position and the frontal recess opens to the middle meatus or suprabullar recess. If the uncinate process inserts at the skull base or middle nasal meatus, the frontal recess opens to the middle meatus via the ethmoidal infundibulum. This blind end is called a terminal cell.

Table 16.1 Paranasal sinuses, nasolacrimal ducts, and their opening to the nasal cavity

Paranasal sinus	Opening
Frontal sinus	Semilunar hiatus (middle meatus), or ethmoidal infundibulum (middle meatus)
Anterior ethmoid sinus	Ethmoidal infundibulum (middle meatus), lateral recess (middle meatus)
Posterior ethmoid sinus	Sphenoethmoidal recess
Sphenoid sinus	Sphenoethmoidal recess
Maxillary sinus	Ethmoidal infundibulum (middle meatus), accessory openings (middle meatus)
Nasolacrimal duct	Anterior edge of the attachment of the niferior nasal concha (inferior meatus)

Surgical Annotation (Frontal Sinus Cranialization for Frontal Fractures and Anterior Skull Base Reconstruction)

Frontal sinus cranialization is required to treat severe frontal fractures that have spread to the posterior table of the frontal sinus with cerebrospinal fluid leakage, as well as to perform

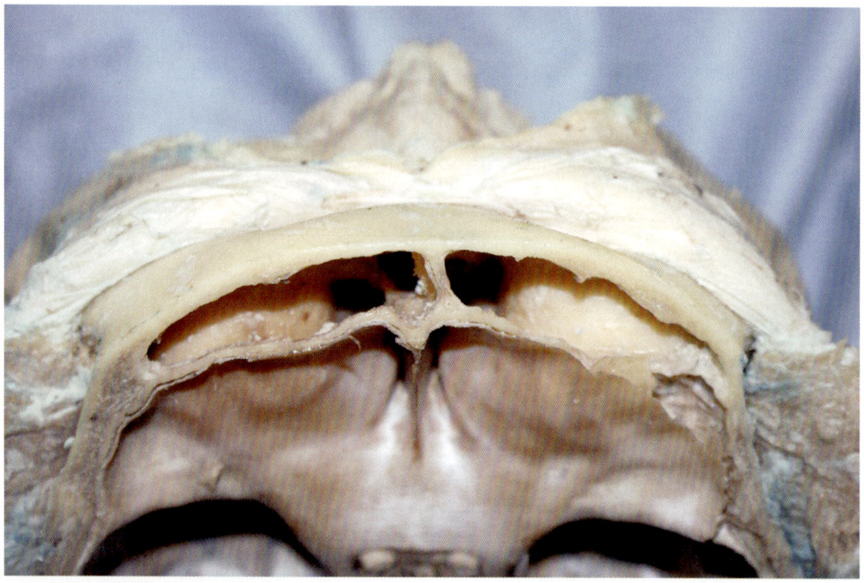

Fig. 16.8 Frontal sinus (cadaver dissection). Calvaria vault and brain were removed.

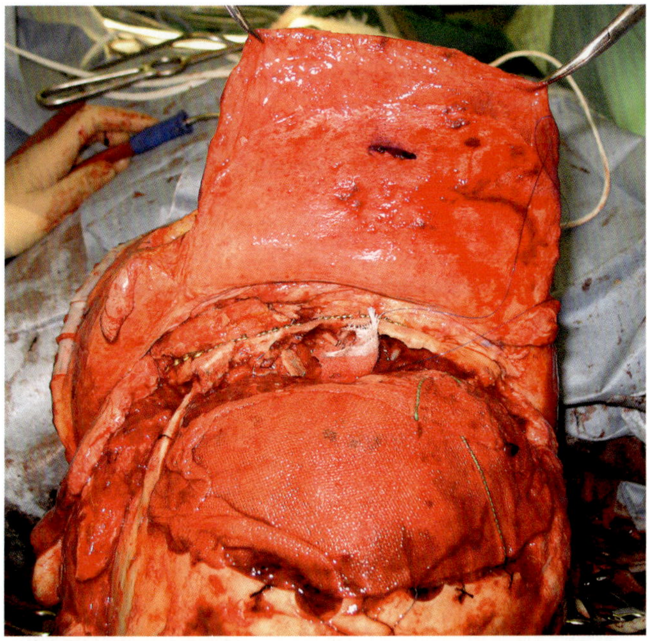

Fig. 16.9 Operative findings of frontal sinus cranialization. Case of a comminuted fracture of the frontal bone. The posterior wall of the frontal sinus and mucosa were removed, and the anterior skull base was reconstructed using a frontal musculoperiosteal flap. In this illustration, the frontal musculoperiosteal flap had just been created.

anterior skull-base tumor resection involving communication between the cranial cavity and nasal cavity (**Fig. 16.9**). Frontal-sinus cranialization allows the frontal sinus to become part of the cranial cavity by removing the posterior table of the frontal sinus. A bicoronal skin incision is usually chosen for the frontal bone approach. A flap for the anterior skull base is then prepared during dissection of the cranial soft tissue. Either a temporal pericranial flap or a frontal pericranial flap is usually selected. On completion of the frontal craniotomy, the posterior table of the frontal sinus and mucosa on the sinus are completely removed. The soft tissue flap is transplanted to the anterior skull base, just above the point at which the frontal sinus meets the frontonasal duct, to disconnect the cranial cavity and nasal cavity.

Frontal sinus cranialization is not needed to treat fractures localized only in the anterior table of the frontal bone. Instead, repositioning and fixation of the fracture is effective. Placement of a drainage tube in the frontonasal duct helps to prevent discharge from pooling in the frontal sinus.[10,11]

Ethmoid Sinus and Sinus around the Frontal Recess

The ethmoid sinus is located in the ethmoidal labyrinth and comprises many small air cells (**Fig. 16.10**). The sinus is adjacent to the medial wall of the orbit, near the orbital plate of the ethmoidal labyrinth laterally and extending to the nasal cavity near the medial wall of the ethmoidal labyrinth medially (**Table 16.2**). The ethmoid sinus usually contains five bony septa called basal lamellae, which separate the sinus in the anteroposterior direction. These lamellae are numbered from anterior to posterior. The first lamella is the septum that continues to the uncinate process. The second lamella arises from the posterior wall of the ethmoidal bulla. The third lamella is the thickest of all five basal lamellae and is uniform in shape. It arises from the middle nasal concha. The fourth lamella continues to the superior nasal concha. Finally, the fifth lamella is the septum supporting the superior nasal concha. The sphenoethmoidal recess is located posterior to the fifth basal lamella (basal lamella of the superior concha).[12] The ethmoid sinus is generally divided by the third basal lamella (basal lamella of the middle turbinate) into two parts: the anterior ethmoid sinus and posterior ethmoid sinus.

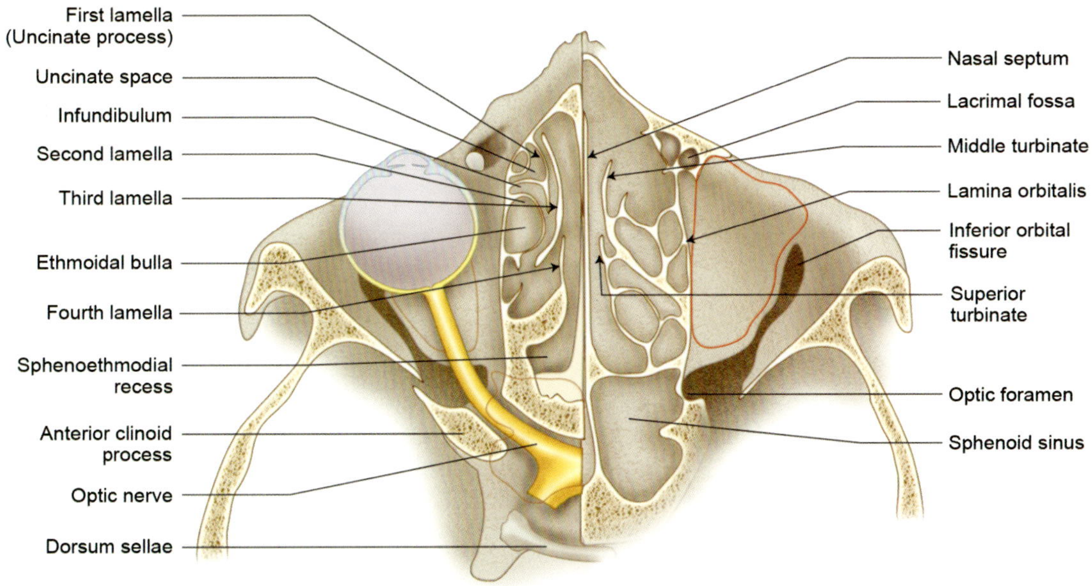

Fig. 16.10 Horizontal section of the right ethmoid sinus.

Table 16.2 Lamellae of the ethmoid sinus

Basal lamellae	Related structure
The first lamella	Uncinate process
The second lamella	Posterior wall of the ethmoidal bulla
The third lamella (basal lamella of the middle turbinate)	Middle nasal concha
The fourth lamella	Superior nasal concha
The fifth lamella	Superior nasal concha

The posterior ethmoid sinus is the air cell that drains to the sphenoethmoidal recess. The posterior sinus sometimes develops within the sphenoid sinus, and the optic nerve and internal carotid artery may thus be exposed within the air cells. These cells constitute the sphenoethmoidal sinus and are sometimes termed Onodi cells.[8] In the anterior ethmoidal sinus, the cells between the second and third basal lamella constitute what is sometimes called the middle ethmoid sinus; however, this term has not been used recently.[9]

The ethmoidal bulla cells, which form the anterior ethmoid sinus, are located relatively posterior to and within the space between the middle nasal concha and uncinate process (i.e., the middle ethmoid sinus). The ethmoidal bulla cells usually open to the lateral recess, which is the space located posterior to the ethmoidal bulla cells. These structures sometimes form the sinus called the lateral recess. The drainage pathway of the frontal sinus passes between the first and second basal lamella and opens to the middle nasal meatus through the ethmoidal infundibulum. The shape of this duct is not a simple tube connecting the frontal sinus and ethmoidal infundibulum but is instead an irregularly shaped cell. Thus, the term *frontonasal duct* is used less frequently today.[9] The air cells located in the superior anterior part of the anterior ethmoidal sinus and surrounding the drainage pathway of the frontal sinus (frontal recess) are called the frontal recess cells. The air cells located around the ethmoidal infundibulum and that open to it are called the infundibular cells.

Anterior to the ethmoidal sinus, some air cells originate from the frontal process of the maxilla. The agger nasi cells, frontal ethmoidal cells, and frontal bulla cells are included in this category. A single agger nasi cell is usually located behind the agger nasi, which is the bulge anterior to the middle nasal concha. By computed tomography, this air cell is detected in more than 90% of cases as the most superficial cell in the coronal section.[13,14] It is an important landmark in the approach to the frontal recess during endoscopic surgery. The air cells facing the lacrimal bone (inferior to the agger nasi cells) are termed the lacrimal cells.

Surgical Annotation

Causes of Bleeding During Ethmoid Sinus Surgery

When performing treatments involving the medial orbital wall, such as fracture repair (medial orbital wall fractures, etc.), tumor resection, or ethmoidal sinus surgery, unexpected massive bleeding sometimes occurs (**Fig. 16.11**). This bleeding is usually caused by damage to the anterior ethmoidal artery or posterior ethmoidal artery. These arteries are branches of the ophthalmic artery, which enters the orbital cavity along with the optic nerve through the optic canal. The artery and nerve then penetrate the medial orbital wall through the anterior and posterior ethmoidal foramens, respectively, which are located on the su-

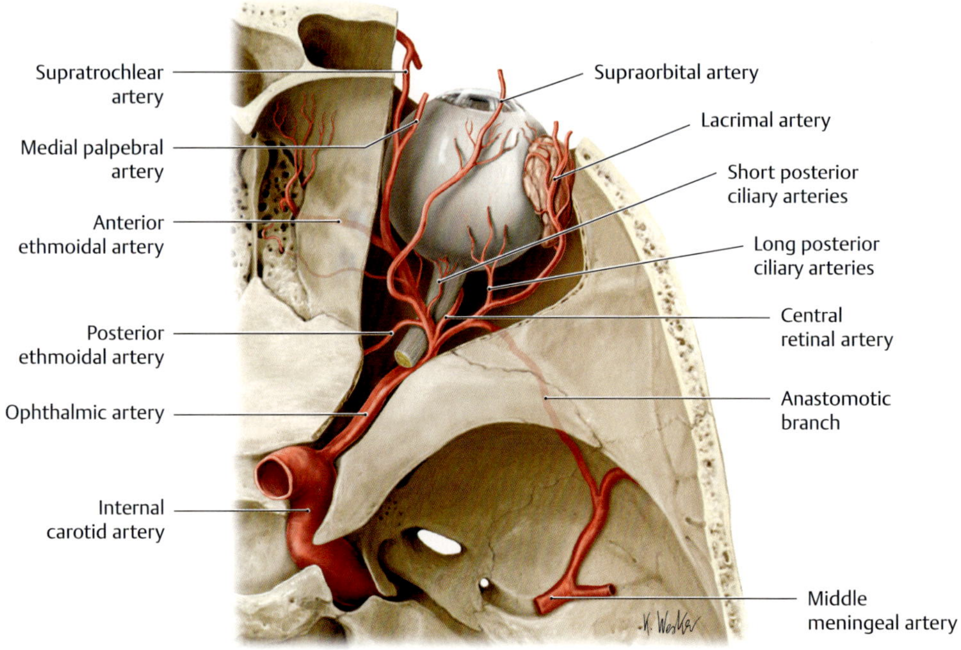

Fig. 16.11 Anterior and posterior ethmoidal arteries. (From THIEME Atlas of Anatomy, Head and Neuroanatomy. © Thieme 2010, Illustration by Karl Wesker).

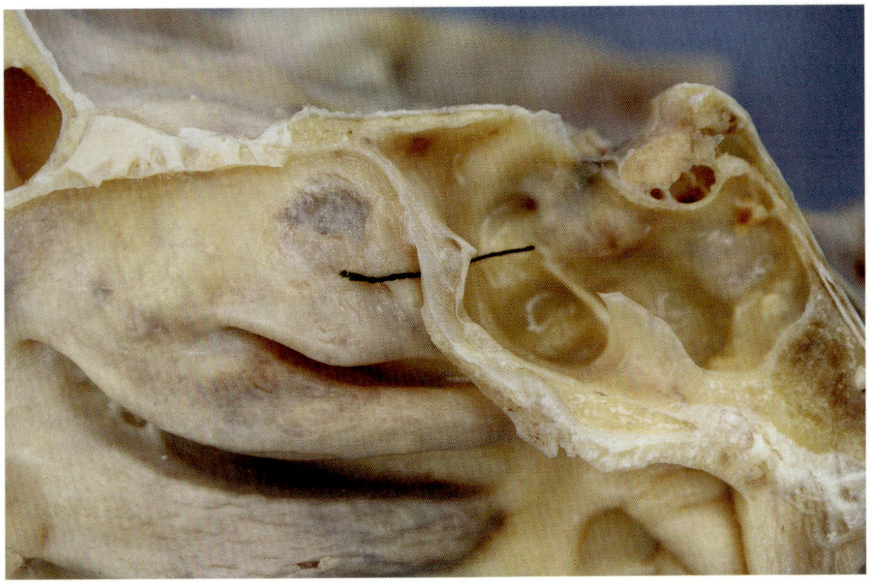

Fig. 16.12 Sagittal section of the right sphenoid sinus. The black string indicates the opening of the sphenoid sinus.

perior part of the medial orbital wall. The anterior ethmoidal artery supplies the anterior and middle ethmoidal air cells and the frontal sinus. After entering the cranium, this artery branches into the meningeal branch and finally enters the nasal cavity through the ethmoidal foramen to supply the nasal cavity. The terminal branch of this artery emerges from the dorsum of the nose between the nasal bone and the lateral cartilage. The posterior ethmoidal artery supplies the posterior ethmoidal air cell after leaving the orbit through the posterior ethmoidal canal and then branches into the meningeal branch after entering the cranium; it finally enters and supplies the nasal cavity.[15]

Sphenoid Sinus

The sphenoid sinus is located posterior to the ethmoidal air cells and is positioned within the body of the sphenoid, forming the posterior roof of the nasal cavity (**Fig. 16.12**). It contains a bony septum that divides the bilateral sinuses. In most cases, the bony septum deviates from the midline. The sinus opens to the sphenoethmoidal recess (the space superior and posterior to the superior nasal concha) through the ostium opening on the anterior wall of the sphenoid sinus. It lies adjacent to important structures in the cranial cavity, including the optic nerve, optic chasm, pituitary gland, internal carotid artery, and cavernous sinus.[3,16]

Maxillary Sinus

The maxillary sinuses are located within the maxilla and have the largest capacity of all the paranasal sinuses (**Fig. 16.13**). They mainly open to the middle nasal meatus at the ethmoidal infundibulum. This opening is called the natural ostium. The maxillary sinuses have one or more accessory openings at their fontanelle in the middle nasal meatus. The shape of these sinuses

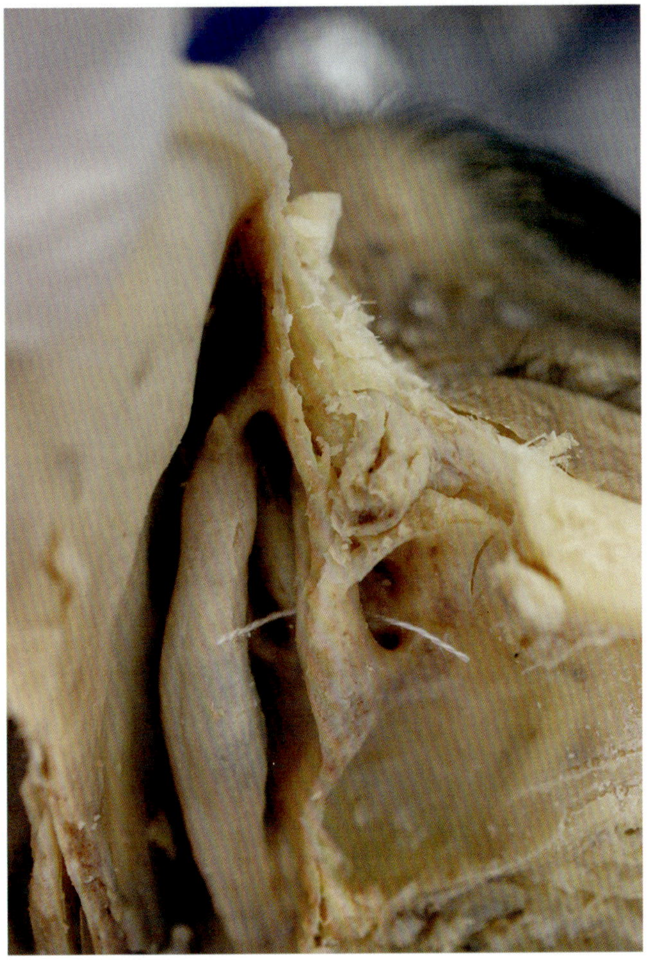

Fig. 16.13 Maxillary sinus (left maxillary sinus, inferior view). The white string indicates the natural ostium of the left maxillary sinus (posterolateral view, after removal of the floor of the maxilla and nasal floor).

is pyramidal, their base is the lateral wall of the nasal cavity, and their apex extends to the zygomatic process. Their roof forms the orbital floor and extends medially to the inferior orbital canal.[1,2] The maxillary sinuses may have septa that divide the sinuses into intercommunicating spaces. The size of these sinuses varies from 9.5 to 20.0 ml; the average is about 15.0 ml.[3] Some important structures are located in the maxillary sinuses. The nasolacrimal duct is located in the anterior part of the medial wall of this sinus. The infraorbital nerve, a branch of the maxillary nerve, passes through a bony wall (the infraorbital canal) in the roof of the maxillary sinus to the maxillary skin. The maxillary nerve gives off three branches: the posterior superior; middle superior; and anterior superior alveolar nerves, which innervate the maxillary teeth. The posterior superior alveolar nerve arises just before the maxillary nerve that enters the infraorbital canal, the middle superior alveolar nerve from the posterior part of the infraorbital canal, and the anterior superior alveolar nerve from just before the nerve coming out from the canal. These alveolar nerves run in the bony wall of the maxillary sinus; infratemporal surface (posterior superior), lateral (middle superior), and anterior surface (anterior superior), respectively; communicate with each other; and innervate the teeth. In the posterior region, the maxilla is contiguous with the lateral pterygoid plate and forms the pterygomaxillary fissure. The pterygopalatine fossa is located inside the fissure and gives off the terminal branches of the maxillary nerve and maxillary artery. The descending palatine artery and greater palatine nerve, which course to the palate, pass through the greater palatine canal in the inferior part of the fossa.[1] This neurovascular complex is extremely important in Le Fort I osteotomy.

Surgical Annotation (Le Fort I Osteotomy and Maxillary Fracture)

The opportunity to treat the inferior meatus surgically (e.g., by LeFort I osteotomy or maxillary sinus drainage for maxillary fractures) sometimes arises in the field of plastic surgery. In such cases, the surgeon must pay attention to two important structures in the inferior nasal meatus. One is the opening of the nasolacrimal duct, which is located at the anterior end of the inferior nasal meatus just below the inferior nasal concha, and the other is the descending palatine artery, which is located within the greater palatine canal, inferior to the maxillary sinus. Obstruction of the nasolacrimal duct may rarely occur after maxillary surgery, usually because of secondary inflammation or sometimes direct injury of the valve of Hasner.[17,18] To open the maxillary sinus, drainage to the inferior meatus also should make enough rearward to the valve of Hasner. The descending palatine artery (**Fig. 16.14**) poses a potential risk of massive

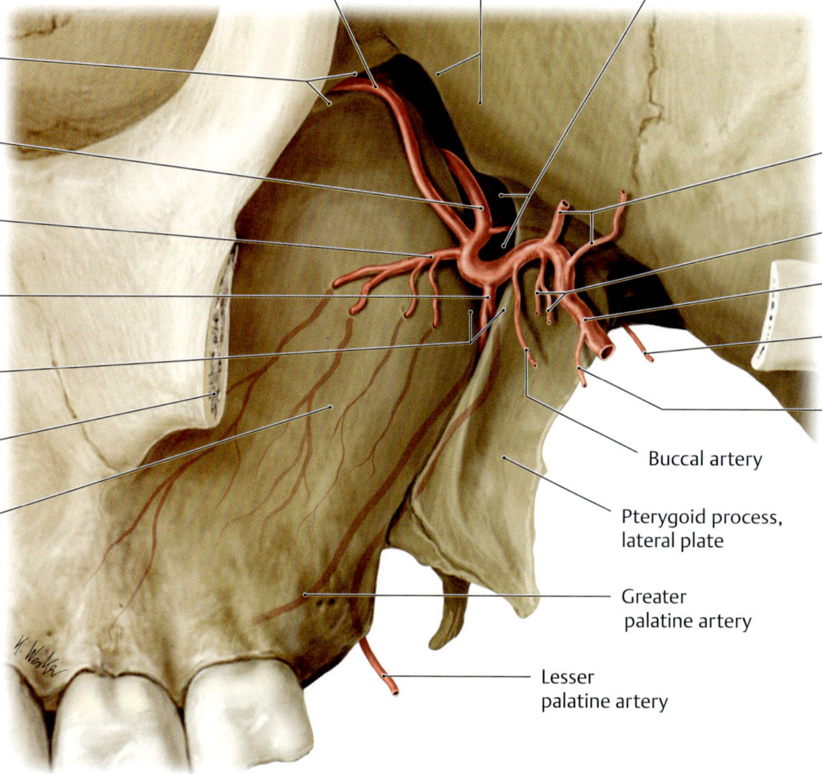

Fig. 16.14 Descending palatine artery. Left lateral view. The descending palatine artery arises from the maxillary artery in the pterygopalatine fossa and descends in the greater palatine canal. The descending palatine artery becomes the greater palatine artery after emerging from the greater palatine foramen at the palate. (From THIEME Atlas of Anatomy, Head and Neuroanatomy. © Thieme 2010, Illustration by Karl Wesker.)

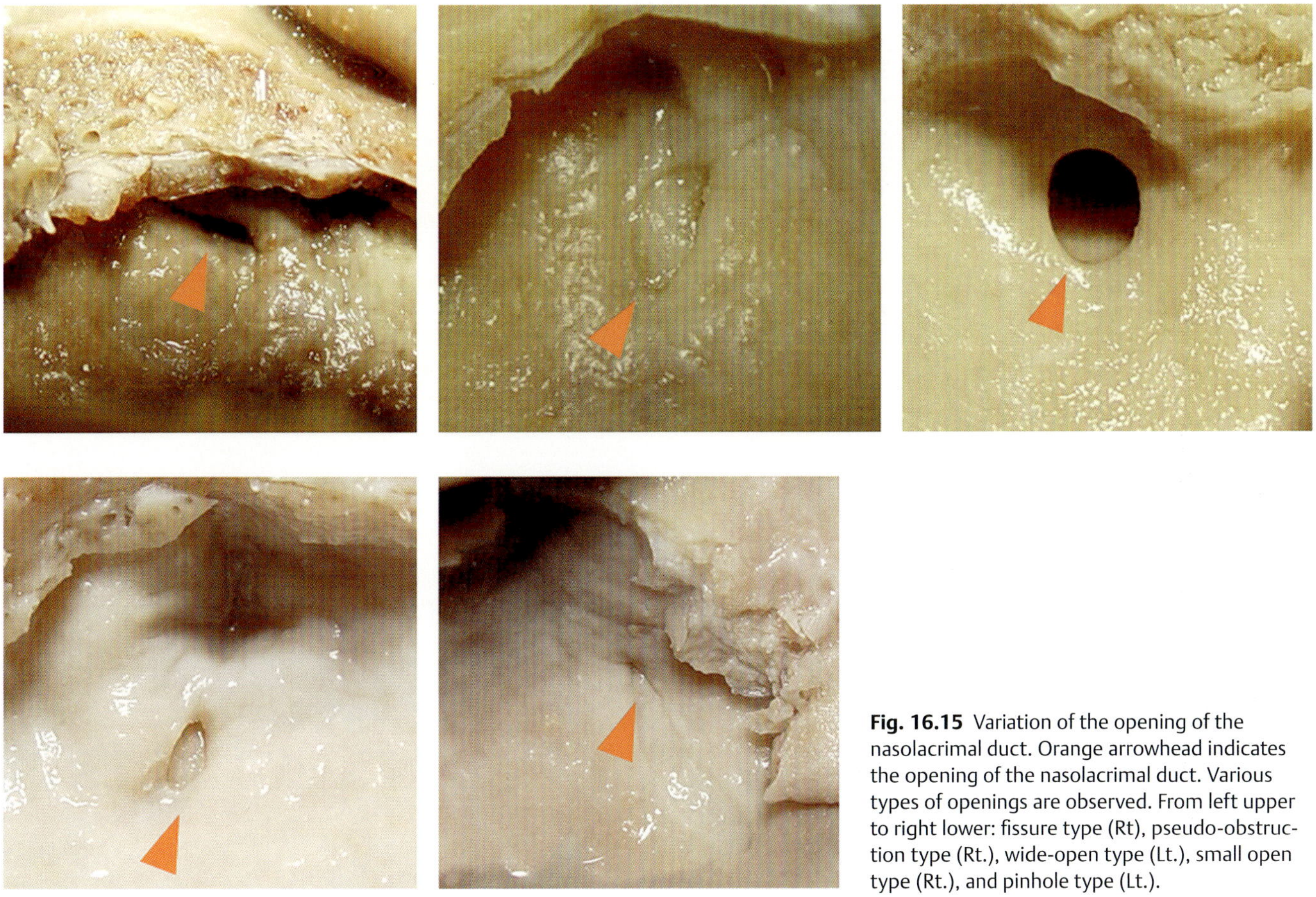

Fig. 16.15 Variation of the opening of the nasolacrimal duct. Orange arrowhead indicates the opening of the nasolacrimal duct. Various types of openings are observed. From left upper to right lower: fissure type (Rt), pseudo-obstruction type (Rt.), wide-open type (Lt.), small open type (Rt.), and pinhole type (Lt.).

bleeding during Le Fort I osteotomy. To avoid damage to the descending palatine artery, osteotomy performed using a chisel or bone saw should be stopped before reaching the artery, and blunt down fracture to the residual posterior part of the maxilla should be performed. Li et al[19] reported that the average distance from the piriform rim to the descending artery was 35.4 mm (range, 31.0–42.0 mm). They found that the greater palatine foramen was located between the second and third molars and that the average distance between the pterygomaxillary fissure and greater palatine foramen was 6.6 mm (range. 2.0–10.0 mm).[19]

Opening of Nasolacrimal Duct (Valve of Hasner)

The nasolacrimal duct opens obliquely on the lateral nasal wall of the inferior nasal meatus, around the anterior edge of the attachment of the inferior nasal concha (**Fig. 16.15**). In our cadaver dissection study,[20] the opening of the nasolacrimal duct was located 36.60 ± 3.92 mm from the anterior edge of the nostril, 19.20 ± 3.21 mm horizontally from the anterior edge of the nostril, and 14.10 ± 3.76 mm vertically from the nasal floor. The shape of the valve reportedly ranges from a round to slit shape, and the frequency of the shape varies among reports. Schaeffer[21] reported that an oval shape was most frequent among Europeans. In contrast, Orhan et al[22] reported a high frequency of the vertical sulcus type. In our study, the fissure type was observed most frequently (**Table 16.3**).[20]

Table 16.3 Variations of the opening of the nasolacrimal duct

Opening of the nasolacrimal duct	Frequency (%)
Wide opening type	17
Small opening type	15
Pinhole type	14
Fissure type	32
Pseudo-obstruction type	22
Obstruction type	0

Source: Tanaka K. An anatomical study of the inferior nasal meatus region of the human nasolacrimal duct. Kurume Igakkai Zasshi 2008;71:38–52.

References

1. Clemente CD, ed. Gray's Anatomy. Philadelphia: Lea & Febiger; 1985
2. Moore KL, Dalley AF, Agur AMR. Clinically Oriented Anatomy. Philadelphia: Lippincott Williams & Wilkins; 2013
3. Lang J. Clinical Anatomy of the Nose, Nasal Cavity and Paranasal Sinuses. New York: Thieme; 1989
4. Blaugrund SM. Nasal obstruction: The nasal septum and concha bullosa. Otolaryngol Clin North Am 1989;22(2):291–306
5. Earwaker J. Anatomic variants in sinonasal CT. Radiographics 1993;13(2):381–415
6. Pérez-Piñas I, Sabaté J, Carmona A, Catalina-Herrera CJ, Jiménez-Castellanos J. Anatomical variations in the human paranasal sinus region studied by CT. J Anat 2000;197(Pt 2):221–227
7. Guyuron B, Uzzo CD, Scull H. A practical classification of septonasal deviation and an effective guide to septal surgery. Plast Reconstr Surg 1999;104(7):2202–2209, discussion 2210–2212
8. Janfaza P, Nadol JB, Galla RJ, Fabian RL, Montgomery WW, eds. Surgical Anatomy of the Head and Neck. Cambridge, MA: Harvard University Press; 2011
9. Stammberger HR, Kennedy DW; Anatomic Terminology Group. Paranasal sinuses:anatomic terminology and nomenclature. Ann Otol Rhinol Laryngol Suppl 1995;167:7–16
10. Ruggiero FP, Zender CA. Frontal sinus cranialization. Oper Tech Otolaryngol—Head Neck Surg 2010;21(2):143–146
11. Strong EB, Pahlavan N, Saito D. Frontal sinus fractures: a 28-year retrospective review. Otolaryngol Head Neck Surg 2006;135(5):774–779
12. Kim SS, Lee JG, Kim KS, Kim HU, Chung IH, Yoon JH. Computed tomographic and anatomical analysis of the basal lamellas in the ethmoid sinus. Laryngoscope 2001;111(3):424–429
13. Wormald PJ. Surgery of the frontal recess and frontal sinus. Rhinology 2005;43(2):82–85
14. Wormald PJ. Three-dimensional building block approach to understanding the anatomy of the frontal recess and frontal sinus. Oper Tech Otolaryngol—Head Neck Surg 2006;17(1):2–5
15. Erdogmus S, Govsa F. The anatomic landmarks of ethmoidal arteries for the surgical approaches. J Craniofac Surg 2006;17(2):280–285
16. Kim HU, Kim SS, Kang SS, Chung IH, Lee JG, Yoon JH. Surgical anatomy of the natural ostium of the sphenoid sinus. Laryngoscope 2001;111(9):1599–1602
17. Osguthorpe JD, Calcaterra TC. Nasolacrimal obstruction after maxillary sinus and rhinoplastic surgery. Arch Otolaryngol 1979;105(5):264–266
18. Serdahl CL, Berris CE, Chole RA. Nasolacrimal duct obstruction after endoscopic sinus surgery. Arch Ophthalmol 1990;108(3):391–392
19. Li KK, Meara JG, Alexander A Jr. Location of the descending palatine artery in relation to the Le Fort I osteotomy. J Oral Maxillofac Surg 1996;54(7):822–827
20. Tanaka K. An anatomical study of the inferior nasal meatus region of the human nasolacrimal duct. Kurume Igakkai Zasshi 2008;71:38–52(in Japanese)
21. Schaeffer JP. Types of ostia nasolacrimalis in man and their genetic significance. Am J Anat 1912;13:183–192
22. Orhan M, Ikiz ZAA, Saylam CY. Anatomical features of the opening of the nasolacrimal duct and the lacrimal fold (Hasner's valve) for intranasal surgery: a cadaveric study. Clin Anat 2009;22(8):925–931

17 External Nose

Hideaki Rikimaru

Introduction

The nose is located in the center of the face and is one of the most impressive features to other people. The shape is a three-dimensionally complex and differs between individual, sex, and race. This complex structure is formed by skin, soft tissue, bone, cartilage, and mucosa, which differ in composition depending on the region of the nose. The vascular supply and innervation of the nose are also intricate. Several vessels and nerves are distributed within the relatively small space of the nose. Thus, it is essential to have a good understanding of the anatomy of the nose for any surgical procedure.

External Anatomy of the Nose

In the lateral view of the skeleton, the uppermost part of the nasal bone connects to the frontal bone by the nasofrontal suture. The midline point on the suture is defined as the *nasion*. The depressed area below the nasion is the nasal root, where the most depressed part is usually located slightly superior to the medial canthal tendon of the eyelid. On the skin, the most depressed point is usually more cranial to the point directly over the bony nasal root because the subcutaneous fat and the mimetic muscles are thick in this area. Heading downward along the nasal ridge, the long straight part protruding anteriorly is the nasal dorsum. The nasal dorsum is narrowest at the intercanthal line, which is the line connecting the bilateral medial canthal tendons that becomes wider as you move down the nose. The junctional point between the upper lateral cartilage and lower lateral cartilage is the supratip breakpoint, which is the inferior border of the nasal dorsum. Below the supratip breakpoint, the highest part of the nose is the nasal tip, and the highest point is the pronasale. The inferior border of the nasal tip is the columellar breakpoint, which is the point corresponding to the angle between the medial crus and middle crus of the lower lateral cartilage. The area superior to the tip defining point in the nasal tip is the supratip lobule and inferior to the point is the infratip lobule. The columella is the inferior margin of the nasal septum, ending in the subnasale (**Fig. 17.1**).

In the inferior view, the shape of the nostril and the length of the columella affect the general shape of the lower nose. In general, the length between the bilateral alar creases and the length from the subnasale to the pronasale are equal. Furthermore, the ratio between the length of the height of the nostril and the length of the infratip lobule is 2:1[1]; however, the shape and proportion of this area vary by race (**Fig. 17.2**).[2,3]

Skin

The characteristics of the nasal skin are distinctly different between its upper and lower parts. The upper part of the skin tends to be thin and mobile. Some wrinkles can be observed during changes in facial expression. Conversely, the skin in the lower part of the nose is thicker and tends to fix to underlying structures. As a result, wrinkles are not observed during changes in facial expression in this area. The skin also plays a role in forming the three-dimensionally complicated nasal structure with the underlying cartilage. The lower part of the skin usually has many exocrine glands, namely, sebaceous and sweat glands. Regarding the thickness of the nasal skin, Lesserd and Daniel reported that it is thickest at the nasofrontal groove at approximately 1.25 mm and thinnest at the rhinion at approximately 0.6 mm.[1,4] This means that the skin is the thinnest in the middle area of the nose (around the rhinion), and becomes thicker above and below this point. The thickness of the skin changes by region with the skin in the columella and along the alar margin usually being thinner.[1] At the nostril apex, there is a soft triangle where the nostril lining skin and lobule skin touch without any subcutaneous structure (**Fig. 17.2**).

Subcutaneous Layer

Lesserd and Daniel also reported that four layers are observed in the soft tissue structures under the skin: the superficial fatty panniculus; the fibromuscular layer; the deep fatty layer; and the periosteum (or perichondrium) (**Fig. 17.3**). The superficial fatty panniculus is the layer consisting of subdermal adipose tissue and interlacing vertical fibrous septa. This layer presents throughout the nose but is concentrated in the glabellar and supratip regions. The fibromuscular layer consists of nasal muscles

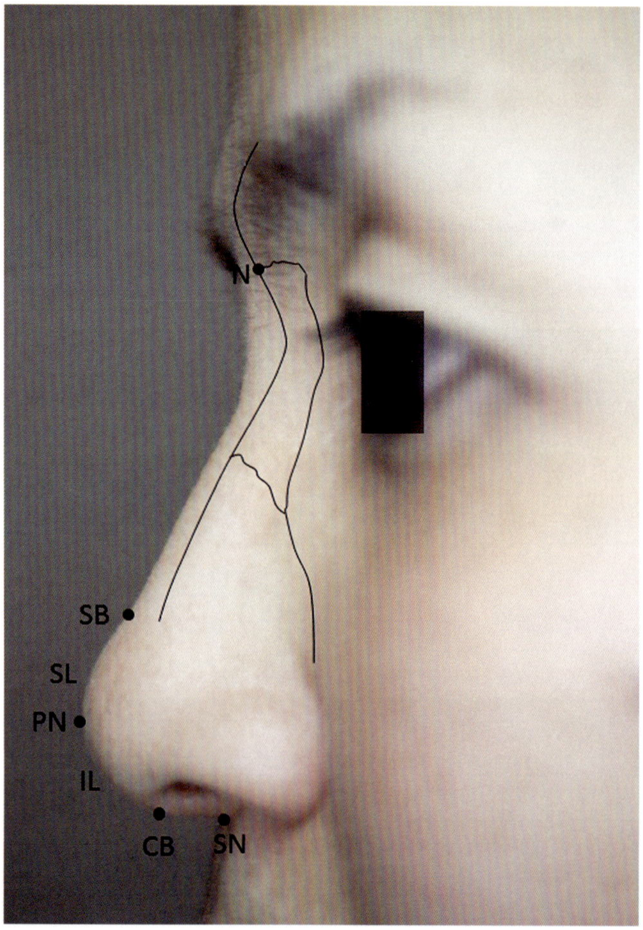

Fig. 17.1 The lateral view of the external nose. CB, Columella breakpoint; IL, infratip lobule; N, nasion; PN, pronasale; SB, supratip breakpoint; SL, supratip lobule; SN, subnasale.

and fibrous layers covering the muscles from superficial and deep aspects. This layer is defined as the nasal superficial musculoaponeurotic system (SMAS) and is continuous with the facial SMAS. The deep fatty layer consists of the loose areolar fat without fibrous septa, which gives mobility to nasal skin.[5]

Muscle Layer of the Nose

The musculature of the nose is categorized functionally into four groups: the elevators; depressors; compressors; and dilators (**Table 17.1**).[1,4,6] The elevators include the procerus, levator labii superioris alaeque nasi, and anomalus nasi muscles. These muscles have a role in lifting and shortening the nose, and also in opening the nasal valve. The depressors include the alar part of the nasalis muscle and depressor septi muscle. These muscles lengthen the nose and dilate the nostril. The compressor includes the transverse part of the nasalis muscle. This muscle also works to lengthen the nose and narrow the nostril. The dilators consist of the dilator naris anterior and posterior muscles and work to dilate the nostril. The zygomatic branch of the facial nerve innervates each of these muscles.

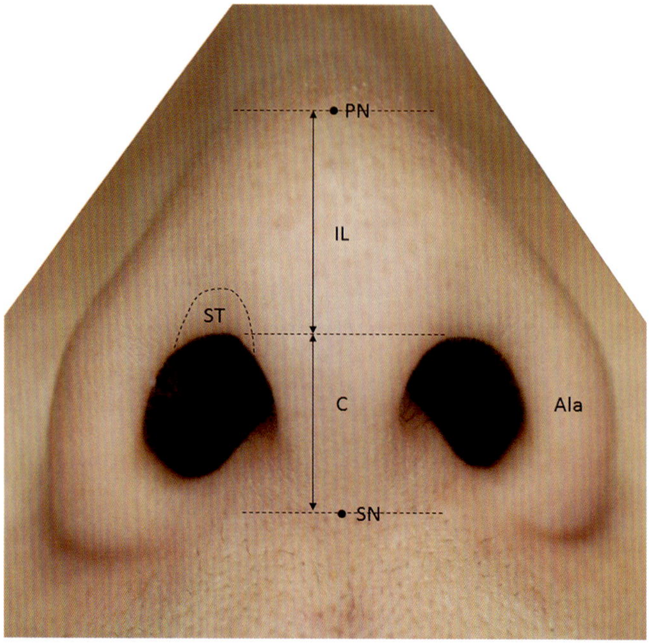

Fig. 17.2 The inferior view of the external nose. C, Columella; IL, infratip lobule; PN, pronasale; SN, subnasale; ST, soft triangle.

Blood Supply of the Nose

Four arteries originating either from the internal carotid or from the external carotid arteries are the main supply for the external nose (**Table 17.2**). The arteries originating from the internal carotid artery are the dorsal nasal and anterior ethmoidal arteries, both of which are branches of the ophthalmic artery. Two arteries, the angular artery and superior labial artery, originate from the facial artery, one of the main branches of the external carotid artery.

The dorsal nasal artery emerges from the orbital cavity to the subcutaneous layer above the medial canthal tendon, which runs obliquely inferomedially and distributes in the upper dorsal part of the nose. The anterior ethmoidal artery, which is also a branch of the ophthalmic artery, emerges from the base between the nasal bone and the lateral nasal cartilage and runs downward to the nasal tip. The angular artery, which is a continuation of the facial artery, has a number of branches, such as the lateral nasal branch to the lower lateral nose. The superior labial artery primarily supplies the nostril sill and columella.

The venous drainage of the nose is carried out by veins with the same name as the arteries they travel with. These finally drain into the facial vein or the cavernous sinus via the ophthalmic vein.

The arterial and venous networks distribute in or above the mimetic muscle layer (fibromuscular layer; nasal SMAS layer). Then, the desirable layer of dissection of the nose is under the fibromuscular layer to preserve the blood circulation of the nasal skin, prevent bleeding, and to reduce edema after surgery. Especially, open rhinoplasty requires extremely accurate treatment about dissection of the layers.

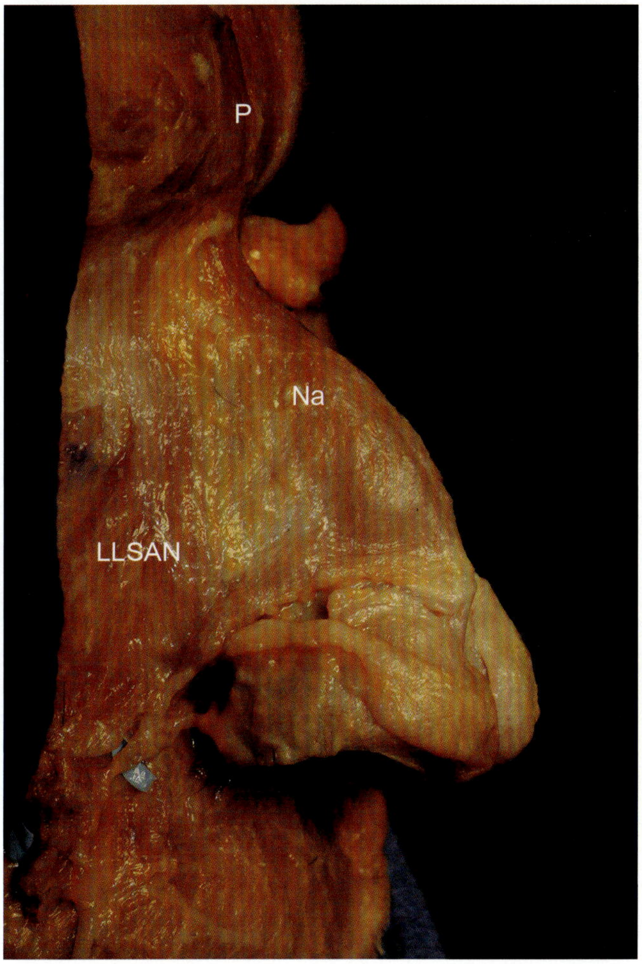

a

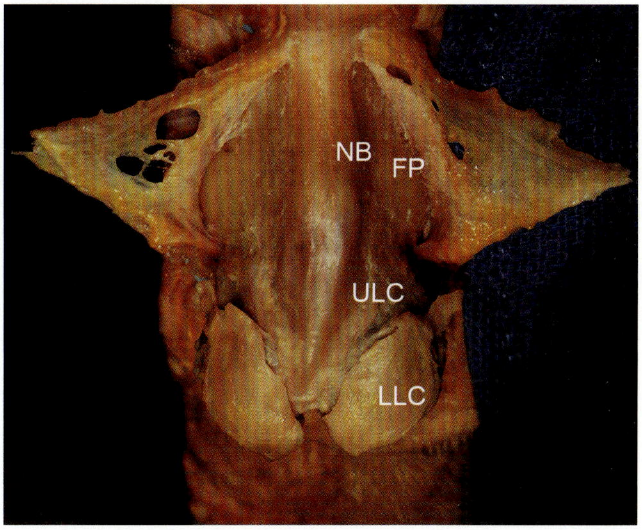

b

Fig 17.3 Soft tissue layers of the external nose. **(a)** The external nose is dissected under the subcutaneous layer. The fibromuscular layer is exposed. LLSAN, Levator labii superioris alaeque nasi, Na, Nasalis; P, Procerus. **(b)** The fibromuscular layer and periosteum are dissected and turned over to the lateral sides. Bony and cartilaginous structures are exposed. FP, Frontal process of the maxilla; LLC, lower lateral cartilage; NB, nasal bone; ULC, upper lateral cartilage.

Table 17.1 Muscles of the nose

Group	Action	Muscles
Elevators	Lifting and shortening the nose	Procerus Levator labii superioris alaeque nasi Anomalous nasi
Depressors	Lengthening the nose and dilating the nostril	Alar part of the nasalis Depressor septi
Compressors	Narrowing the nostril	Transverse part of the nasalis
Dilators	Dilating the nostril	Dilator naris anterior and posterior

Table 17.2 Blood supply of the nose

Artery	Origin	Distribution
Dorsal nasal artery	Ophthalmic artery	Upper dorsal part
Anterior ethmoidal artery	Ophthalmic artery	Nasal tip
Branches of the angular artery	Facial artery	Lower lateral nose
Superior labial artery	Facial artery	Nostril and columella

Table 17.3 Sensory innervation of the nose

Nerve	Origin	Distribution
Supratrochlear nerve	Ophthalmic nerve	Upper part of the nose
Infratrochlear nerve	Ophthalmic nerve	Upper part of the nose
Anterior ethmoidal nerve	Ophthalmic nerve	Distal dorsum and nasal tip
Infraorbital nerve	Maxillary nerve	Distal nose (ala, columella, etc.)

Sensory Innervation of the Nose

Four nerves, the supratrochlear, the infratrochlear, the anterior ethmoidal, and the infraorbital nerves provide sensory innervation to the external nose (**Table 17.3**). The supratrochlear and infratrochlear nerves originate from the ophthalmic division of the trigeminal nerve, emerging from the medial orbital rim and traveling to the subcutaneous layer to be distributed to the upper part of the nose. The anterior ethmoidal nerve emerges from between the nasal bone and lateral nasal cartilage, and is distributed to the distal dorsum and the nasal tip. Injury of the anterior ethmoidal nerve causes sensory disturbance to the nasal tip. The infraorbital nerve is a branch of the maxillary division of the trigeminal nerve that runs inferomedially to the ala after emerging from the infraorbital foramen, and distributes in the distal nose, including the ala and columella.

Bony and Cartilaginous Structures of the Nose

The bony and cartilaginous frame of the nose can be divided into three parts according to structure (**Fig. 17.4**). Pairs of nasal bones form the upper part and frontal processes of the maxilla, the middle part is made of pairs of upper lateral cartilages, and the lower part consists of lower lateral cartilages.

In the upper part, the paired nasal bones and frontal processes of the maxilla form the pyramidal vault in horizontal section. The paired nasal bones are rectangular shaped bone and fuse in the midline. In the lateral view, the nasal bone changes the angle of the ridgeline at approximately the upper one-third point, defined as the nasofrontal groove. The nasal bone is also fused with the frontal bone superiorly by the frontonasal suture and with the frontal process of the maxilla by the nasomaxillary suture. The inferior border joins to the upper lateral cartilage. At the internal surface, the nasal bone connects with the structures forming the nasal septum, such as the nasal spine of the frontal bone, the perpendicular plate of the ethmoid, and the cartilage of the nasal septum. The nasal bone is generally thicker and narrower in the superior region and thinner and wider inferiorly. The bone varies in form and size in different individuals. However, Lessard and Daniel reported that the average length from the nasofrontal suture line to the inferior border is 25.1 mm.[4] The frontal process of the maxilla is the upward projection of the maxilla and fuses with the frontal bone superiorly, with the nasal bone medially, and the lacrimal bone laterally. The levator labii superioris alaeque nasi and orbicularis oculi muscles attach to the process. The medial canthal tendon attaches to the frontal process at the narrowest part of the nose. The line connecting the bilateral medial canthal tendona is the intercanthus line. Taking the inter canthus line as a reference, the nasofrontal suture is ~10.7 mm above, the nasofrontal groove is ~5.8 mm above, and the inferior border of the nasal bone is ~14.4 mm below the line.[4]

In the middle part of the nose, the upper lateral cartilage makes up the hard structure. At the transition zone between the nasal bone and upper lateral cartilage, nasal bone overlaps the cartilage (the nasal bone lies on the upper lateral cartilage), and they connect to each other by dense connective tissue. The overlapping area is called the keystone area, which forms a cres-

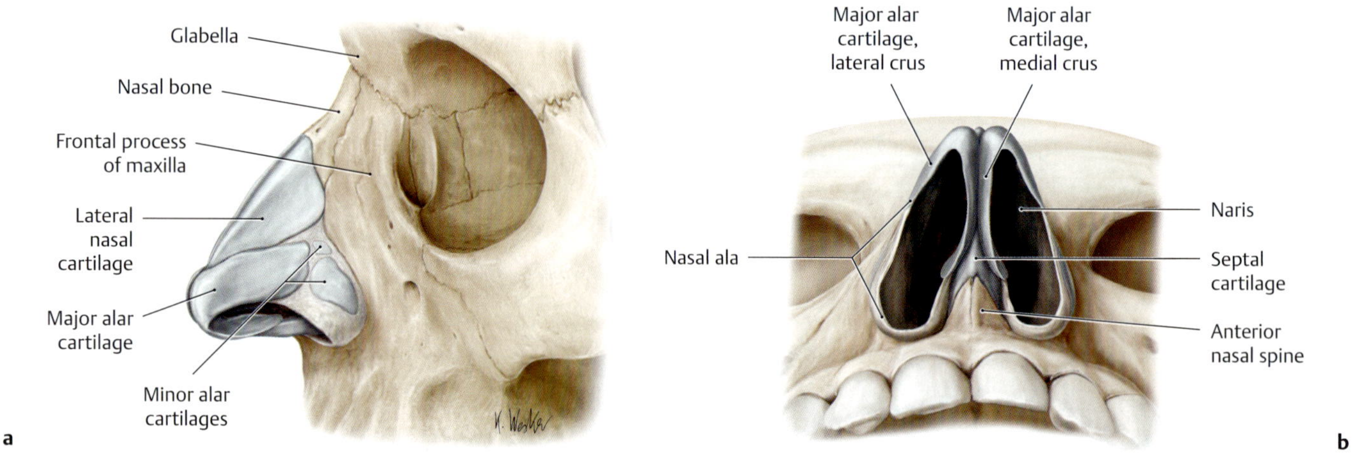

Fig. 17.4 Bony and cartilaginous structures of the external nose. **(a)** Left lateral view. **(b)** Inferior view. (Modified from THIEME Atlas of Anatomy, Head and Neuroanatomy. © Thieme 2010, Illustrations by Karl Wesker.)

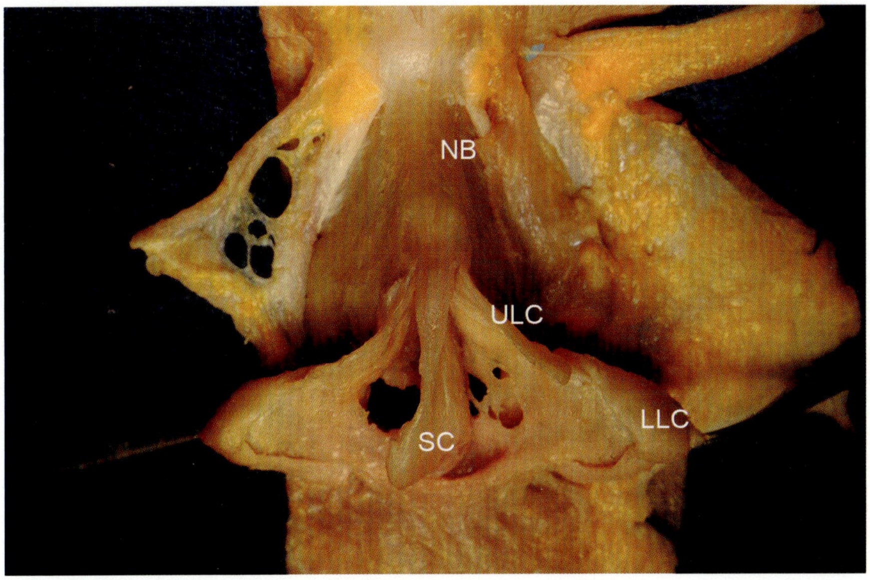

Fig. 17.5 The upper lateral cartilage. Bilateral upper lateral cartilages and cartilaginous regions of the nasal septum integrate as a unified structure, but a linear gap appears between the upper lateral cartilage and the septal cartilage, which is less than two-thirds of the area. LLC, Lower lateral cartilage; NB, Nasal bone; SC, Septal cartilage; ULC, Upper lateral cartilage.

cent shape in a concave upward direction, widest in the midline, decreasing in width laterally.[7] In the upper region of the upper lateral cartilage, including an overlapping area, the bilateral upper lateral cartilages and the cartilaginous part of the nasal septum integrate as a unified structure, but a linear gap appears between the upper lateral cartilage and the septal cartilage that constitutes less than two-thirds of the area (**Fig. 17.5**). Some people consider the upper lateral cartilages to be winglike extensions of the septal cartilage.[8–10] At the lowest part, the upper lateral cartilage connects with the lateral crus of the lower lateral cartilage, which is referred to as the scroll.[9] In most cases, these two cartilages overlap in various shapes, and this connection bears a major tip-supporting mechanism.[11]

In the lower part, a pair of lower lateral cartilages, the alar cartilages, are the supporting structures and affect greatly the shape of the lower nasal structure (**Fig. 17.6**). The lower lateral cartilage can be divided into three crura—the medial, middle, and lateral crura—all three of which intimately correlate to the outer shape of the nose.[12,13] The medial crus consists of the columella and is divided into two segments; the footplate and columella segments. The cartilage is curved convex toward the medial side as a whole, just like a section of cut cylinder, and it curves laterally in the frontal view and posteriorly in the lateral view between the two segments. The footplate segment forms the bulge in the base of the columella, and the columella segment forms the columella. The bilateral cartilages in the columella segment are open in the frontal view. Inappropriate dissection of the columella during open rhinoplasty can cause unexpected bifidity. At the upper border of the columella segment, the columella segment transits to the middle crus, a region known as the columella–lobular junction. In this region, the cartilage is curved posteriorly to some degree in the lateral view, which is referred to as rotation angle.[1,12] The middle crus is the part corresponding to the shape of the surrounding tip area, including the nasal tip and soft triangle. The middle crus is also divided into two segments: the lobular and domal segments. The lobular segment is relatively straight, but bilateral cartilages adjoin the posterior and anterior parts. The domal segment is the region where the cartilage curves drastically in the inferolateral direction on the frontal view and posteriorly on the lateral view.

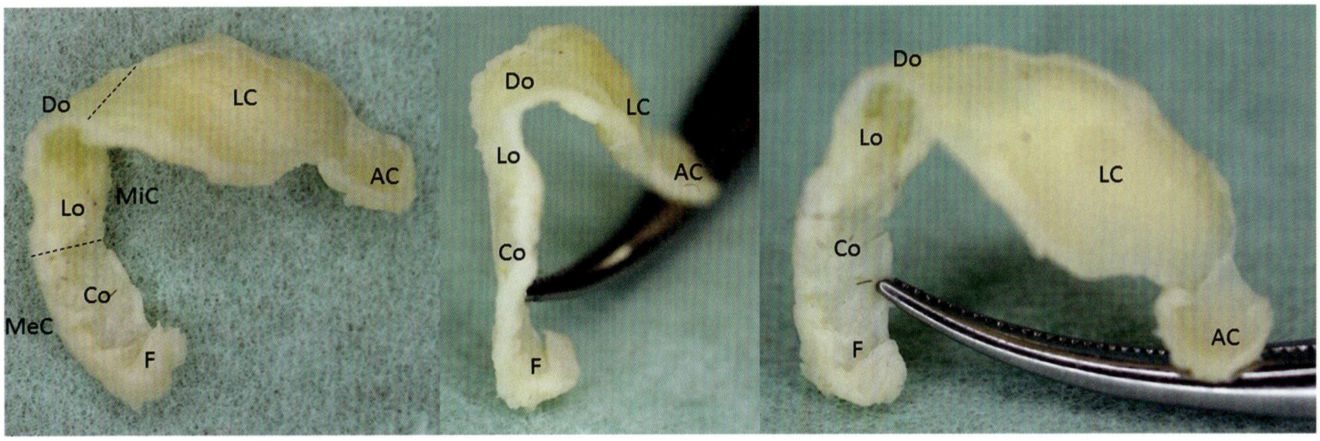

Fig. 17.6 The left alar cartilage (lower lateral cartilage). AC, accessory cartilage; Co, columella segment; Do, domal segment in the middle crura; F, footplate segment; LC, lateral crura; Lo, lobular segment in the middle crura; MiC, middle crura; MeC, medial crura.

The bent part forms the high canopy of the nares. Daniel (1992) described the length of the lobular segment as correlating significantly with tip shape, and the domal segment corresponds to the shape of the soft triangle of the lobule. Lateral to the domal segment is the domal junction, where the transition from the middle crus to the lateral crus is found. The region is located at the border between the tip and ala, with the tip defining points falling on the domal junction line.[12] The lateral crus is located in the alar and is the largest part of the lower lateral cartilage. This region affects the shape, size, and position of the ala. The lateral crus connects to the pyriformis through some accessory cartilages located lateral to the crus.[12] The lower lateral cartilage, accessory cartilage, and the ligaments supporting these cartilages form a ring surrounding the nostril and have an important role in the shape of the nostril.[14,15]

Tip Support Mechanism

The nasal tip lies on the bilateral lower lateral cartilages and is thus supported by the soft elastic pillars. Regarding the supporting system of the nasal tip, Anderson advocated the tripod concept.[16] This system postulates the tip supporting structure as a trigonal pyramid with bilateral lower lateral cartilages and their connection to the surrounding tissues. One pillar of the trigonal pyramid is almost perpendicular and consists of the combination of the bilateral medial crus of the lower lateral cartilages. The other two pillars are sloped and mainly consist of the lateral crus of the lower lateral cartilage. There are also some other structures contributing to the support of the nasal tip, including the ligament connecting the bilateral middle crua, the ligament connecting the bilateral medial crua, the connection between the lateral crus and caudal end of the upper lateral cartilage, known as the scroll area, the membranous septum, the length of the medial crus, the fat pad beneath the columella, and the lateral crus itself.

Conversely, Janeke and Wright and others have reported four kinds of tip-supporting structures, the junction between the lower and upper lateral cartilages, the lateral sesamoid cartilage complex (connection between lower lateral cartilage and the pyriformis), the junction between the medial crus and caudal septum (connection between the caudal septum and the bilateral medial crus), and the interdomal sling (connection between the bilateral middle crus).[17–20] The balance of these three pillars greatly affects the shape of the base of the nose.

References

1. Oneal RM, Beil RJ Jr, Schlesinger J. Surgical anatomy of the nose. Clin Plast Surg 1996;23(2):195–222
2. Farkas LG, Kolar JC, Munro IR. Geography of the nose: a morphometric study. Aesthetic Plast Surg 1986;10(4):191–223
3. Leong SC, Eccles R. A systematic review of the nasal index and the significance of the shape and size of the nose in rhinology. Clin Otolaryngol 2009;34(3):191–198
4. Lessard ML, Daniel RK. Surgical anatomy of septorhinoplasty. Arch Otolaryngol 1985;111(1):25–29
5. Letourneau A, Daniel RK. The superficial musculoaponeurotic system of the nose. Plast Reconstr Surg 1988;82(1):48–57
6. Griesman BL. Muscles and cartilages of the nose from the standpoint of a typical rhinoplasty. Arch Otolaryngol HeadNeck Surg 1944;39(4):334–341
7. Natvig P, Sether LA, Gingrass RP, Gardner WD. Anatomical details of the osseous-cartilaginous framework of the nose. Plast Reconstr Surg 1971;48(6):528–532
8. Basmajian JV, Grant JCB. Grant's Method of Anatomy: By Regions, Descriptive and Deductive. Baltimore, MD: William & Wilkins, 1972
9. McKinney P, Johnson P, Walloch J. Anatomy of the nasal hump. Plast Reconstr Surg 1986;77(3):404–405
10. Anderson KJ, Henneberg M, Norris RM. Anatomy of the nasal profile. J Anat 2008;213(2):210–216
11. Lam SM, Williams EF III. Anatomic considerations in aesthetic rhinoplasty. Facial Plast Surg 2002;18(4):209–214
12. Daniel RK. The nasal tip: anatomy and aesthetics. Plast Reconstr Surg 1992;89(2):216–224
13. Sheen JH, Sheen AP. Aesthetic Rhinoplasty. 2nd ed. St. Louis: Mosby; 1987
14. Farkas LG, Deutsch CK, Hreczko TA. Asymmetries in nostrils and the surrounding tissues of the soft nose—a morphometric study. Ann Plast Surg 1984;12(1):10–15
15. Stevens MR, Emam HA. Applied surgical anatomy of the nose. Oral Maxillofac Surg Clin North Am 2012;24(1):25–38
16. Anderson JR. A reasoned approach to nasal base surgery. Arch Otolaryngol 1984;110(6):349–358
17. Bernstein L. Applied anatomy in corrective rhinoplasty. Arch Otolaryngol 1974;99(1):67–70
18. Janeke JB, Wright WK. Studies on the support of the nasal tip. Arch Otolaryngol 1971;93(5):458–464
19. Han SK, Lee DG, Kim JB, Kim WK. An anatomic study of nasal tip supporting structures. Ann Plast Surg 2004;52(2):134–139
20. Rohrich RJ, Hoxworth RE, Thornton JF, Pessa JE. The pyriform ligament. Plast Reconstr Surg 2008;121(1):277–281

18 Auricle and External Acoustic Meatus

Noritaka Komune, Junichi Fukushima, and Albert L. Rhoton, Jr.

Introduction

The external ear is formed by the auricle, external acoustic meatus, and tympanic membrane. The auricle is a concave structure that directs sound waves into the external acoustic meatus. It is also cosmetically important and its anatomical structures are extremely complicated and delicate.

The external ear is a focus of otologic and plastic surgery, but it is also important in neurologic and lateral skull-base surgery. Surgery resulting in cosmetic and functional satisfaction relies not only on the surgeon's skill and use of advanced technologies but also on their complete understanding of the area's microsurgical anatomy, which makes surgery gentler and safer.

This chapter examines the microsurgical anatomy of the auricle and external acoustic meatus in cadaveric dissections and organizes the results in the following sections: (1) bone structure, (2) auricle, (3) cartilaginous skeleton of the auricle, (4) external acoustic meatus, (5) muscles, (6) neural innervation, (7) vascular supply, and (8) fascial structure. Finally, there is a short description of clinical considerations.

Bone Structure

The temporal bone consists of five components: squamous, tympanic, petrous, mastoid, and styloid parts (**Fig. 18.1a**). The bony canal of the external acoustic meatus is composed of three parts of the temporal bone: squamous, tympanic, and mastoid. The anterior and inferior bony walls are formed by the tympanic part. The superior and posterior bony walls are formed by the squamous and mastoid parts, and the squamomastoid suture can be identified (**Fig. 18.1b**). The tympanic part produces three sutures: tympanosquamous, tympanomastoid, and petrotympanic. The tympanosquamous suture, between the squamous and tympanic parts, is continuous medially with the petrotympanic and petrosquamous fissures (**Fig. 18.1b**). Additionally, two spines are identified in the bony portion of the meatus: endomeatal and suprameatal spines. The suprameatal spine (Henle's spine) is situated at the upper and posterior part of the orifice of the external acoustic meatus. The endomeatal spine is formed by a projection of the tympanosquamous suture into the canal.

The posterior root of the zygomatic arch of the squamous part forms the roof of the external acoustic meatus. At the anterior edge of this roof, the postglenoid process is positioned between the mandibular fossa and anterior wall of the external acoustic meatus. The tympanosquamous suture runs between the postglenoid process and the tympanic part of the temporal bone.

The edge of the tympanic membrane is thickened to form a fibrocartilaginous ring (tympanic annulus) attached to the tympanic sulcus, an incomplete ring of the tympanic bone that is interrupted by the notch of Rivinus. Above the superior end of the tympanic sulcus, the tympanic annulus becomes a fibrous band. The tympanic membrane within the notch of Rivinus, above the anterior and posterior malleolar folds extending to the lateral process of the malleus, is called the pars flaccida. This part is closely related to the anterior and posterior canal for the chorda tympani and the petrotympanic suture.

Auricle

The auricle is the lateral-most part of the external ear and is composed mainly of cartilage and skin. It is divided into two surfaces: lateral and medial.

The lateral surface is covered by a thin layer of skin, which is formed mainly by the perichondrium and an extremely fine subcutaneous layer. On this surface, the marginal edge is formed mainly by the helix, which is a smooth and round arch. The helix starts at the crus of the helix, passes anterosuperiorly, turns posteriorly and then inferiorly, and finally ends at the helical tail, which is continuous with the lobule. The scaphoid fossa is located just anterior to the helix along most of its length (**Fig. 18.2a,b**).

Next to the entrance of the external acoustic meatus, a well-defined hollow, the concha, leads into the meatus. This hollow has two parts: the cymba and the cavum conchae, separated by the crus of the helix. The antihelix, which has a Y shape, passes upward anterior to the posterior rim of the helix and divides into superior and inferior crura, separated by the triangular fossa. The root of the inferior crus of the antihelix forms the sharp rim of the concha and separates it from the triangular fossa. The superior crus of the antihelix forms the anterior border of the scaphoid fossa. The tail of the antihelix joins the antitragus. The inferior crus, tragus, and antitragus overhang the concha, making it look smaller. The well-defined notch between the tragus and antitragus is called the intertragic notch.

The skin of the medial surface is thicker than that of the lateral surface. On the medial surface, the prominences and sulci follow an obviously inverse pattern to that on the lateral surface (**Fig. 18.2c**). From the medial view, the concha and fossa on the lateral surface are seen as eminences, and the crura are seen as grooves. Eminences include the scaphoid, triangular, and conchal eminences. The antihelix on the lateral surface forms a depression on the medial surface called the antihelical fossa.

The most inferior part of the auricle is the lobule. The lobule is soft, formed mainly by fatty tissue between two cutaneous layers. The main defining feature of this area is the lack of cartilage, which makes the reconstruction of the lobule difficult because of postoperative retraction.

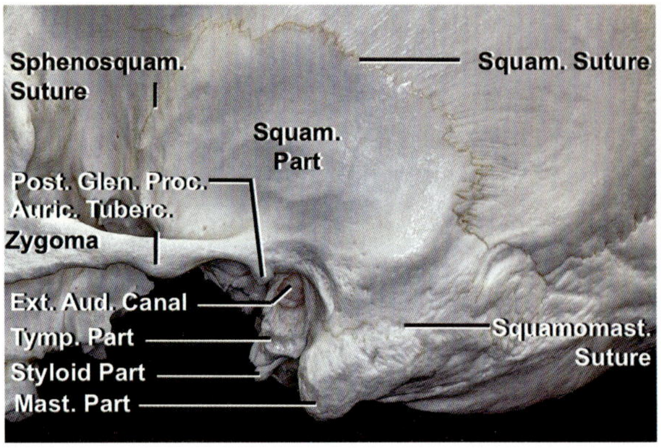

a

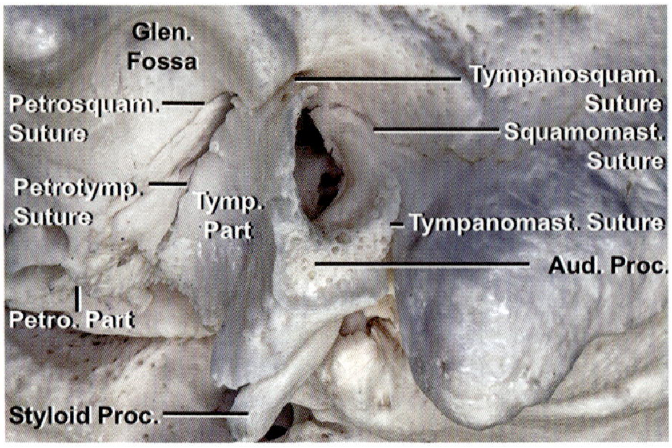

b

Fig. 18.1 Osseous anatomy and relationships of the external acoustic canal. **(a)** Lateral view. **(b)** Oblique view from anterior, laterally and inferiorly. Aud., Auditory; Ext., external; Glen., glenoid; Mast., mastoid; Petro., petrous; Petrosquam., petrosquamous; Petrotymp., petrotympanic; Proc., process; Sphenosquam., sphenosquamous; Squam., squamous; Squamomast., squamomastoid; Tymp., tympanic; Tympanomast., tympanomastoid; Tympanosquam., tympanosquamous.

Cartilage

The entire auricle except the lobule has elastic cartilage as its framework (**Fig. 18.3**). This cartilage allows the auricle to be flattened, bent, and folded. Repair of cartilage defects and reconstruction of the auricle remain challenging because the cartilage is a unique tissue without its own vascularization. A thin, adherent layer of perichondrium covers the auricular cartilage and can be separated from it; however, this perichondrium is more adherent in some lesions to the fossae.

The cartilage is strikingly similar to the surface of the auricle. Convexities on the lateral surface of the auricle include the helix, antihelix, superior and inferior crura of the antihelix, crus of helix, tragus, and antitragus. Concavities include the triangular fossa, cymbal and cavum conchae, and scaphoid fossa. The depressions and elevations on the lateral surface are aligned with the elevations and depressions on the medial surface.

From the surface of the auricle, some cartilaginous structures that are not seen are the incisura terminalis, ponticulus, antitragohelicina fissure, cauda of the helix, cartilage of the external acoustic meatus, and spine of the helix. The incisura terminalis separates the tragal lamina, which is the vertical curved plate of the tragus, and the cartilage of the external acoustic meatus from the main auricular cartilage. The lower part of the helix continues downward as a process called the cauda of the helix. The cauda of the helix is separated from the antitragus by a deep fissure, the antitragohelicine fissure. The spine of the helix is the anterior extremity of the crus of the helix. The ponticulus is the vertical ridge crossing the eminence of the concha on the medial surface. A deep groove can be identified on the medial surface between the eminences of the triangular fossa and concha. This deep groove is called the transverse sulcus of the antihelix and corresponds to the antihelix and its inferior crus on the lateral surface.

The cartilage of the external acoustic meatus forms a semicanal that extends medially from the lateral lamina of the tragus. This cartilaginous semicanal is usually interrupted by two vertical fissures in the anterior portion of the cartilage (Santorini fissures). These fissures can allow infections and malignant tumors to extend between the external acoustic meatus and parotid gland.

The cartilage of the auricle is attached to the auditory process, which is the lateral edge of the tympanic part of the temporal bone and has an extremely rough surface (**Fig. 18.1b**), and fixed to the skull by three ligaments: anterior, superior and posterior. The anterior ligament attaches the helix and tragus to the zygomatic process. The superior ligament attaches the spine of the helix to the superior margin of the bony external auditory canal. Furthermore, the posterior ligament is located between the medial surface of the concha and the mastoid process.

External Acoustic Meatus

The external acoustic meatus extends from the bottom of the concha to the tympanic membrane, forming an S shape that is divided into cartilaginous and bony portions (**Fig. 18.4**). First, it extends medially and slightly anteriorly and superiorly, then it turns medially and slightly posteriorly (cartilaginous part), and finally passes medially, anteriorly and slightly inferiorly (bony part). Pulling the auricle posteriorly and superiorly makes the canal straight and provides better visualization of the tympanic membrane.

The external canal has two narrow portions. One is close to the inner end of the cartilaginous portion (cartilage-bony junction), and the other is the isthmus in the osseous portion. The isthmus is the narrowest point along the canal and is located not at the cartilage-bony junction but in the bony portion.

The cartilaginous portion is continuous with the cartilage of the auricle and attaches to the auditory process, where the cartilage is attached medially to the bony part with dense connective tissue (**Fig. 18.1b**). The posterior and superior part of the cartilaginous part actually lacks cartilage but is filled with fibrous tissue.

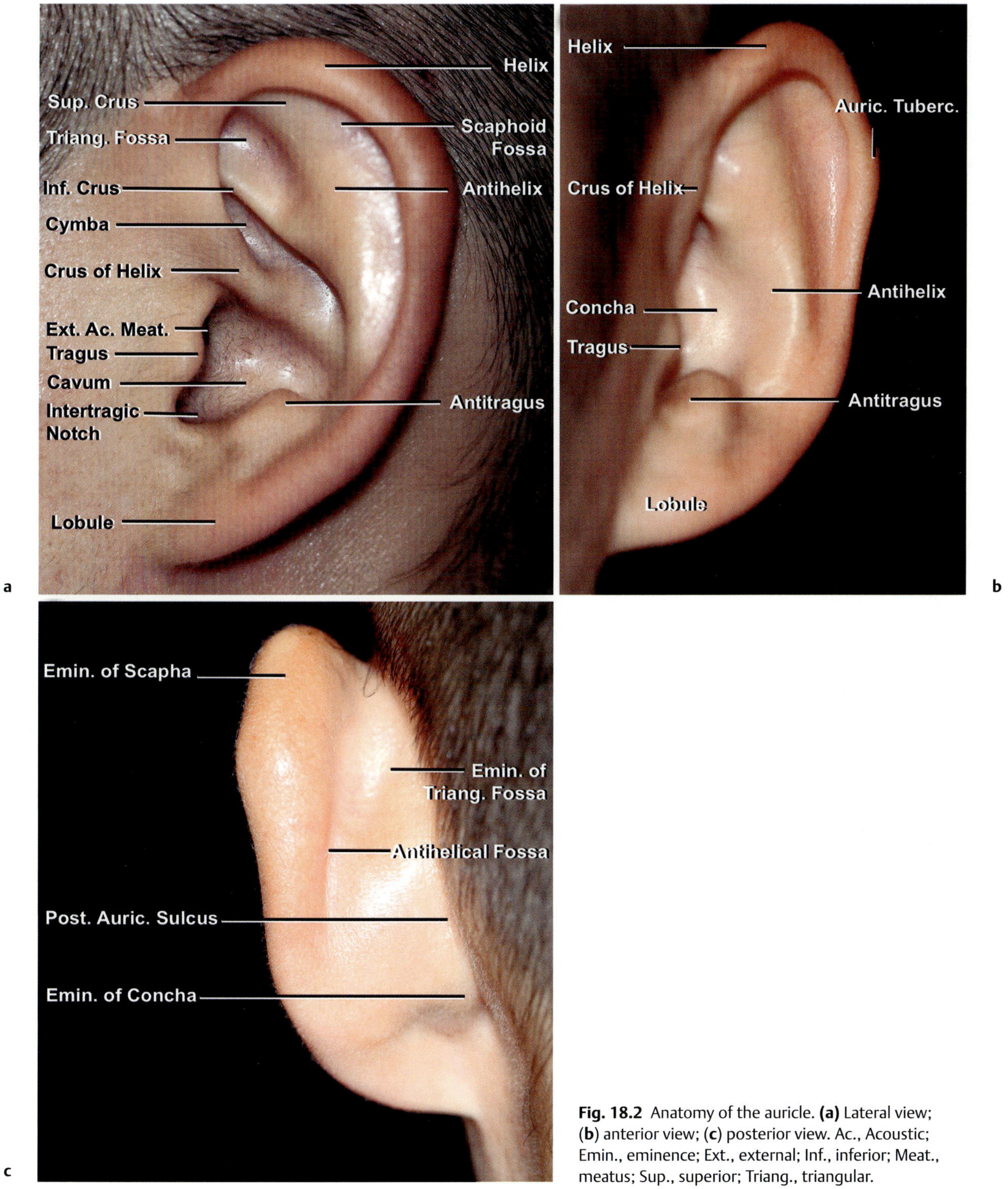

Fig. 18.2 Anatomy of the auricle. **(a)** Lateral view; (**b**) anterior view; (**c**) posterior view. Ac., Acoustic; Emin., eminence; Ext., external; Inf., inferior; Meat., meatus; Sup., superior; Triang., triangular.

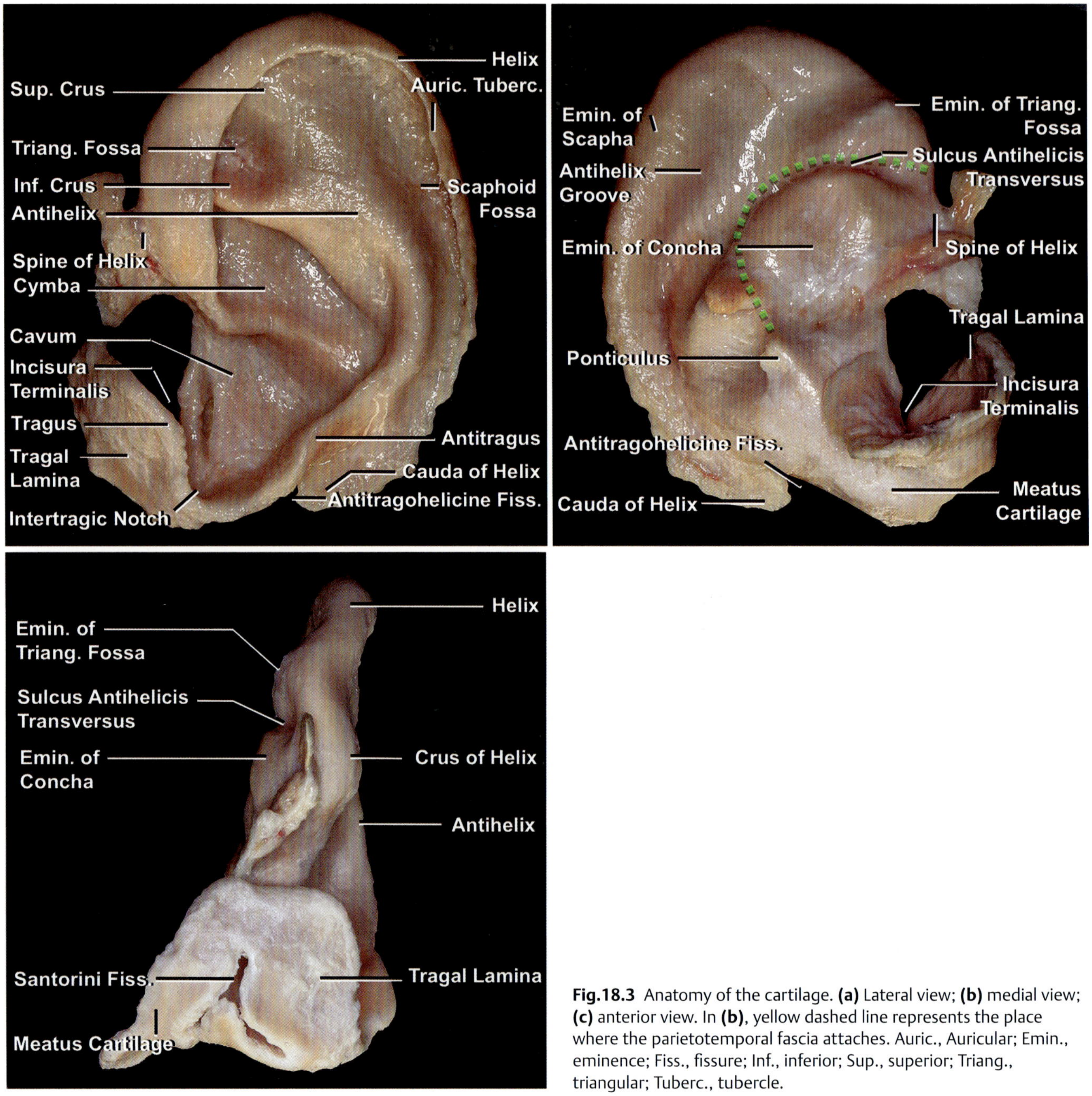

Fig.18.3 Anatomy of the cartilage. **(a)** Lateral view; **(b)** medial view; **(c)** anterior view. In **(b)**, yellow dashed line represents the place where the parietotemporal fascia attaches. Auric., Auricular; Emin., eminence; Fiss., fissure; Inf., inferior; Sup., superior; Triang., triangular; Tuberc., tubercle.

The bony portion is narrower than the cartilaginous portion. The conically shaped tympanic membrane is located at the medial end of the meatus and is titled anteroinferiorly. The angle between the tympanic membrane and the anteroinferior bony wall (anterior tympanomeatal angle) is acute and often obstructed by the bony eminence of the anterior wall.

The tympanic membrane is composed of three layers. The lateral epithelial layer is continuous with the skin of the external acoustic meatus. The middle fibrous layer is called the lamina propria, which is not identified in the pars flaccida. The medial mucosal layer is continuous with the mucosa of the middle ear cavity.

The skin covering the meatus is visibly thin, though slightly thicker on the cartilaginous portion than the bony portion, and it adheres closely to the cartilaginous and osseous portions of the meatus. The skin of the bony portion has no hair or glands. In the cartilaginous part, the subcutaneous tissue has hair follicles and ceruminous and sebaceous glands, which secrete the yellowish brown earwax.[1,2] In the auricle, the sebaceous glands are predominant in the concha and triangular fossa; ceruminous glands are located around the orifice of the external acoustic meatus.[3,4]

In three regions, the skin is more firmly adherent to the bony canal: (1) supra meatal spine (Henle's spine), (2) tympanomastoid suture, and (3) endomeatal spine and tympano-

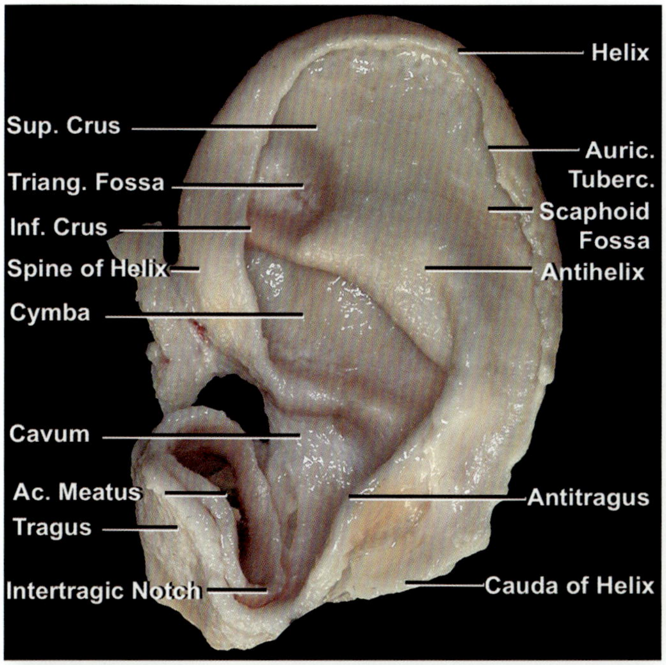

a

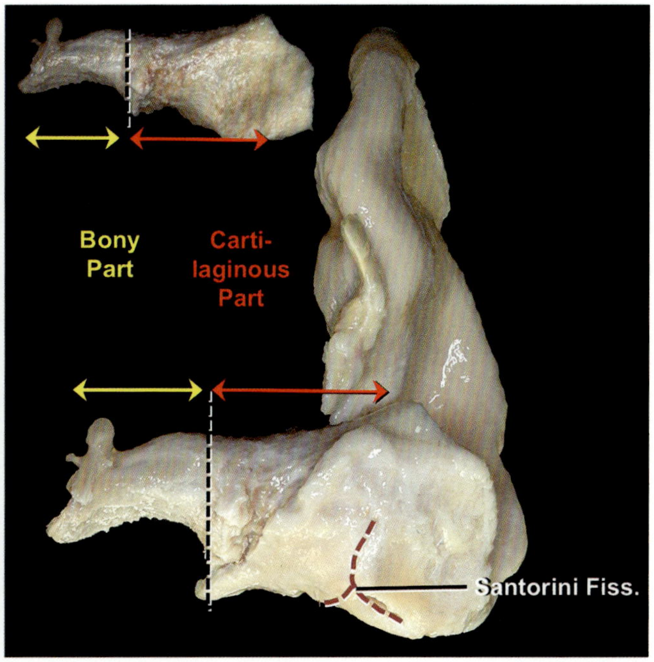

b

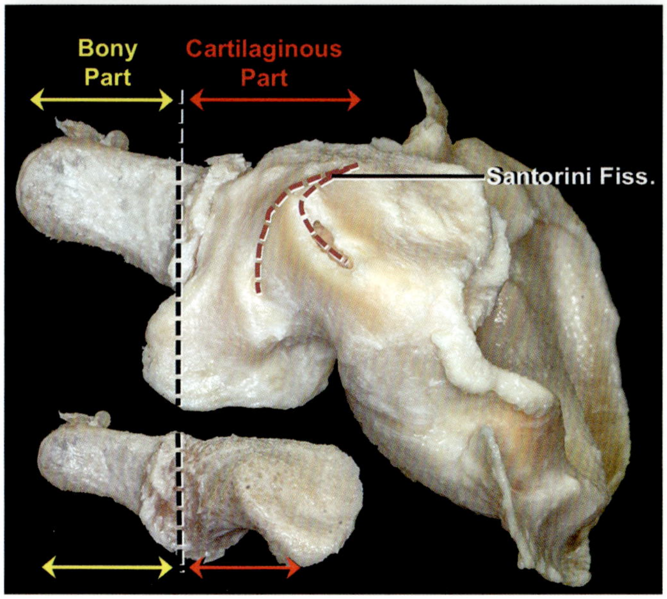

c

Fig. 18.4 Anatomy of the external acoustic meatus. **(a)** Lateral view; **(b)** anterior view; **(c)** inferior view. Ac., Acoustic; Auric., auricular; Fiss., fissure; Inf., inferior; Sup., superior; Triang., triangular; Tuberc., tubercle.

squamous suture. These sutures and spines make elevating a tympanomeatal flap from the bony canal difficult.

Muscle and Facial Nerve

The muscles and ligaments that attach to the auricle are divided into two types: extrinsic and intrinsic (**Fig. 18.5**). The extrinsic muscles include the posterior, superior, and anterior auricular muscles. These muscles are small but hold the auricle firmly in place. The intrinsic muscles include the helicis major, helicis minor, tragicus, antitragicus, transverse auricular, oblique auricular, pyramidal auricular, and incisurae helicis muscles (**Table 18.1**). These intrinsic muscles contribute to creating the complex folded configuration of the cartilage. In humans, the auricular muscles are considered vestigial remnants and thus useless structures.

Theoretically, the superior, posterior, and anterior auricular muscles function to pull the auricle, upward, backward, and forward, respectively; however, these muscles are generally too weak to do so. In our dissection, we did not identify the helicis major, incisurae helicis, and pyramidal auricular muscles.

The superior auricular muscle arises from the galeal aponeurosis, which is continuous with the temporoparietal fascia, and inserts into the area around the spine of the helix. The posterior auricular muscle usually has two or three fascicles and is supported by the posterior auricular ligament. These muscles and

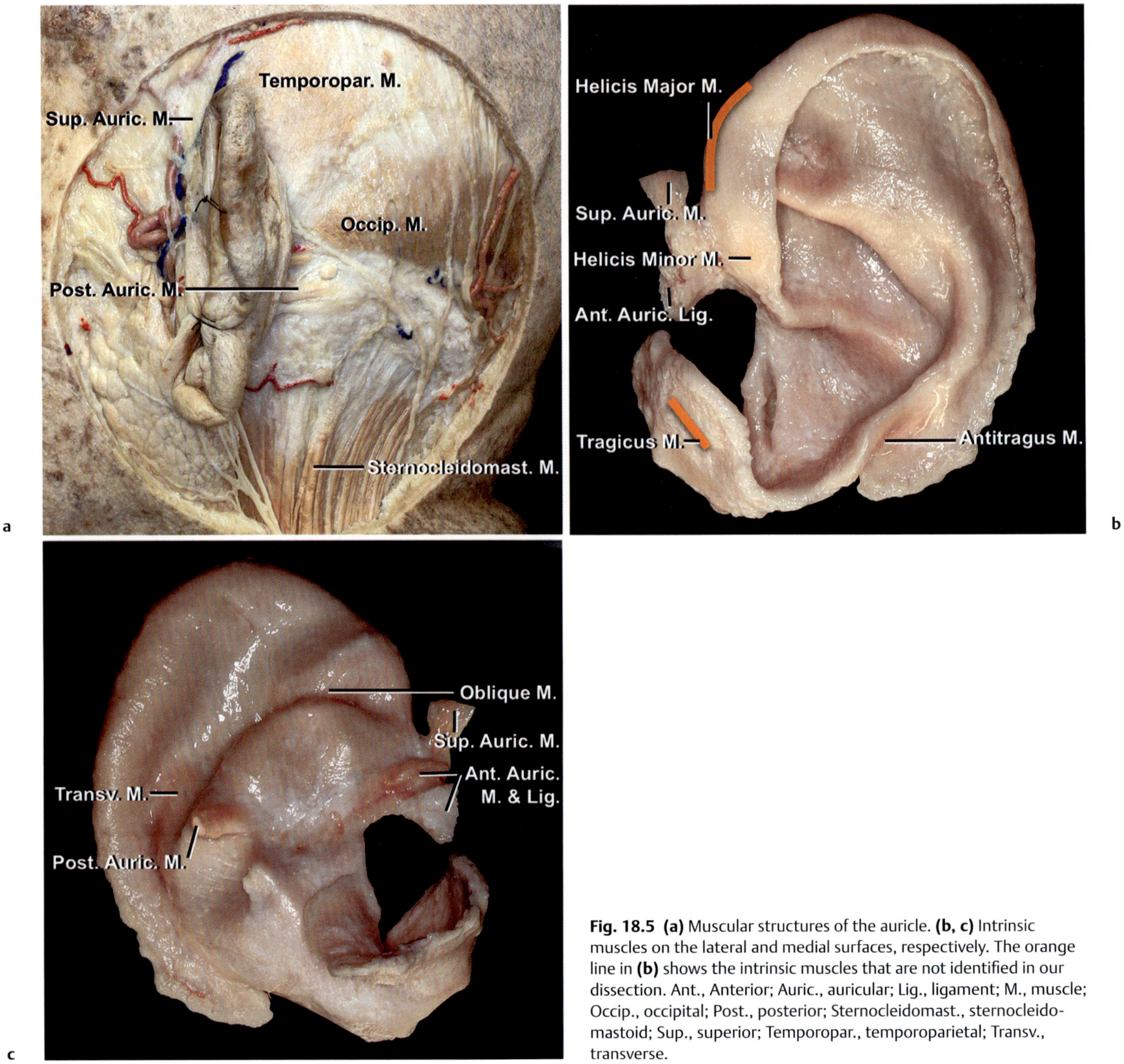

Fig. 18.5 **(a)** Muscular structures of the auricle. **(b, c)** Intrinsic muscles on the lateral and medial surfaces, respectively. The orange line in **(b)** shows the intrinsic muscles that are not identified in our dissection. Ant., Anterior; Auric., auricular; Lig., ligament; M., muscle; Occip., occipital; Post., posterior; Sternocleidomast., sternocleidomastoid; Sup., superior; Temporopar., temporoparietal; Transv., transverse.

Table 18.1 Origin and insertion of the auricular muscles

Muscles	Origin	Insertion
Lateral surface		
Helicis major	Helix	Spine of helix
Helicis minor	Spine of helix	Crus of helix
Tragicus	Tragus	Tragus
Antitragicus	Antitragus	Antitragus
Pyramidal	Tragus	Spine of helix
Medial surface		
Transverse auricular	Eminence of concha	Eminence of scaphoid fossa
Oblique auricular	Eminence of triangular Fossa	Eminence of concha
Incisurae helicis	Tragus	Antitragohelicine fissure

ligament arise from the mastoid periosteum and are attached to the eminence of the cymbal concha and the ponticulus. The posterior auricular ligament supports this muscle and runs parallel to it. The anterior auricular muscle attaches to the zygomatic arch and temporoparietal fascia at the anterior end, and the spine of the helix at the posterior end. This muscle is supported by the anterior auricular ligament, which tethers the tragus and the spine of the helix to the zygomatic arch and temporoparietal fascia. In addition to these three extrinsic muscles, the temporoparietal muscles and part of the occipital muscle are also attached to the medial surface of the auricle by a fibrous ligament, which is part of the temporoparietal fascia.

Innervation

Both cranial and cervical nerves are involved in the sensory innervation of the auricle (**Fig. 18.6**). Four cranial nerves contribute to the innervation of this region: trigeminal, facial, glossopharyngeal, and vagus nerves. Two branches of the cervical plexus are involved: the lesser occipital and great auricular nerves.

The auriculotemporal nerve is a branch of the mandibular nerve, which is the third division of the trigeminal nerve.[5] It arises as two roots from the posterior division of the mandibular nerve and encircles the middle meningeal artery before forming a single trunk. It runs between the neck of the mandible and the sphenomandibular ligament and enters the retromandibular region of the parotid gland posterior to the temporomandibular joint and mandibular neck. It gives off parotid branches and turns superiorly to give off anterior branches to the auricle, which innervate the anterosuperior parts of the lateral surface. It then crosses over the root of the zygomatic process of the temporal bone, parallel to the superficial temporal artery. It penetrates the superficial muscular aponeurotic system (SMAS) and passes upward superficial to the temporoparietal fascia. The fibers of the superior root of this nerve pass through the otic ganglion without synapsing and supply cutaneous sensation to the anterior region of the auricle, external acoustic meatus, outside of the tympanic membrane and skin in the temporal region. The branch innervating the anterior part of the external acoustic meatus and outside of the tympanic membrane passes into the petrotympanic fissure in the glenoid fossa. The glossopharyngeal nerve gives off the parasympathetic fibers that form the tympanic nerve. This nerve enters the tympanic cavity and forms the tympanic plexus with the internal carotid nerve, which is composed of sympathetic fibers, on the promontory in the middle ear cavity. This plexus gives off the lesser petrosal nerve, which synapses in the otic ganglion, and its postganglionic fibers form the inferior root of the auriculotemporal nerve, which provides sympathetic innervation to the scalp, and parasympathetic innervation to the parotid gland.

Four cervical branches, the transverse cervical, greater, and lesser occipital and supraclavicular nerves exit the posterior edge of the sternocleidomastoid muscle at the nerve point. These nerves arise from the cervical nerve plexus formed by the ventral ramus of the C2 and C3. The lesser occipital nerve penetrates the postauricular fascia, where the fasciae of the occipital and sternocleidomastoid muscles attach tightly to the superior nuchal line, divide into the auricular and the occipital branches, and communicate with the greater occipital, postauricular, and great auricular nerves.

The great auricular nerve ascends from the nerve point and plays a major role in the sensory innervation of the auricle. This nerve divides into three types of branches. The most anterior branches innervate the preauricular area. Branches of the second type pass through the lobule and innervate the inferior and posterosuperior parts of the lateral surface of the auricle. The third type of branches passes under or behind the lobule and supplies the medial surface of the auricle and the skin over the mastoid tip.

The vagus nerve, when it exits the intrajugular part of the jugular foramen, gives off the auricular branch, also called Arnold's nerve. A branch of the glossopharyngeal nerve then joins Arnold's nerve, which passes along the anterolateral edge of the jugular fossa and enters the mastoid canaliculus. It travels in the temporal bone and crosses the facial nerve, giving off a tiny branch to the facial nerve, which divides into two branches. One joins the posterior auricular nerve, and the other passes through the tympanomastoid fissure, located between the mastoid process and the tympanic part of the temporal bone, to innervate the posterior wall of the external acoustic meatus and skin around the meatal entrance.

The posterior auricular and frontal branches of the facial nerve innervate the auricular muscles. The posterior auricular nerve arises just after the facial nerve exits the stylomastoid foramen. This nerve passes backward and upward along the anterior surface of the mastoid process. The auricular branch of the vagus and the great auricular and lesser occipital nerves give off branches that join the posterior auricular nerve. This nerve gives off the two main branches that innervate the occipital and auricular regions and the occipital, posterior auricular, and intrinsic muscles on the medial surface of the auricle. In our dissection, the occipital branch passed medial to the posterior auricular muscles and gave off tiny branches to the occipital region and posterior auricular muscle. The branches to the occipital region course between the fascicles of the posterior auricular muscle passing along the superior nuchal line. The frontal and posterior auricular branches innervate the anterior auricular and posterior auricular muscles, respectively.

Vascular Supply

The arterial supply of this area is derived from branches of the external carotid artery (**Fig. 18.7**). The venous drainage follows the arteries. The external jugular vein, maxillary vein, and pterygoid venous plexus are responsible for venous drainage. The external carotid artery gives off occipital and posterior auricular branches and finally divides in the parotid gland into two terminal branches: maxillary and superficial temporal. These four arteries play an important role in the vascularization of the external ear.

The three main arteries supplying the auricle are the posterior auricular, superficial temporal, and occipital arteries. These vessels form a complex network between the skin and perichondrium of the auricle. The posterior auricular artery passes around the mastoid process, gives off the mastoid branch to the

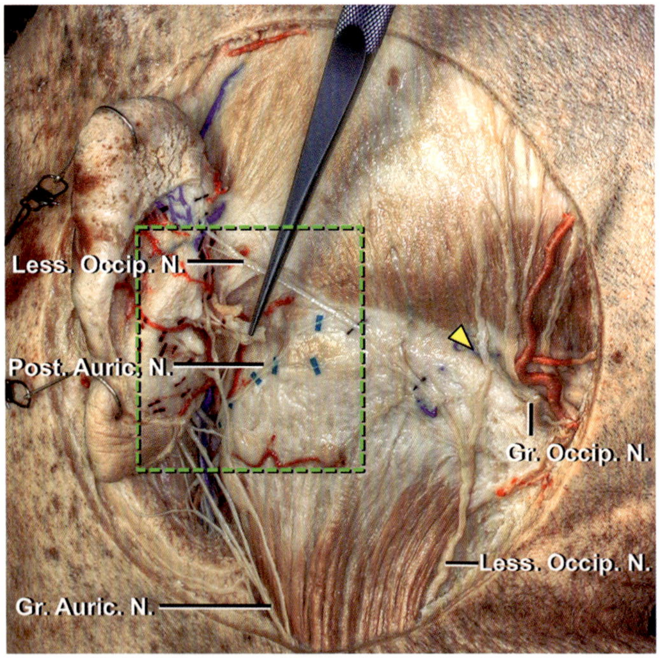

a

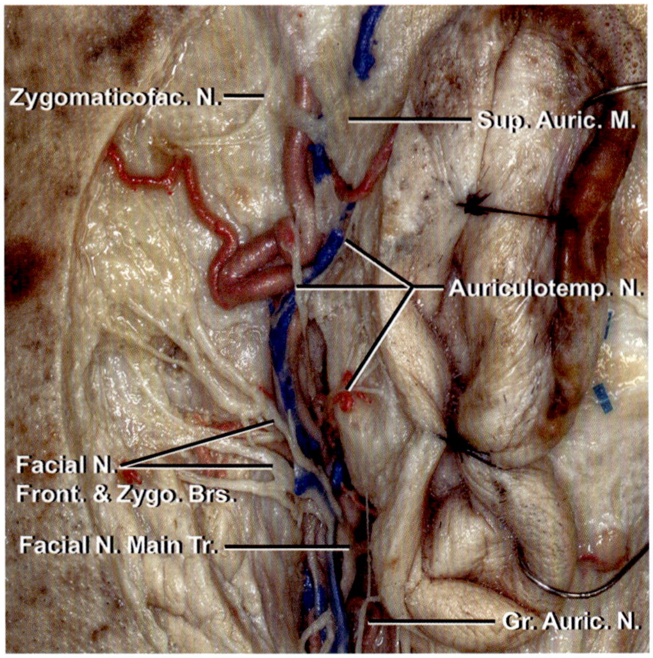

b

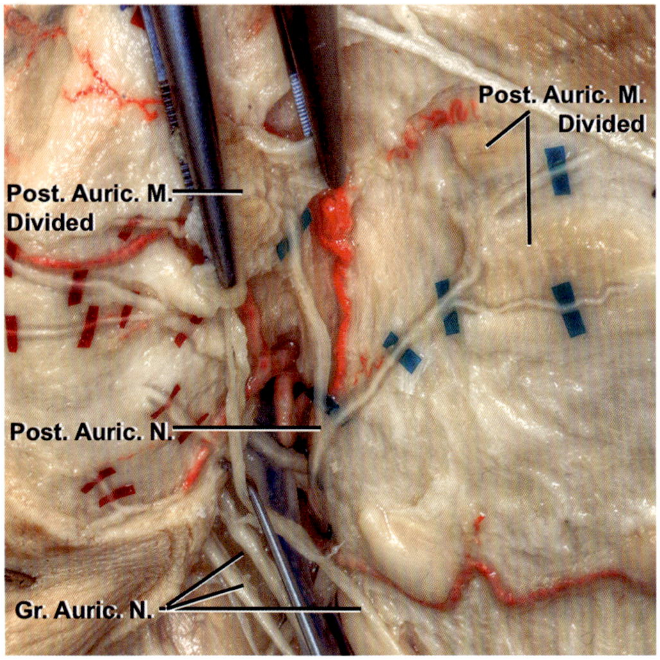

c

Fig. 18.6 Innervation of the auricle. **(a)** Posterolateral view. The green dashed area is enlarged in **(c)**. **(b)** Anterolateral view. **(c)** Course of the postauricular nerve. The yellow arrow in **(a)** shows the anastomosis of the lesser and greater occipital nerves. The red, blue, and black fabric enhances the course of the great auricular, facial, and lesser occipital nerves, respectively. Auric., Auricular; Auriculotemp., auriculotemporal; Front., frontal; Gr., great; Less., lesser; M., muscle; N., nerve; Occip., occipital; Post., posterior; Sup., superior; Tr., trunk; Zygo., zygomatic; Zygomaticofac., zygomaticofacial.

skin on the mastoid process, and passes superiorly to supply the medial surface of the auricle through three main branches: superior, middle, and inferior.

These branches perforate the cartilage to anastomose with the arterial network on the lateral surface. The superficial temporal artery gives off the anterior auricular branches, which include superior, middle, and inferior auricular arteries that supply the lateral surface of the auricle from the helix to the lobule. There are also perforating branches that penetrate the cartilage from the regions of the antitragus, cymbal conchae, and triangular fossa to supply the medial surface of the auricle. The superior auricular artery's typical course connects the superior temporal artery and the posterior auricular arterial network. The auricular branch of the occipital artery supplies the medial surface of the auricle, especially around the eminence of the concha.

The external acoustic meatus is supplied mainly by three arteries: posterior auricular, superficial temporal, and maxillary. The auricular branches of the superficial temporal artery supply the anterior region and the roof of the external acoustic meatus. The auricular branches of the posterior auricular artery penetrate the cartilage of the auricle and supply the posterior por-

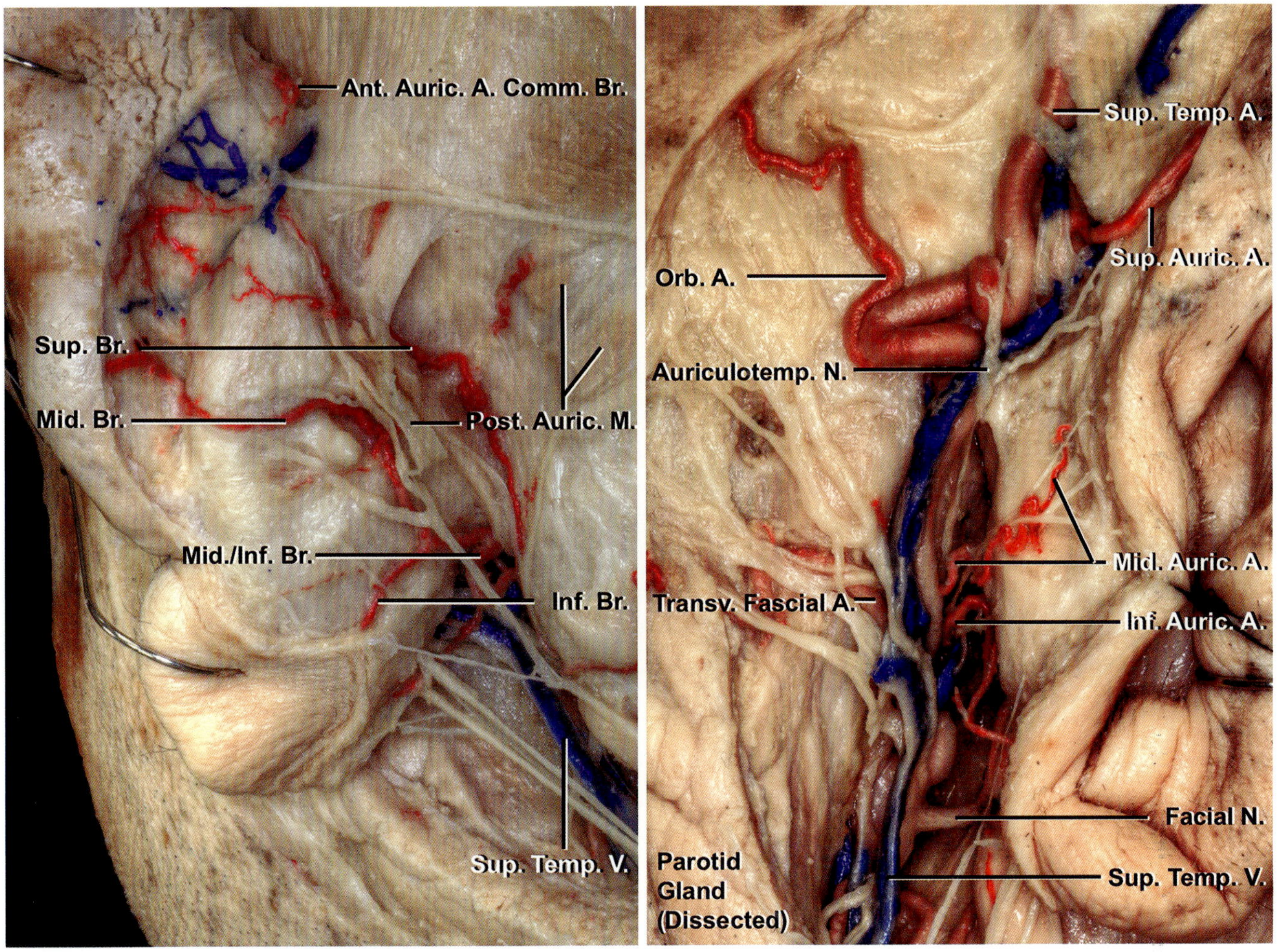

Fig. 18.7 Vascular supply of the auricle. **(a)** Medial surface of the auricle. **(b)** Lateral surface of the auricle. A., Artery; Ant., anterior; Auric., auricular; Auriculotemp., auriculotemp; Br., branch; Comm., communicating; Inf., inferior; M., muscle; Mid., middle; N., nerve; Orb., orbital; Post., posterior; Sup., superior; Temp., temporal; Transv., transverse; V., vein.

tion of the canal. The deep auricular branch arises from the first portion of the maxillary artery and ascends in the parotid gland behind the temporomandibular joint to pierce the cartilaginous or bony portion of the external acoustic meatus to supply the anterior wall of the meatus and the outer surface of the tympanic membrane.

Aydin et al[6] demonstrated the lymphatic drainage pattern of the auricle. The lymphatic drainage pattern closely follows the vascular supply. Their study with lymphoscintigraphies showed that the injection sites of the technetium-99–labeled nanocolloid within the territory of the superficial temporal artery drained along the superficial temporal vein to the parotid sentinel lymph nodes. The sites within the territory of the posterior auricular artery drained along the posterior auricular vein to the extraparotid sentinel lymph nodes. This drainage pattern has a parallel relationship with embryonic development. The anterior three hillocks derived from the mandibular arch correspond predominantly to the territories of the superficial temporal artery. On the other hand, the posterior three hillocks derived from the hyoid arch correspond to the territories of the posterior auricular artery.

Fascial Layers

The skin of the lateral surface of the auricle is tightly adherent to the perichondrium covering the cartilage framework without the interposition of fatty tissue (**Fig. 18.8**). Vessels and nerves pass within an extremely thin layer between the skin and perichondrium. The skin covering the anterior surface of the lamina of the tragus and the area between the antitragus and helical tail located above the lobule is thicker than that covering the other area of the lateral surface and slides over the cartilage.

In contrast, the skin of the medial surface is loosely adherent to the cartilage with interposition of adipose tissue, which is composed of two layers: superficial and deep. The superficial layer is firm with large fat cells. The deep layer overlying the

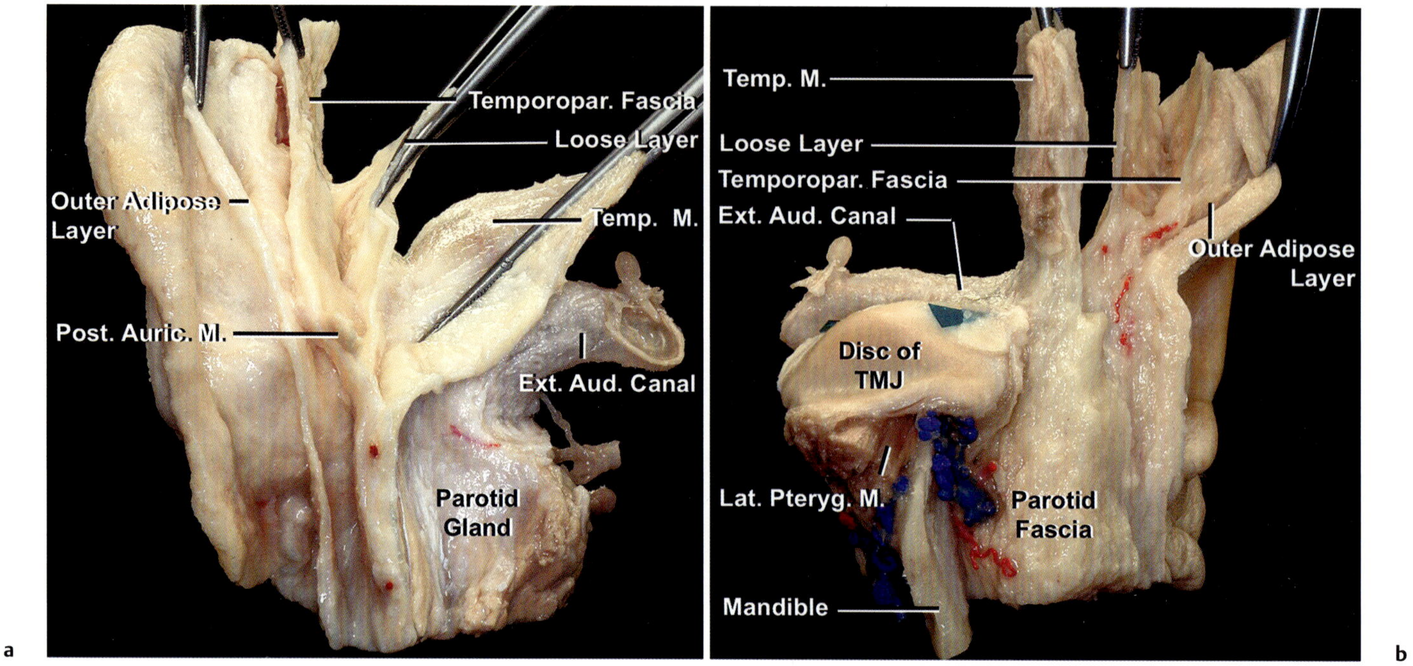

Fig. 18.8 Fascial layers of the auricle. **(a)** Anterior view. **(b)** Posterior view. Blue fabric shows the periosteum of the glenoid fossa covering the auricular disc of the temporomandibular joint. Aud., auditory; Auric., auricular; Ext., external; Lat., lateral; M., muscle; Post., posterior; Pteryg., pterygoid; Temp., temporal; Temporopar., temporoparietal; TMJ, temporomandibular joint.

perichondrium is thin and loose. The nerves, vessels, and lymphatics pass through this adipose tissue, mainly between its two layers. The subcutaneous vascular network also passes more superficially. The skin extends over the helical rim with the transition of its structure from one type to the other.

Generally, the soft tissue of the face is divided into five basic layers: (1) skin, (2) subcutaneous, (3) musculoaponeurotic layers, (4) areolar tissue, and (5) deep fascia/periosteum.[7,8] In the parietotemporal region, the temporal muscle layer is located between the fourth and fifth layers. Davidge et al[9] reviewed previous studies on the layers of the temporoparietal area and proposed, based on the terminologica anatomica,[10] that the layers of fascia in the temporoparietal region are (1) skin and subcutaneous tissue, (2) temporoparietal fascia, (3) loose areolar tissue plane, (4) superficial leaflet of temporal fascia, (5) temporal fat pad of temporal fascia, (6) deep leaflet of temporal fascia, (7) fat pad deep to temporal muscle, (8) temporal muscle, and (9) pericranium. These layers are closed related to the fasciae of the auricle. Our dissection showed the relationship between the auricular and cranial fascial layers is shown.

The temporoparietal fasciae include the superior auricular and parietotemporal muscles and are continuous with the frontal muscle anteriorly, occipital muscle posteriorly, and galea aponeurotica superiorly. This layer attaches around the auricle along the transverse sulcus and ponticulus. Furthermore, it fuses with the superficial layer of the adipose layer of the auricle. Thus, the auriculocephalic sulcus corresponds to the junction of the temporoparietal fascia on the cranial surface and the superficial adipose layer of the auricle. The temporoparietal fascia is tightly adherent to the surface of the mastoid process and is continuous with the strong, heavythick fibrous fasciae, called the superficial mastoid fascia.[11] Datta and Carlucci[11] examined the facial layers around the mastoid process. In this region, the temporoparietal fascia gets thicker and more fibrous and is better vascularized. The areolar layer in the parietotemporal region is continuous with the deep mastoid fascia. In our dissection, these fasciae attached tightly to the superior nuchal line and posterolateral surface of the mastoid process.

The superficial fascia of the temporal muscle (superficial temporal fascia) is one of the two fascia layers covering the temporal muscle and is tightly attached to the anterior border of the zygomatic arch and anterior ligament of the auricle, which attaches to the posterior root of the zygomatic process. Loose areolar tissue is located between the superficial temporal and temporoparietal fasciae. On the posterolateral surface of the mastoid process, these layers are fused with thick fibrous tissue. This areolar layer covers the perichondrium of the cartilage of the auricle on the medial surface of the auricle. The anterior auricular muscle is in a different layer from the temporoparietal fascia and was related to the looser areolar layer on the cranial side in our dissection.

Two adipose layers are present on the medial surface of the auricle between the anterior surface of the lamina of the tragus and the anterior surface of the helix. The outer adipose layer and parietotemporal fascia are fused together and attached to the zygomatic process. The anterior auricular ligament, which arises from the spine of the helix, is also attached to the zygomatic process.

In the area between the cartilage of the tragus and the posterior border of the platysma, which is included in the SMAS, is a diffuse area of the ligamentous attachment, described as the platysma auricular fascia.[12] In this area, the layers from subcutaneous to deep cervical are attached as a retaining ligament and are difficult to separate into layers. This ligamentous region is named by a variety of authors, including Furnas, Stuzin et al, and Loré, as the platysma auricular ligament, parotid cutaneous ligament, and tympanoparotid fascia (Loré's fascia), respectively.[7,12,13]

The deep cervical fascia is attached from the superior nuchal line of the occipital bone to the mastoid process of the temporal bone, and extends to the inferior border of the body of the mandible. This fascia encloses the sternocleidomastoid muscle and binds its anterior edge to the mandible. It also encloses the parotid gland under the parotidomasseteric fascia, and together they extend superiorly and posteriorly to attach to the zygomatic arch, auricle, and mastoid process. A thick fibrous band is located inferior to the auricle, where it firmly tethers the parotid grand to the auricle and the sternocleidomastoid. This fibrous layer extends upward and medial to the parotid gland to the styloid process forming the stylomandibular ligament.

Clinical Considerations

Reconstruction of deformities of the auricle is one of the main concerns of plastic and otologic surgeons. Deformities of the auricle are classified into two groups: congenital and acquired. Previous studies presented a classification of congenital anomalies of the auricle: anotia, microtia, prominent ear, and so forth.[14–16] These classifications utilized embryologic, anatomical, functional, and clinical elements to identify the anomalies of the ear. Appropriate surgical planning for reconstruction depends on the classification of the abnormality. Acquired deformities of the auricle are also difficult to reconstruct. Because of its location, the auricle is vulnerable to deformities caused by external trauma. Furthermore, deformities can also be caused by surgery for malignancies of the lateral skull base. Defects or damages affecting the cartilage are more difficult to reconstruct than skin-only defects. The postauricular flap, used to repair defects of the auricle, is constructed of skin from the posterior ear, which has an abundant vascular supply, and its location ensures that the postoperative scar is hidden behind the auricle. This flap in the postauricular region from the medial surface of the auricle to the superficial mastoid surface has been used in a variety of applications in cosmetic and otologic surgery.

The posterior auricular artery has been reported to be a donor artery for the middle cerebral artery bypass, although it is usually too small for this use.[17,18] Preoperative angiography may reveal that the posterior auricular artery is large enough to use for bypass.

The anatomy of the external ear is complex. It is important to understand the microsurgical anatomy of the external ear to obtain satisfactory cosmetic and functional surgical results. The external ear is important in cosmetic, general, and otologic surgery, as well as neurologic and lateral skull-base surgery.

References

1. Perry ET, Shelley WB. The histology of the human ear canal with special reference to the ceruminous gland. J Invest Dermatol 1955; 25(6):439–451
2. Shelley WB, Perry ET. The physiology of the apocrine (ceruminous) gland of the human ear canal. J Invest Dermatol 1956;26(1):13–22
3. Morris H, McMurrich JP. Morris's Human Anatomy: A Complete Systematic Treatise by English and American Authors. 4th ed. Philadelphia: P. Blakiston's Son & Co.; 1907
4. Shiffman MA. Advanced Cosmetic Otoplasty Art, Science, and New Clinical Techniques. Berlin, New York: Springer; 2013
5. Joo W, Yoshioka F, Funaki T, Mizokami K, Rhoton AL Jr. Microsurgical anatomy of the trigeminal nerve. Clin Anat 2014;27(1):61–88
6. Aydin MA, Okudan B, Aydin ZD, Ozbek FM, Nasir S. Lymphoscintigraphic drainage patterns of the auricle in healthy subjects. Head Neck 2005;27(10):893–900
7. Stuzin JM, Baker TJ, Gordon HL. The relationship of the superficial and deep facial fascias: relevance to rhytidectomy and aging. Plast Reconstr Surg 1992;89(3):441–451
8. Mendelson BC. Advances in the understanding of the surgical anatomy of the face. In: Eisenmann-Klein M, Neuhann-Lorenz C, eds. Innovations in Plastic and Aesthetic Surgery. New York: Springer Verlag; 2007:141–145
9. Davidge KM, van Furth WR, Agur A, Cusimano M. Naming the soft tissue layers of the temporoparietal region: unifying anatomic terminology across surgical disciplines. Neurosurgery 2010; 67(3, Suppl Operative):120–130
10. Federative Committee on Anatomical Terminology, International Federation of Associations of Anatomists. Terminologia Anatomica International Anatomical Terminology. 2nd ed. Stuttgart: Thieme; 2011
11. Datta G, Carlucci S. Reconstruction of the retroauricular fold by 'nonpedicled' superficial mastoid fascia: details of anatomy and surgical technique. J Plast Reconstr Aesthet Surg 2008;61(Suppl 1): S92–S97
12. Furnas DW. The retaining ligaments of the cheek. Plast Reconstr Surg 1989;83(1):11–16
13. Loré JM, Wabnitz R. An Atlas of Head and Neck Surgery. Vol 2. 3rd ed. Philadelphia: Saunders; 1988
14. Tanzer RC. The constricted (cup and lop) ear. Plast Reconstr Surg 1975;55(4):406–415
15. Rogers BO. Microtic, lop, cup and protruding ears: four directly inheritable deformities? Plast Reconstr Surg 1968;41(3):208–231
16. Melnick M, Myrianthopoulos NC, Paul NW. External ear malformations: epidemiology, genetics, and natural history. Birth Defects Orig Artic Ser 1979;15(9):i–ix, 1–140
17. Horiuchi T, Kusano Y, Asanuma M, Hongo K. Posterior auricular artery-middle cerebral artery bypass for additional surgery of moyamoya disease. Acta Neurochir (Wien) 2012;154(3):455–456
18. Tokugawa J, Nakao Y, Kudo K, et al. Posterior auricular artery-middle cerebral artery bypass: a rare superficial temporal artery variant with well-developed posterior auricular artery: case report. Neurol Med Chir (Tokyo) 2013;(Oct):21

19 Mandible and Masticatory Muscles

Kyung-Seok Hu and Yang Hun Mu

Introduction

The mandible provides support for the teeth and attachment of the maxillofacial muscles and with the temporal bone, forms the temporomandibular joint (TMJ). Tributaries of the inferior alveolar neurovascular bundle, passing through the mandibular canals, are distributed to the skin of the chin and mandibular teeth. An impingement of the mandibular canal can result in sensory disorders of the mandibular teeth and skin of the chin.

The masticatory muscles consist of the masseter, temporalis, and medial and lateral pterygoids, and these are innervated by the mandibular nerve. The masticatory muscles and their associated neurovascular and fascial systems are important in various surgical approaches.

Mandible

The mandible is the only bone of the lower jaw. It consists of an arch-shaped body and two quadrilateral rami (**Fig. 19.1**). The mandible provides support for the mandibular teeth; provides for attachment of muscles, including facial, masticatory, and infrahyoid muscles; and is the lower component for the TMJ. The bone also provides passage for the inferior alveolar nerve and vessels supplying the mandibular teeth and lower face.

Body

The body of the mandible is U-shaped and convex anteriorly. It has external and internal surfaces and an alveolar part (tooth-bearing portion). The inferior border of the body continues with the ramus, and together they form the mandibular base.

External Surface of the Body of the Mandible

During development, half-sides of the mandible are fused by a mandibular symphysis in the midline (**Fig. 19.2**). A vague median ridge at the upper external surface in an adult mandible can indicate the fused site. The ridge bifurcates at the lower external surface, and the mental protuberance lies between them and is triangular-shaped. Two mental tubercles and the small central depression between them lie on the base of the mental protuberance.

The mental protuberance and tubercles constitute the chin (i.e., the mentum). The mental foramen is usually located below the interval between the premolar teeth or second premolar, approximately on the midpoint between upper and lower border of the mandible. The mental neurovascular bundle emerges from the mental foramen after passing through a canal inside the mandible (mandibular canal). The bundle emerges backward, and thus the posterior rim of the foramen is smooth, whereas the anterior rim is more distinct. The exact position of the mental foramen and the course of the neurovascular bundle within it are important during dental implant procedures.

The external oblique line is faint and ascends posteriorly from the mental tubercle to the anterior border of the ramus of the mandible. The line is distinct farther backward and continuous with the sharp anterior border of the ramus.

Surgical Annotation. Harvesting Bone from the Chin

Alveolar bone resorption resulting from tooth loss reduces supporting bone for the dental implant placement. To enhance vertical bone dimensions, the mandibular symphysis area is recommended as the donor site for the autogenous bone graft. An osteotomy should be made away from the apex of the root of the incisors. It is suggested that the surgical site of the osteotomy be located 5 mm from the dental roots.[1]

Additionally, encroachment of the mental foramen by the osteotomy results in insensitivity on the chin. According to dentition, the mental foramen lies below the premolar area, especially in the interval between these teeth. Superficially, the mental foramen lies about 2 cm below the corner of the mouth and slightly lateral to it. The distance between the bilateral mental nerves is about 45 mm.[2] Regarding the anterior loop (mandibular canal anterior to mental foramen (**Fig. 19.3**), the safe area might be narrower than the interval between the mental foramina.

The cortical plate on the chin is thick further downward. Anatomical research in Asians has demonstrated that the maximum volume of graft block can be harvested from the rectangular site from the mandibular symphysis with a height of 1 to 1.5 cm and a width of 4.0 cm centered at the midline.[1]

Internal Surface of the Body of the Mandible

An oblique mylohyoid line extends from the area below the mandibular third molar as far forward as the midline and gives attachment to the mylohyoid (**Fig. 19.4**). The concave area below the line is a submandibular fossa providing space for the submandibular gland. The line is faint further forward and ends by widening into a concave sublingual fossa for the sublingual gland. The mylohyoid groove from the ramus lies below the mylohyoid line at the posterior end of the mylohyoid line. The digastric fossa lies near the midline on each side on the internal

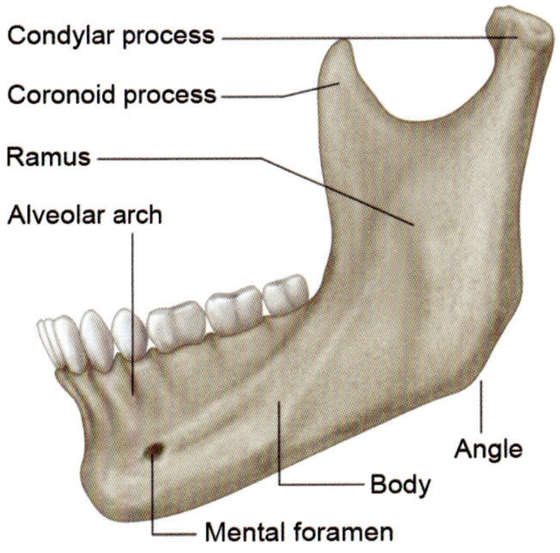

Fig. 19.1 Body and ramus of mandible.

surface of the mandible and gives attachment to the anterior belly of digastric.

Mental spines lie near the internal aspect of the mandibular symphysis on both sides. Although it sometimes merges into a single tubercle or is absent, the spine usually divides into two parts: an upper part for attachment to genioglossus and a lower part for attachment to geniohyoid.

Alveolar Part

The upper border between the internal and external surfaces of the mandible forms the alveolar part, giving support for the mandibular teeth. It contains the alveoli (alveolar sockets) for seven to eight mandibular teeth on one side. The alveolar part consists of the buccal and lingual plates, which are located on the external

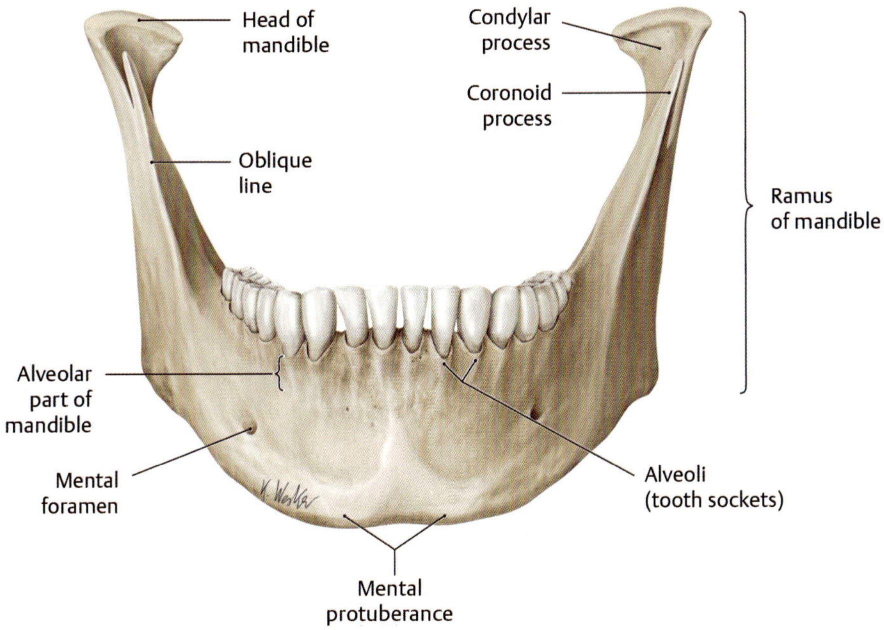

Fig. 19.2 External surface of mandible. (From THIEME Atlas of Anatomy, Head and Neuroanatomy. © Thieme 2010, Illustration by Karl Wesker.)

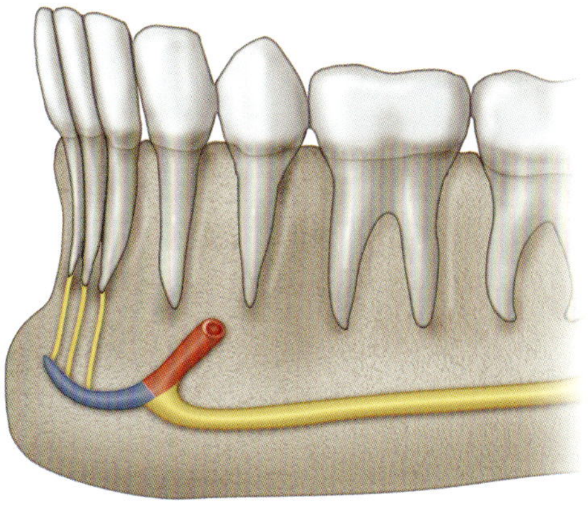

Fig. 19.3 Anterior loop of the mandibular canal. The yellow portion of thick canal represents the mandibular canal, and the red represents the anterior loop of the mandibular canal proceeding toward the mental foramen. The blue portion presents the incisive canal. The yellow small lines in the anterior region indicate the incisive nerves innervating the incisive teeth.

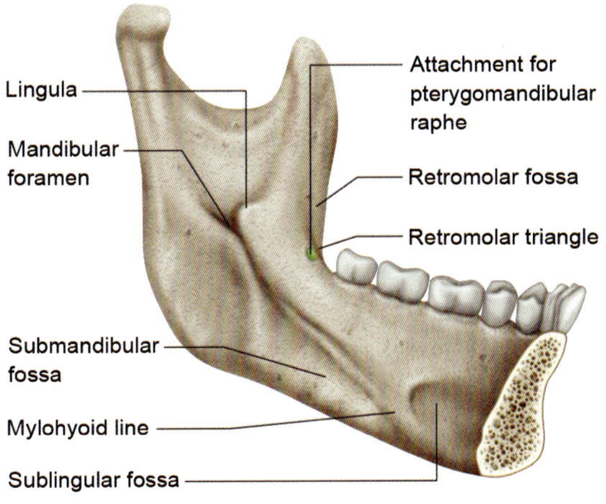

Fig. 19.4 Internal surface of mandible.

and internal aspects of the bone, and interdental and interradicular septa, which separate each tooth and root, respectively.

Ramus

The ramus of the mandible is a broad square-shaped part extending backward and upward from behind the body (**Fig. 19.5**). It consists of lateral and medial surfaces, four borders (superior, inferior, anterior, and posterior), condylar, and coronoid processes. The ramus provides entrance and passage for the inferior alveolar bundle (mandibular foramen and canal), attachment for masticatory muscles, and the condylar process for articulation at the TMJ.

Surfaces and Borders

The lateral surface is smooth except where the masseter attaches to its lower part. The medial surface of the ramus is more complicated. The mandibular foramen, the opening of the mandibular canal, is located at the point just above a center of the ramus. The anterior portion of the foramen is partially covered by a sharp triangular spine, the lingula. The tip of the needle should be placed at the vicinity of the lingula during an inferior alveolar nerve block (**Fig. 19.6**). The ligula lies about 1 cm above the occlusal plane.

The mylohyoid groove extends forward and downward from the lowermost part of the mandibular foramen. The anterior end of the groove lies below the mylohyoid line. Nerve and vessels proceed on the groove and distribute to the mylohyoid, which is the main muscle forming the floor of the mouth. The medial pterygoid muscle attaches to a rough surface behind and below the mylohyoid groove.

The external oblique ridge continues along the anterior border of the ramus on its lateral surface. From the tip of the anterior border (coronoid process), a ridge descends on the medial side of the process to the area posterior to the third molar region. This ridge, the temporal crest, constitutes a small triangular depression (retromolar fossa) with the external oblique line.

The joining of the mandibular base and the posterior border of the ramus forms the angle of mandible. A portion of the mandibular base anterior to the angle is slightly curved superiorly and is called the premasseteric notch. The facial artery passes beneath the premasseteric notch; thus, the pulsation of the artery can be palpated here.

The superior border bears a sharp, triangular coronoid process and a round and claviform condylar process. The mandibular notch is an incisure with a sharp superior edge between two distinct processes. Nerve and vessels to the masseter on the lateral surface of the ramus pass though the mandibular notch.

Surgical Annotation: Identifying the Mandibular Foramen

With a thumb on the anterior border of the ramus fits on the concave line of the border, the line through the distal end of the thumbnail and the interproximal point of the two premolars on the opposite side passes through the vicinity of the mandibular foramen. This line is usually used for an inferior alveolar nerve block.

Coronoid Process

The coronoid process is thin, triangular shaped, and protects upward. Its anterior border is a continuum of the external oblique ridge, and the mandibular notch limits its posterior border. The

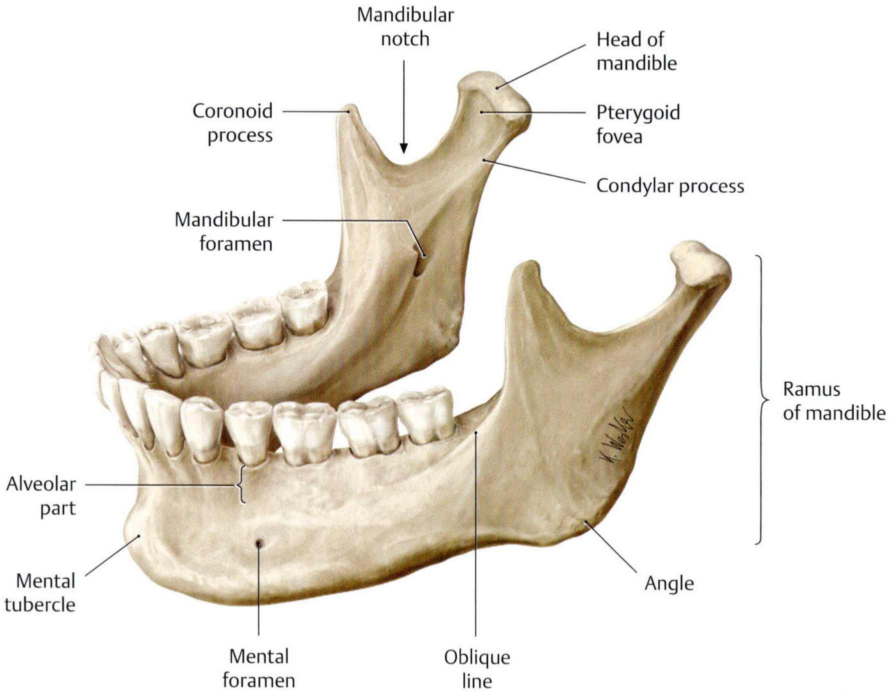

Fig. 19.5 Internal surface of ramus of mandible. (From THIEME Atlas of Anatomy, Head and Neuroanatomy. © Thieme 2010, Illustration by Karl Wesker.)

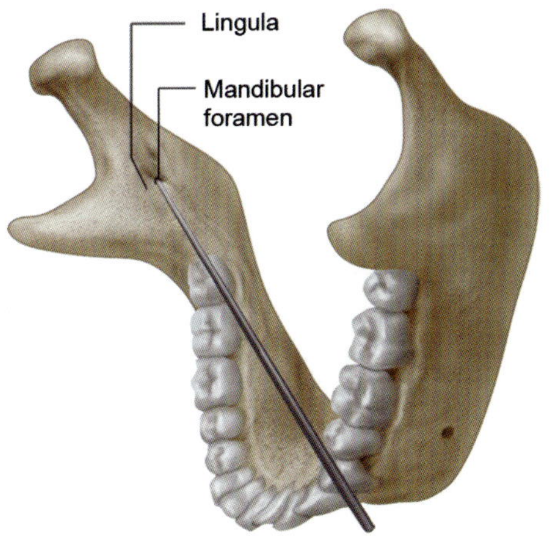

Fig. 19.6 Passage of needle to mandibular foramen for inferior mandibular block.

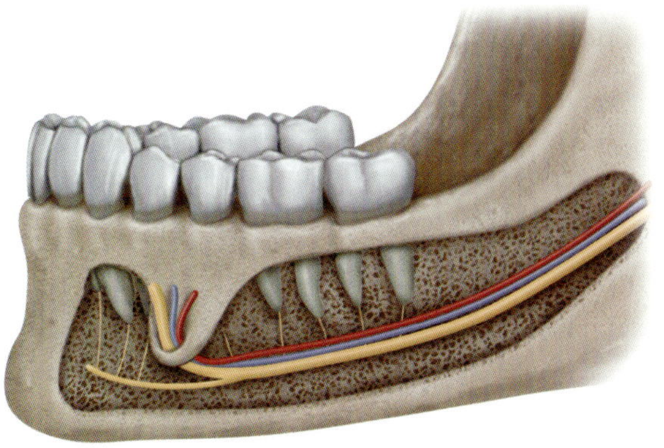

Fig. 19.7 Arrangement of inferior alveolar neurovascular bundle. Yellow represents the inferior alveolar nerve, mental nerve, and incisive nerve. Red and blue represent the inferior alveolar artery and vein, respectively.

temporalis is attached to the anterior, posterior, and medial borders of the coronoid process.

Condylar Process

The condylar process consists of the articular head and the neck. The articular head participates in articulation with the mandibular fossa of the temporal bone. The pterygoid fovea is a small fossa on the anterior surface of the neck and gives attachment to the upper head of the lateral pterygoid. Since the head of the condylar process is larger than its neck and the condylar process acts as an axis of jaw joint, the condylar process is frequently fractured with trauma.

Mandibular Canal

The mandibular canal is the bony canal extending from the mandibular foramen to the mental foramen. The canal runs downward and forward within the ramus then runs horizontally within the body under the tooth-bearing portion. The canal is closer to the external surface (labial cortical plate) farther forward. In the anterior end of the canal, it extends anterior to the mental foramen and curves back to the foramen, forming the anterior loop.

The inferior alveolar nerve and vessels enter the mandibular canal through the mandibular foramen. The trunk of the inferior alveolar nerve divides into mental and incisive nerves. The former exits through the mental foramen and innervates the skin of the chin. The latter passes medially within the mandible and innervates the incisors. The bony passage of the incisive nerve is called the incisive canal.

The neurovascular bundle from the inferior alveolar nerve and vessels to the teeth is within numerous tiny canaliculi between the canal and the alveolar part. Radiographically, the mandibular canal's upper border is less distinct compared with its lower border.

Damage to the Mandibular Canal

The inferior alveolar nerve innervates all mandibular teeth, and the mental nerve supplies sensation of the skin and mucosa of the chin. Intrusion of an instrument or dental implant can result in a sensory disorder of the teeth distal to the injury site.[1] Therefore, an injury of the inferior alveolar nerve within the mandibular canal causes partial or complete numbness of the chin area.

Additionally, the mental nerve is a branch from the inferior alveolar nerve, and its sensory component is conveyed through the buccal portion of the inferior alveolar nerve. The foramen is located below the premolars in about half the cases.[2] The position of the mental foramen varies among races and individuals. Therefore, its position on radiography should be performed before surgical intervention on the premolar area.

The inferior alveolar nerve lies below the inferior alveolar vessels, and the artery is located lingual to the vein in most cases (**Fig. 19.7**).[1] Therefore, transient numbness can result indirectly from the compression of, for example, a hematoma.

Some surgeons try to overcome limitation of a fixture placement because of the mandibular canal by altering angulation or position of the fixture; however, some difficult situations (more than 10%) occur in which the mandibular canal follows midway or a lingual one-third passage within the mandible.[1] The buccolingual position should be evaluated radiographically before intervention.

Masticatory Muscles

The main masticatory muscles consist of the masseter, temporalis, and medial and lateral pterygoids. The masseter lies on the external surface of the ramus of the mandible and the temporalis is located in the temporal fossa. The two pterygoid muscles and the tendon of temporalis are located in the infratemporal fossa (**Fig. 19.8a–c**).

The four muscles are derived from the first pharyngeal arch and are innervated by the mandibular division of the trigeminal nerve. The maxillary artery from the external carotid artery and supplementary branches from the facial or superficial temporal arteries supply blood to the masticatory muscles. The masticatory muscles produce movements of the mandible at the TMJ; elevate the mandible (masseter, temporalis, medial pterygoid); pull down (lateral pterygoid), protrude (lateral pterygoid) and retract it (temporalis). They also act together to provide complicated side-to-side movements. Functionally, the infrahyoid muscles, including the digastric, stylohyoid, geniohyoid, and myohyoid muscles, participate in accessory mastication functions such as opening the mandible. The four masticatory muscles innervated by the mandibular nerve are commonly regarded as principal movers of the jaw.

Masseter

The masseter has been commonly described as a muscle arising from the maxillary process of the zygomatic bone and the zygomatic arch and inserting into the angle and the lower part of the lateral surface of the ramus of the mandible. The main action of the masseter is to occlude the teeth by elevating the mandible.

Actually, the masseter consists of three layers; superficial, middle, and deep layers. Although the fibers of the three layers mostly pass downward and backward, detailed directions of the muscle fibers are slightly different according to the layer. The superficial layer arises from the maxillary process of the zygomatic bone and the anterior two-thirds of the zygomatic arch and inserts into the angle and its neighboring portion of the external surface of the ramus. The origin of the middle layer lies posterior to the superficial layer. The middle layer arises from the medial aspect of the anterior two-thirds of the zygomatic arch and the lower border of the posterior one-third of the arch and inserts into the central part of the ramus. The direction of the superficial layer is anterior to the middle one, and thus the superficial layer participates more in protraction of the mandible. The deep layer arises from the deep surface of the zygomatic arch and inserts into the upper part of the ramus and the

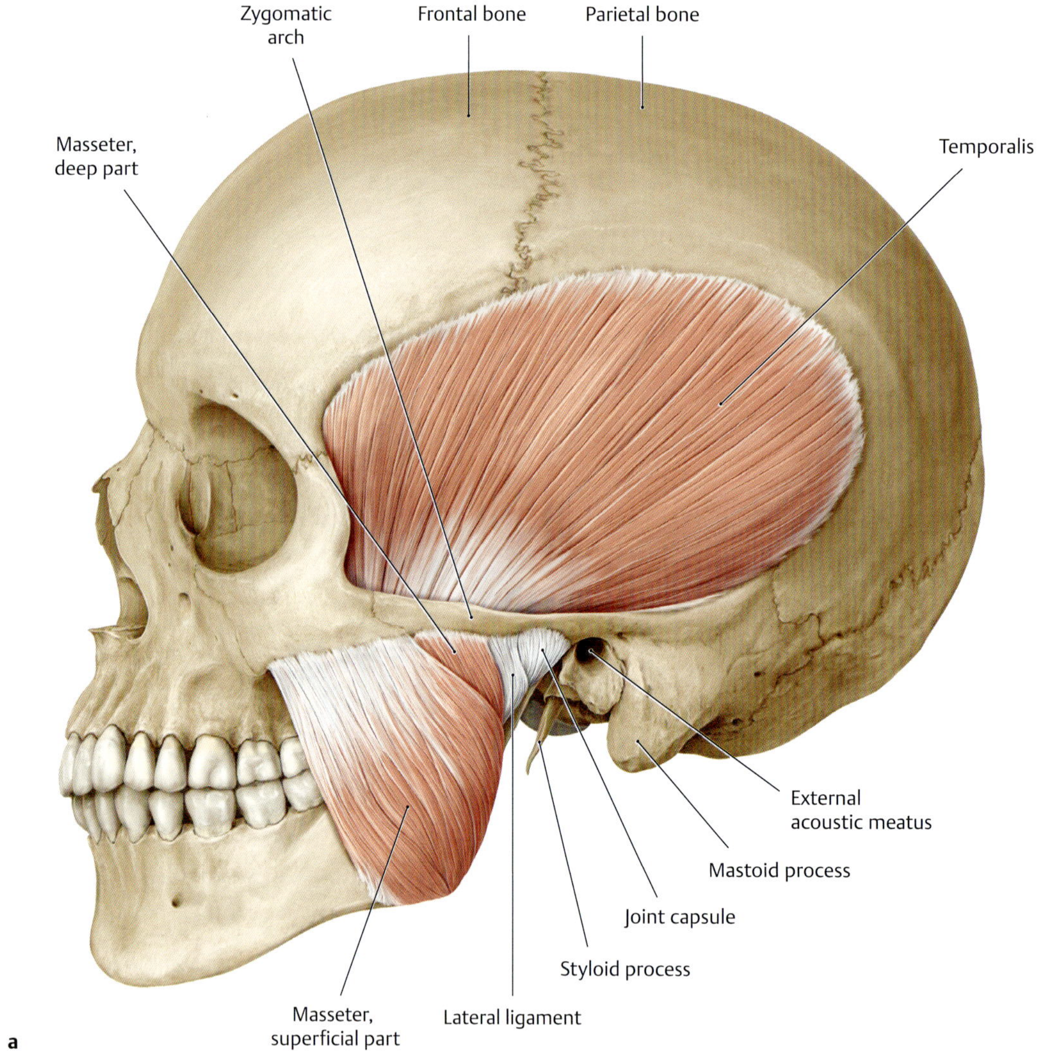

Fig. 19.8 Four masticatory muscles; masseter, temporalis, medial, and lateral pterygoids. **(a)** Masseter with temporalis muscle.

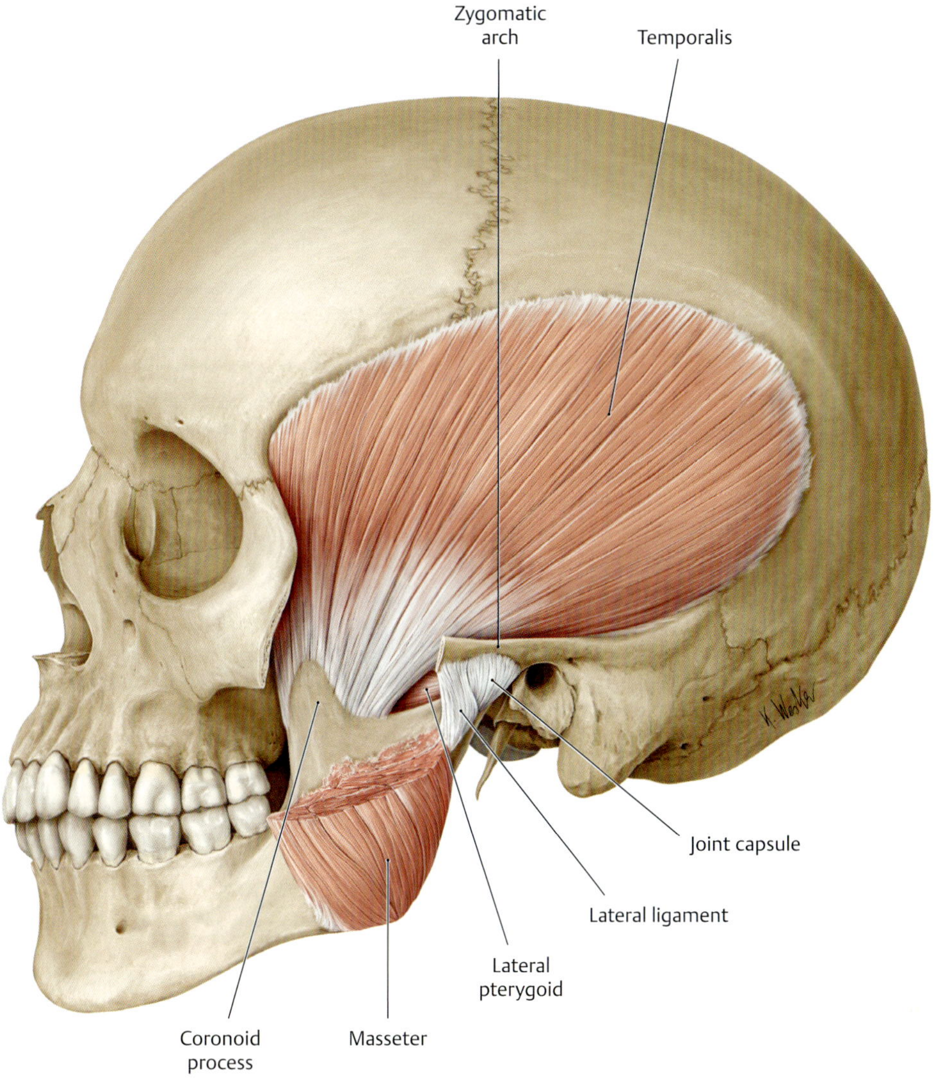

b

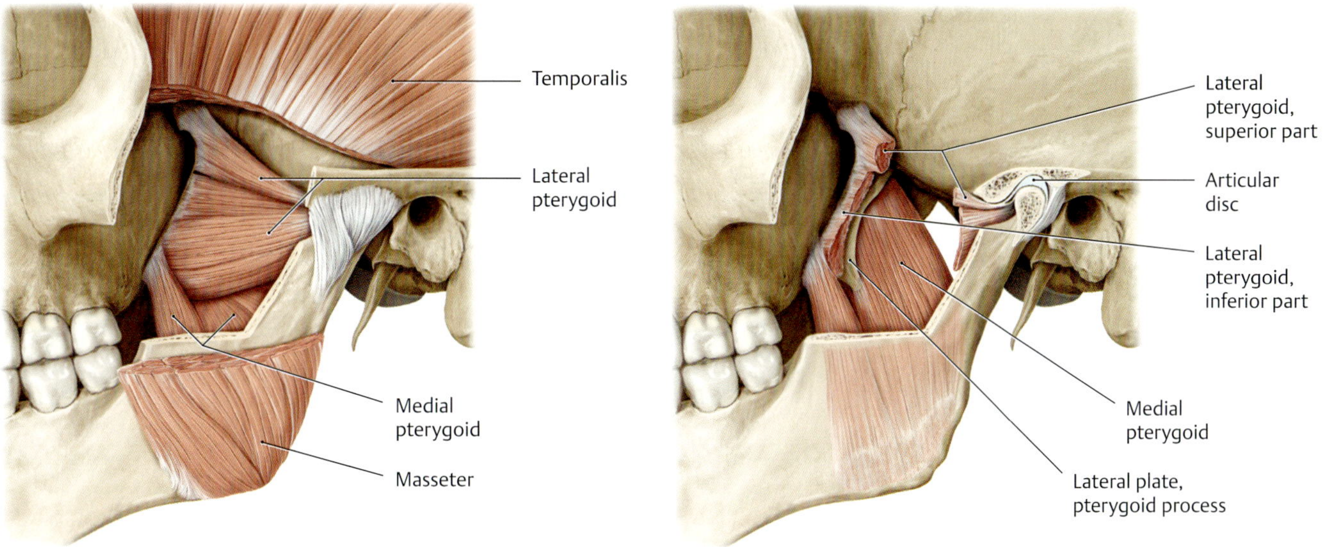

c

d

Fig. 19.8 (*continued*) **(b)**Temporalis muscle (masseter and zygomatic arch are removed). **(c)** Lateral pterygoid muscle (coronoid process of mandible is removed). **(d)** Medial pterygoid muscle (lateral pterygoid muscle is removed). (From THIEME Atlas of Anatomy, Head and Neuroanatomy. © Thieme 2010, Illustrations by Karl Wesker.)

coronoid process. Some parts of the middle and deep layers are involved in retraction of the mandible. The temporalis and buccinator muscles lie deep to the masseter. Most of the buccal branches, some zygomatic branches of the facial nerve, and facial vein cross over the masseter. The parotid gland overlaps the posterior part of masseter.

Vascular Supply of the Masseter

The maxillary artery gives rise to the masseteric artery, which supplies the masseter. The main trunk of the maxillary artery proceeds anteriorly and medial to the mandibular condyle within the infratemporal fossa. It gives off the masseteric artery near the lateral pterygoid and the artery leaves the infratemporal fossa with the masseteric nerve through the mandibular notch. Several branches from the facial artery and the transverse temporal artery are located on the external surface of the masseter; they supply blood to the anterior and superior parts of the masseter, respectively. The facial artery gives off the premasseteric artery passing upward along the anterior border of the masseter. The transverse facial artery arises from the superficial temporal artery and also supplies the masseter. It usually travels anteriorly between the parotid duct and the zygomatic arch.

Various Masseteric Branches

Knowledge of the arterial distribution to masseter is crucial in preventing vascular complications during various surgical procedures, such as masseter flap formation, reduction of the mandibular angle, parotidectomy, and ramus osteotomy. Although the massteric artery from the maxillary artery is delineated primarily as a main vessel distributing masseter, the muscle can be supplied by several other arterial branches from the external carotid artery (**Fig. 19.9**).[3] (1) The transverse facial artery from the superficial temporal artery gives off masseteric branches that cross transversely over the muscle. Its intramuscular branches to the masseter are distributed to a broad posterior area of the muscle. (2) The external carotid artery and superficial temporal artery give rise to direct masseteric branches to the angular and articular portions of the masseter. The facial artery directly gives off the masseteric branch as it emerges on the external surface of the mandible after turning upward. It is distributed to the anterior lower portion of the muscle. The facial artery gives off the premasseteric artery running along the anterior border of masseter, and it also gives rise to a small masseteric branch supplying blood to the anterior midportion of the muscle. (3) The deep temporal artery, another tributary of the maxillary artery, also supplies a branch to the masseter and specifically to its anterior upper portion.

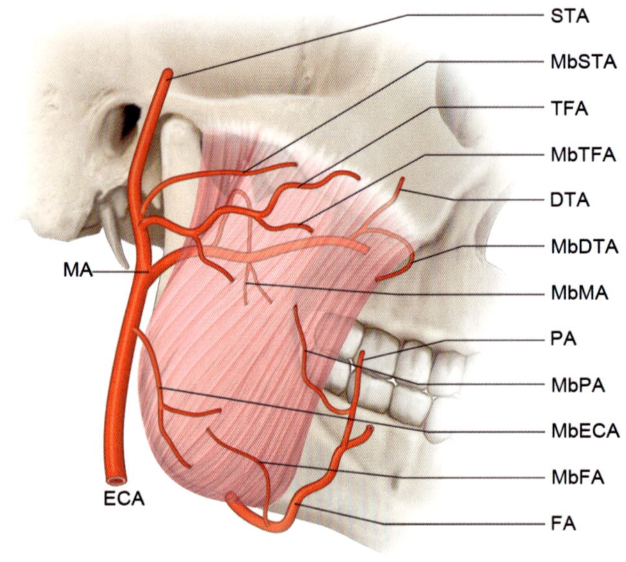

Fig. 19.9 Arteries to the masseter muscle. DTA, deep temporal artery; ECA, external carotid artery; FA, facial artery; MA, maxillary artery; PA, premasseteric artery; STA, superficial temporal artery; TFA, transverse facial artery. Masseteric branches from ECA(MbECA), STA(MbSTA), TFA(MbTFA), DTA(MbDTA), MA(MbMA), PA (MbPA), and FA (MbFA).

Innervation of the Masseter

The masseteric nerve of the mandibular nerve innervates the masseter. The masseteric nerve passes though the mandibular notch and is accompanied by the masseteric artery. The proximal part of the masseteric nerve is located between the mandibular notch and the attachment of the masseter (submasseteric tissue space). Abscess resulting from infection of the mandibular third molar tooth has been known to invade the submasseteric tissue space and irritate the masseteric nerve with resultant muscle spasm and trismus (pathologic limitation of jaw opening).

Intramuscular Innervation to Masseter

The masseteric nerve runs downward and forward between the middle and deep layers of masseter and is divided into four twig groups: anterosuperior, anteroinferior, posterosuperior, and posteroinferior groups (**Fig. 19.10**).[4]

The superficial, middle, and deep layers of the masseter are mostly innervated by the anteroinferior, posterosuperior, and posteroinferior groups, respectively. The anteroinferior group provides perforating branches to the superficial layers, and its termination lies mostly on the inferior midportion of the masseter. The inferior midportion might be an efficient site for botulin injection.

Temporalis

The temporalis is a fan-shaped masticatory muscle that arises from the temporal fossa and the inner surface of the temporal fascia. The muscle's tendon converges and passes to the infratemporal fossa between the zygomatic arch and the lateral side of the skull. The tendon of temporalis attaches to the medial surface, apex, and apical border of the coronoid process. Temporalis elevates and its posterior fibers retract the mandible. Directions of the muscle fibers of temporalis vary according to their location. The muscle fibers of temporalis are arranged more horizontally posteriorly. The anterior parts of temporalis are arranged more vertically. Some fibers of its anterior parts arise from the inner surface of the zygomatic bone. These fibers strongly elevate the mandible by pulling the coronoid process

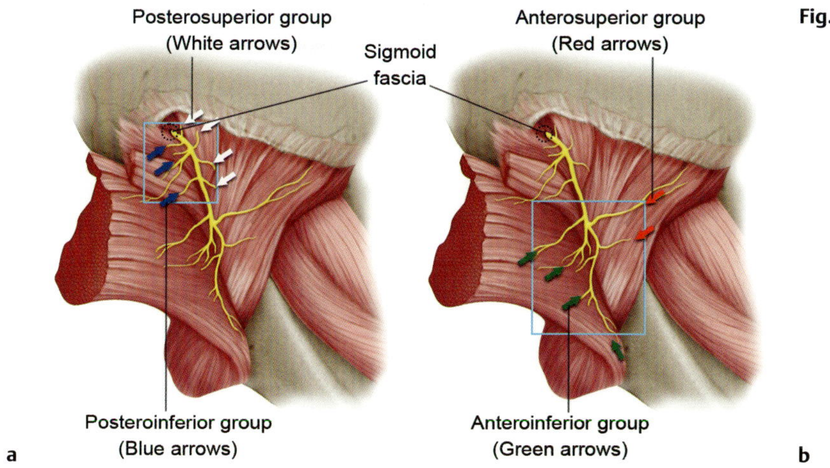

Fig. 19.10 Four groups of masseteric nerves.

upward. The posterior more horizontal parts of temporalis also participate in closing the mouth by rotating the mandible toward the maxilla on the axis of the jaw joint.

Significant structures, including the superficial temporal vessels, the auriculotemporal nerve, and temporal branches of the facial nerve, lie on the temporalis and the temporal fascia.

Vascular Supply

Artery

The maxillary artery gives rise to the anterior and posterior deep temporal arteries on the lateral pterygoid. The deep temporal arteries ascend on the lateral pterygoid and infratemporal crest of the sphenoid bone and then enter temporalis with the deep temporal branches of the mandibular nerve. The superficial temporal artery gives rise to the middle temporal artery just above the zygomatic arch and enters the temporalis after piercing the temporal fascia. The anterior deep temporal artery supplies blood to the anterior portion of temporalis and the posterior deep temporal artery supplies the posterior parts. The middle temporal artery is distributed to the midportion of the temporalis. The frontal branch of the superficial temporal artery ascends on temporalis upward and forward.

Superficial Temporal Artery Over the Anterior Temporalis

The anterior portion of temporalis lies over the temple near the pterion. Various surgical interventions near this area include face lift procedures, the injection of filler material, the injection of botulin toxin for aesthetic purposes, and the injection of anesthetics for the treatment of headaches. Therefore, knowledge of the superficial temporal artery and its topography is important to the clinician.

The superficial temporal artery branches from the external carotid artery in the preauricular area at a distance of 2 to 5 cm from the Frankfurt line (line through the lowermost point of the orbit to the uppermost part of the portion), and it passes forward and upward over the temporalis (**Fig. 19.11**). Because the frontal branch lies within the temporal fascia or between the temporoparietal fascia and temporal fascia, a surgical approach can be safely performed deep to the temporalis.

The artery divides into several frontal branches as it passes over the temporalis. Usually, one or two will reach the border between the temporalis and frontalis (the frontal belly of occipitotemporalis) about 2 cm (approximately the width of the thumb) above the eyebrow. The pulsation of the frontal branch can easily be detected by palpation at its branching point from the superficial temporal artery and as it enters frontalis. Therefore, the surgeon can predict its course by palpation of the branching points because the frontal branch rarely bifurcates except between muscles.

Veins

The veins of the temporal, frontal, and parietal areas converge as the sentinel vein. The medial temporal vein and its continuum (i.e., the superior temporal vein) drain to the retromandibular vein, the anterior and posterior branches of which drain to

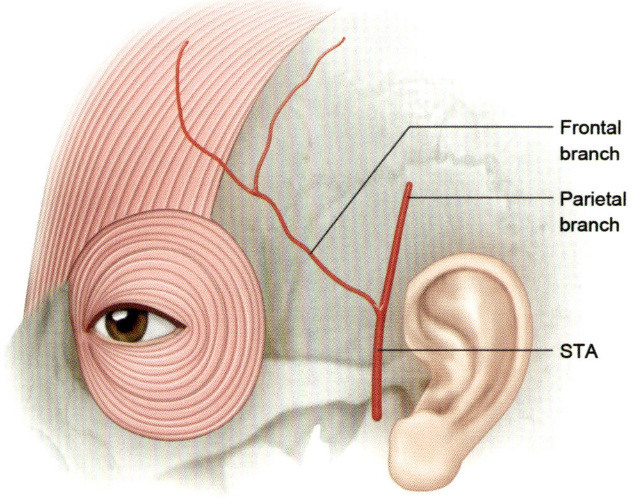

Fig. 19.11 Superficial temporal artery (STA) passing over temporalis.

the external and internal jugular veins, respectively. The blood flow in the sentinel vein can actually flow toward both the infraorbital space and the thoracic area via the valveless venous vessels of the head and neck.

The medial zygomaticotemporal vein has been observed in the vicinity of the temporal branch of the facial nerve during endoscopic procedures aimed at lifting the upper face. The sentinel vein is easily identified on direct or endoscopic view during facelift procedures and is readily detected in recumbent patients or in conscious patients using a Valsalva maneuver.

The sentinel vein pierces the parietotemporal fascia, which is part of the superficial musculoaponeurotic system (SMAS) in about 17% of cases.

Innervation

The deep temporal nerve branches from the mandibular nerve and innervates the temporalis. The deep temporal nerve consists of two or three branches. The branches of the deep temporal nerve pass between the infratemporal crest and upper border of the lateral pterygoid. They enter temporalis with the deep temporal arteries. Sometimes the anterior branch of the deep temporal nerve branches from the buccal nerve and the posterior branch branches from the masseteric nerve.

Fasciae of the Temporal Region

The auriculotemporal nerve, temporal branches of the facial nerve, and superficial temporal vessels are involved in various surgical interventions of the temporalis or temporal region, regardless of their distribution to the temporalis. The anatomy of the fasciae of temporalis is therefore important in the preservation of these neurovascular structures. The temporal fascia is a dense aponeurotic layer covering the temporalis and providing attachment for the surface for the muscle. Its uppermost portion merges with the periosteum at the superior temporal line. The temporal fascia divides into superficial and deep sublayers, which attach to the medial and lateral margins of the zygomatic arch, respectively. The adipose tissue (superficial temporal fat pad) lies between them, and they surround branches of the superficial temporal artery and zygomaticotemporal nerve. Hence, placement of an instrument deep to the temporal fascia can provide a safe surgical approach for manipulating zygomatic arch fractures (Gillies approach).[5]

The temporoparietal fascia lies superficial to the temporal fascia. It is on the same plane as the superficial musculoaponeurotic system (SMAS) blending with the galea aponeurotica. The space between the temporoparietal fascia and the temporal fascia encloses the loose connective tissue with adipose tissue (temporoparietal fad pad), continuing with a subgaleal loose connective tissue plane of the scalp. The auriculotemporal nerve, facial nerve branches, and superficial temporal vessels are located within or slightly deep to the temporoparietal fascia. Surgeons can use this fascia as a landmark to avoid facial nerve damage. Clinically, the temporoparietal fascia is called the superficial temporal fascia, and the temporal fascia is called the deep temporal fascia.

Medial Pterygoid

The medial pterygoid is a square-shaped masticatory muscle that consists of two heads that arise superficial and deep to the lower head of the lateral pterygoid. The deep head of the medial pterygoid arises from the medial surface of the lateral pterygoid plate of the sphenoid bone. The superficial head arises from the maxillary tuberosity and pyramidal process of the palatine bone. Two heads descend backward and attach to the medial surface of the ramus and the angle of the mandible. The posteroinferior direction of the medial pterygoid and its action of elevating the mandible are similar to those of the masseter. When two pterygoid muscles of one side act together, they rotate the mandible forward and medially to the opposite side.

The lateral pterygoid, the sphenomandibular ligament, maxillary artery, the inferior alveolar artery and vessels, and the lingual nerve are located between the lateral side of the medial pterygoid and the medial surface of the ramus of the mandible. Insertion of the medial pterygoid reaches upward to the mandibular foramen and forward to the mylohyoid line.

Vascular Supply and Innervation

The maxillary artery provides several pterygoid branches supplying blood to the medial and lateral pterygoid muscles. The buccal artery from the maxillary artery also gives off branches to the medial pterygoid. A part of the facial artery proceeds medial to the ramus of the mandible between the submandibular gland and the medial pterygoid along the inferior border of the mandible. Some branches are derived from the facial artery here and are distributed to the medial pterygoid at its insertion near the angle of the mandible. The mandibular nerve gives rise to the nerve to the medial pterygoid.

Medial Pterygoid and Mandibular Angle Reduction

Both the medial pterygoid and masseter lie downward and backward 70 degrees from the mandibular base, and they insert onto the medial and lateral surfaces of the angle of the mandible, respectively. Their insertions are located near the gonion (the most posteroinferior point of the angle of the mandible) by a distance of 2 cm.[6] Therefore, the medial pterygoid is an important landmark for mandibular angle reduction. Injury to the arteries approaching the angle is a complication during mandibular angle reduction. According to most anatomy textbooks, the main branch supplying the medial pterygoid derives from the maxillary artery after passing over the condylar process of the mandible; however, the facial artery provides other branches to the angular portion of the medial pterygoid.[7] The artery gives off the ascending palatine artery medial to the angle of the mandible. It also gives off muscular branches before emerging on the superficial aspect of the mandible. There are also small muscular branches arising directly from the facial artery and traveling to the angular portion of the medial pterygoid (**Fig. 19.12**). Therefore, surgeons approaching the angle of

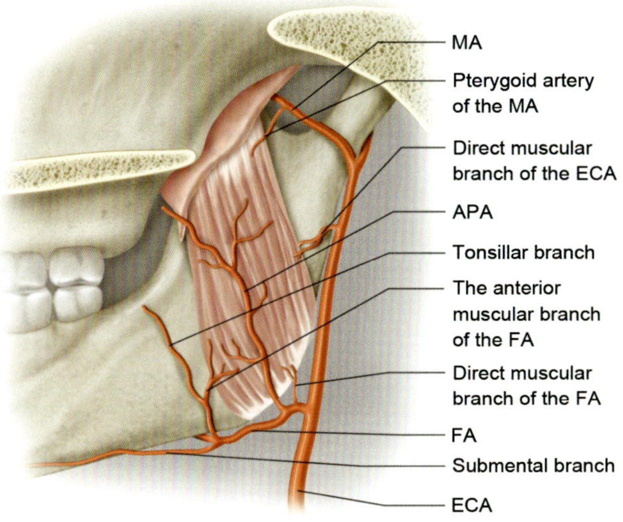

Fig. 19.12 Arteries to medial pterygoid muscle. APA, ascending palatine artery; ECA, external carotid artery; FA, facial artery; MA, maxillary artery.

the mandible should be aware not only of the main trunk of the facial artery but also of the muscular branches to the masseter and medial pterygoid muscles.

Lateral Pterygoid

The lateral pterygoid is a horizontally arranged muscle within the infratemporal fossa muscle and comprises upper and lower heads. The upper head arises from the infratemporal surface and crest of the greater wing of the sphenoid bone, and the lower head arises from the lateral surface of the lateral pterygoid plate. The two heads of the lateral pterygoid run backward, and their muscle fibers converge to be inserted into the pterygoid fovea, a depression on the anterior side of the neck of the mandible. Characteristically, some muscle fibers of the upper head attach to the capsule of the TMJ and the anterior border of the articular disc. Because the TMJ is located lateral to the lateral pterygoid plate, the bellies of the two heads proceed outward, and the muscular fibers of the upper head attach to the medial border of the disc. The lateral pterygoid pulls the neck of the mandible forwards and the condyle of the mandible moves not only forward, but it also downward along the anterior slope of the mandibular fossa.

The rami of the mandible, the masseter, the superficial head of the medial pterygoid, and the tendon of temporalis are superficial to the medial pterygoid and to most of the maxillary artery. The sphenomandibular ligament, the middle meningeal artery, and the mandibular nerve trunk are deep to the muscle.

Function of Lateral Pterygoid: Side-to-Side Movement

The main jaw depressor is not the lateral pterygoid; rather, it is the infrahyoid muscles (e.g., digastric and geniohyoid).[5] Protrusion of the mandible by the lateral pterygoid is limited to an assisting movement for jaw opening and alone is not significant. The most important function provided by the lateral pterygoid is lateral excursion, side-to-side movement of the mandible. The ipsilateral medial and lateral pterygoids pull the mandible medially. The slight but strong medial movement of the jaw is crucial in food grinding. Spasm of the lateral pterygoid can occur in cases of TMJ dysfunction; in such cases, tenderness might be palpated posterior to the maxillary tuberosity.

Vascular Supply and Innervation

The maxillary artery crosses the lateral pterygoid anterosuperiorly. The lateral pterygoid is a landmark for demarcation of the maxillary artery. The proximal portion of the maxillary artery behind the muscle is the mandibular part, the midportion on the muscle is the pterygoid part, and the distal portion in front of the muscle is the pterygopalatine part. The mandibular part of the artery gives off the pterygoid arteries distributed to the lateral pterygoid as the artery crosses it. The ascending palatine artery branches from the facial artery and also supplies the lateral pterygoid. The mandibular nerve gives rise to the nerve to the lateral pterygoid.

Spatial Relations of Lateral Pterygoid to Mandibular Nerves

Many branches from the mandibular nerve have a spatial relationship with the lateral pterygoid.[5] The deep temporal nerves and masseteric nerve run along the infratemporal crest and the upper border of the upper head of the lateral pterygoid. The buccal nerve passes between the upper and lower heads of the muscle. The lingual nerve and inferior alveolar nerve pass below the lower head. The nerve to the lateral pterygoid arises directly from the mandibular nerve or from the buccal nerve passing between the two heads of the muscle. The nerve, after arising directly from the mandibular nerve, enters the deep part of the lateral pterygoid and innervates the medial part of the lower head. The nerve branches from the buccal nerve are distributed to the upper head and lateral part of the lower head. The buccal nerve, after passing through the lateral pterygoid, terminates as a cutaneous nerve supplying the cheek.

References

1. Hu KS, Yun HS, Hur MS, Kwon HJ, Abe S, Kim HJ. Branching patterns and intraosseous course of the mental nerve. J Oral Maxillofac Surg 2007;65(11):2288–2294
2. Song WC, Kim SH, Paik DJ, et al. Location of the infraorbital and mental foramen with reference to the soft-tissue landmarks. Plast Reconstr Surg 2007;120(5):1343–1347
3. Kwak HH, Hu KS, Hur MS, et al. Clinical implications of the topography of the arteries supplying the medial pterygoid muscle. J Craniofac Surg 2008;19(3):795–799
4. Kim DH, Hong HS, Won SY, et al. Intramuscular nerve distribution of the masseter muscle as a basis for botulinum toxin injection. J Craniofac Surg 2010;21(2):588–591
5. Standring S. Gray's Anatomy : The Anatomical Basis of Clinical Practice. 40th ed. Edinburgh: Churchill Livingstone; 2008:530–539
6. Yang SJ, Hu KS, Kang MK, Youn KH, Kim HJ. Topography and morphology of the medial pterygoid muscle for the surgical approach of the mandibular ramus. Korean J Phy Anthropol. 2007;20(3): 157–167
7. Won SY, Choi DY, Kwak HH, Kim ST, Kim HJ, Hu KS. Topography of the arteries supplying the masseter muscle: Using dissection and Sihler's method. Clin Anat 2012;25(3):308–313

20 Oral Cavity and Pharynx

Joe Iwanaga, Shinya Mikushi, and Haruka Tohara

Introduction

The oral cavity is the entrance of the upper digestive tract, continuing into the oropharynx; it is divided into two regions (**Fig. 20.1**). The first region is the oral vestibule, located external to the dental arch. The second region is the oral cavity proper, located internal to the dental arch. The components of the oral cavity include the upper and lower lip mucosa, teeth and gingiva, alveolar mucosa, buccal mucosa, tongue, hard and soft palate, floor of the mouth, and uvula. The palate is the roof of the mouth and separates the oral and nasal cavities. The pharynx is located at the posterior aspect of the oropharyngeal isthmus. Two important functions involving the oral cavity and pharynx are mastication and swallowing. Multiple muscles work together to send a bolus of food to the esophagus. Other major functions are occlusion and aesthetics. The oral cavity and pharynx contain an abundant supply of blood vessels and nerves in a constricted space, providing a particular challenge for clinicians undertaking surgical procedures. In this chapter, we explain the details of the clinical anatomy of oral cavity and pharynx to promote better understanding for clinical practice.

Oral Vestibule

The oral vestibule is the region surrounded by the lip (buccal) mucosa, mucobuccal fold, alveolar mucosa, gingiva, and upper and lower dental arches. Its shape in the axial plane is that of a horseshoe, and it is separated from the oral cavity proper when the upper and lower teeth are in occlusion. Mucosal folds that run from the central incisor region of the alveolar mucosa to the lip mucosa are the frenulum of the upper and lower lips (**Fig. 20.2**). Mucosal folds that run from the molar region of the alveolar mucosa to the buccal mucosa are called buccal frenula. The parotid duct runs from the parotid gland, passes in front of the masseter muscle, enters into the buccal fat pad, and then reaches the parotid papilla located in the buccal mucosa (**Fig. 20.3**). A small triangle (the retromolar triangle) lies just behind the most distal molar and a small ridge in the retromolar region (the retromolar pad) (**Fig. 20.4**). The lingual nerve branches off the mandibular nerve and occasionally crosses over the retromolar triangle.[1] The external oblique ridge, which begins lateral to the retromolar pad, continues on to the anterior border of the ramus. When the mandible opens and closes, or when the lips suck, the bone movement and muscle contraction change the form of the oral vestibule. The lower part of the oral vestibule in particular is affected by the superior pharyngeal constrictor muscle, masseter muscle, buccinator muscle, orbicularis oris muscle, mentalis muscle, and coronoid process; the upper part is affected by the orbicularis oris muscle, buccinator muscle, medial pterygoid muscle, levator anguli oris muscle, nasal muscle, depressor septi muscle, and infrazygomatic crest. If the superior labial frenulum is located in a high position on the gingiva, the right and left maxillary incisor teeth may exhibit a median diastema, and frenoplasty is often required.

The orbicularis oris muscle and buccinator muscle are present beneath the mucous membranes of the labial and buccal mucosae. In the mandible, there are two mental foramina, just inferior to the apex of the second premolars, through which the

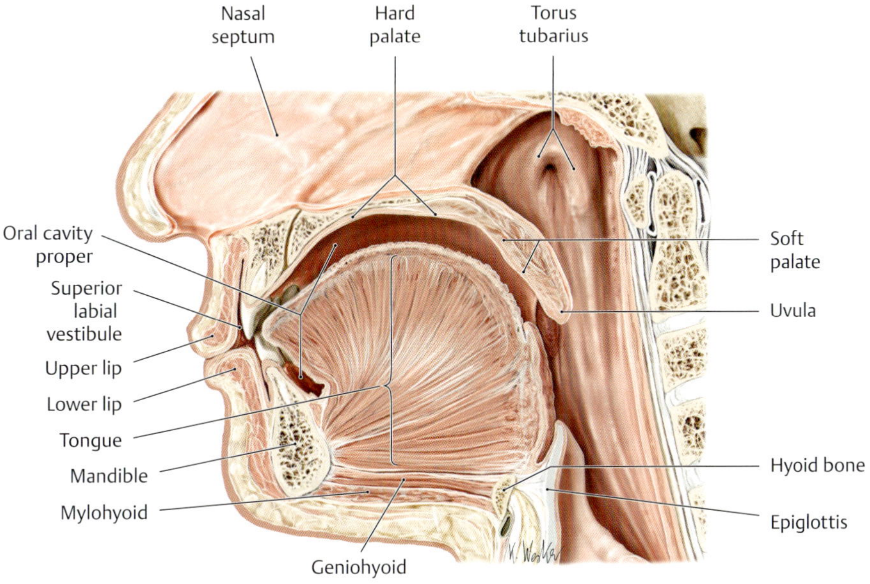

Fig. 20.1 Midsagittal plane of the oral cavity and pharynx. (From THIEME Atlas of Anatomy, Head and Neuroanatomy. © Thieme 2010, Illustration by Karl Wesker.)

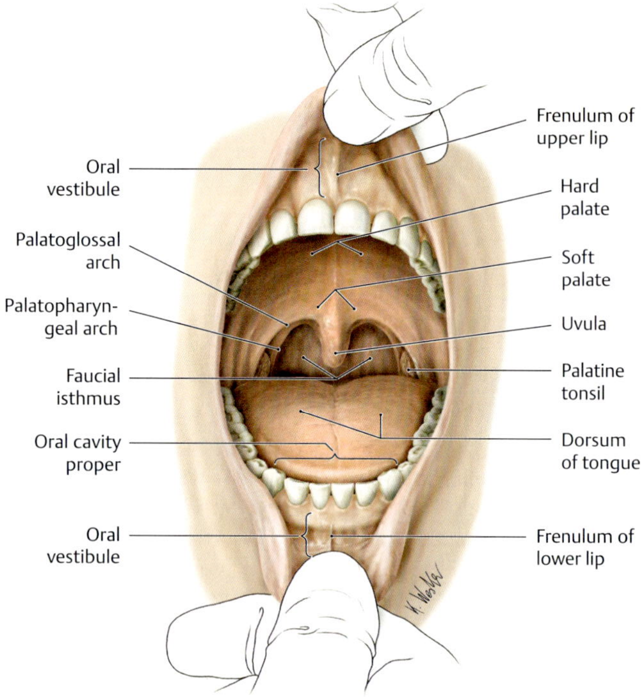

Fig. 20.2 Frenulum of the upper and lower lips. (From THIEME Head and Neck Anatomy for Dental Medicine. © Thieme 2010, Illustration by Karl Wesker.)

mental nerves, arteries, and veins emerge. The vertical distance from the margin of the mandible to the mental foramen is reported to be approximately 12 mm.[2] Surgical procedures in the premolar region should be undertaken carefully. When teeth are lost, the alveolar bone proper resorbs and the thickness of the mandible decreases, so the mental foramina sometimes open just below the alveolar mucosa; nerves exiting the foramina are then easily compressed by dentures. Recent developments in imaging have revealed that accessory mental foramina exist around the mental foramen in approximately 10% of cases[3,4] (**Fig. 20.5**) and that the accessory mental nerve branches off from these accessory foramina.

Teeth and Periodontal Tissues

The teeth consist of a crown, the surface of which is covered by enamel, a hard translucent tissue, and the root, which is covered by cementum. Within the crown and root is a layer of dentin surrounding a central pulp cavity. The apical foramen is a hole at the tip of the root, through which the dental pulp, blood vessels, and lymph vessels enter and exit the dental pulp chamber. The root is surrounded by the periodontal ligament (**Fig. 20.6**). Enamel is the hardest tissue in the human body; at the same time, it is a fragile and breakable tissue. The enamel is approximately 96% inorganic matter called hydroxyapatite; it reaches a maximum thickness of 2.5 mm over the cusps and is quite thin at the cervical margins. After crown formation is complete, no additional enamel forms, but the enamel of young people is easily demineralized and remineralized. Dentin is a yellowish tissue composed of hydroxyapatite (70%), collagen (20%), and water (10%). Dentin is more flexible than enamel, so it acts as a buffer to prevent the enamel from fracturing. Additionally, if inflammation occurs in the dental pulp as a result of dental caries or traumatic injury after the start of occlusal function, secondary dentin will form inside the dentin. The cementum covers the surface of the dentin of the root and is covered by the periodontal ligament, which consists of fibrous connective tissue that is 0.15 to 0.38 mm thick. Sharpey's fibers, which

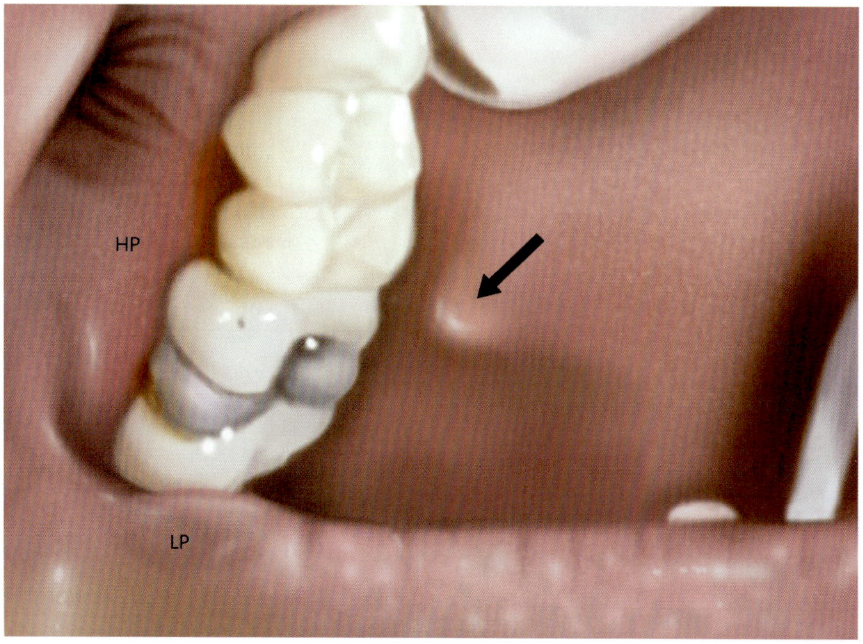

Fig. 20.3 The left parotid papilla (the orifice of the parotid duct) is indicated by the black arrow. HP, Hard palate; LP, lower lip.

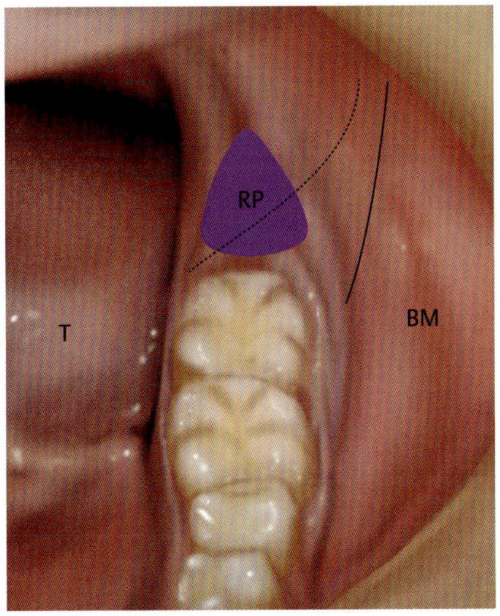

Fig. 20.4 The left retromolar region. Yellow region, retromolar pad; dotted line, internal oblique ridge; solid line, external oblique ridge. BM, Buccal mucosa; RP, retromolar pad; T, tongue.

emerge from the cementum, penetrate the periodontal ligament and enter the alveolar bone. The main roles of the periodontal ligament are to support the teeth, control sensitivity, and provide a blood supply. The activity of the periodontal ligament and the number of fibers it contains decrease with age. Dental pulp is a soft tissue that includes blood vessels, nerve fibers, lymph vessels, and connective tissue. It is divided into two parts, the coronal pulp and the radicular pulp, which communicate at the cervical region. The radicular pulp of anterior teeth is single; but for posterior teeth, there are multiple areas of radicular pulp. Both coronal pulp and radicular pulp become thinner as dentin deposition continues with aging. The apical foramen becomes narrower because of deposition of cementum.

The number of human adult permanent teeth is 32, and these are each surrounded by alveolar bone. Alveolar bone is divided into two parts: alveolar bone proper, which is adjacent to the cementum, and supporting bone. The alveolar bone proper resorbs along with the loss of teeth. There are eight kinds of permanent teeth: central incisor, lateral incisor, canine, first premolar, second premolar, first molar, second molar, and third molar (wisdom teeth) from the midline to posterolateral. The mesial and distal tooth surfaces are those closest to and farthest from the midline, respectively. The term *labial* is used for incisors and canine teeth, and *buccal* is used for premolar and molar teeth. *Palatal* denotes the inside surface of maxillary teeth, and *lingual* denotes the inside surface of mandibular teeth (**Fig. 20.7**). These designations are used to describe the precise location of small carious lesions. The deciduous teeth total 20, and they are called deciduous central incisor, deciduous lateral incisor, deciduous canine, first deciduous molar, and second deciduous molar from median to posterolateral. Deciduous teeth begin to erupt 6 to 8 months after birth. The deciduous central incisor erupts first, and the deciduous dentition finishes erupting at approximately 2 years of age. Then deciduous teeth begin to be replaced by permanent teeth at age 6 to 7 years. The permanent dentition is complete by the age of 13, except for the third molar, for which the age of eruption differs between individuals. The upper teeth are innervated by three superior nerves arising from the maxillary nerve: the posterior superior alveolar nerve, the middle superior alveolar nerve, and the anterior

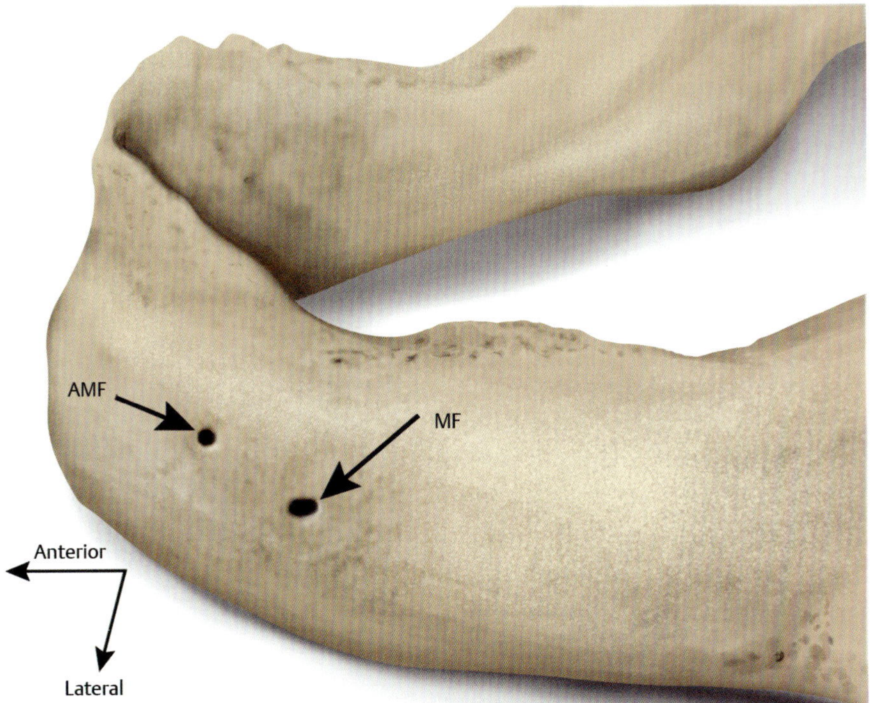

Fig. 20.5 Lateral view of the left mandible. AMF, Accessory mental foramen; MF, mental foramen.

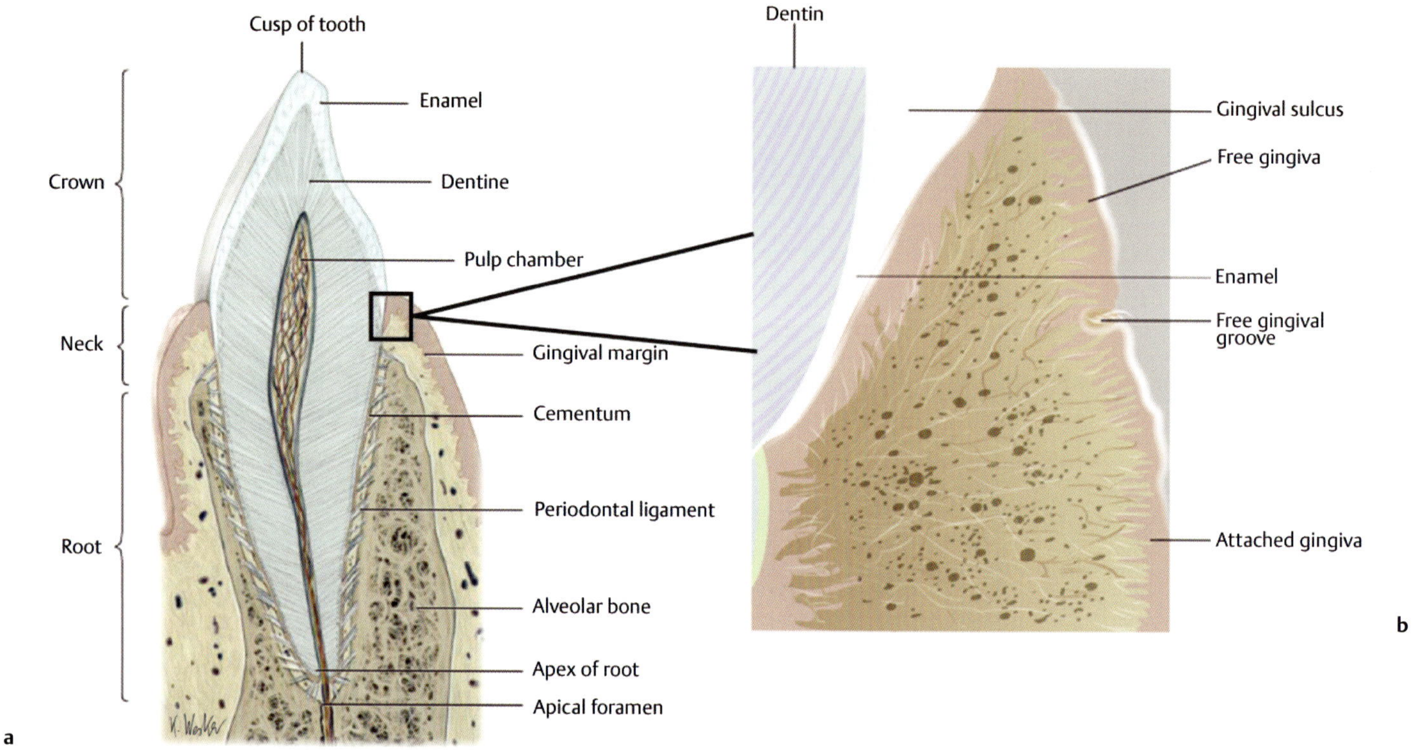

Fig. 20.6 (a) Longitudinal section of the incisor tooth and periodontal tissues. (Modified from THIEME Atlas of Anatomy, Head and Neck Anatomy for Dental Medicine. © Thieme 2010, Illustration by Karl Wesker.) **(b)** Magnified view of the rectangular zone in **(a)** showing the periodontal tissues of the neck region.

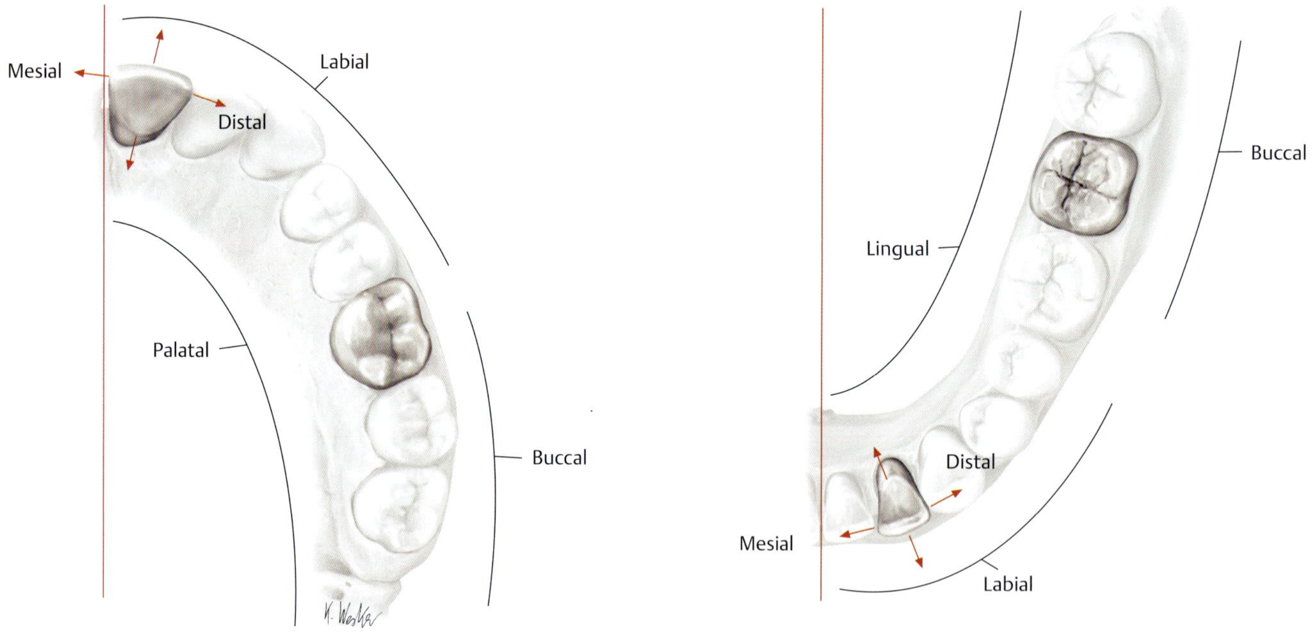

Fig. 20.7 Designation of surfaces of the teeth. **(a)** Inferior view of the maxillary teeth. **(b)** Superior view of the mandibular teeth. (Modified from THIEME Head and Neck Anatomy for Dental Medicine. © Thieme 2010, Illustrations by Karl Wesker.)

Table 20.1 Innervation of the oral mucosa

	Upper jaw	Dominant nerve	Lower jaw part	Dominant nerve
Labial or buccal mucosa	Anterior part	Infraorbital nerve, anterior superior alveolar branch	Anterior	Mental nerve
	Middle part	Buccal nerve	Middle	Buccal nerve
	Posterior part		Posterior	
Labial or buccal gingiva	Anterior part	Infraorbital nerve, anterior superior alveolar branch	Anterior	Mental nerve
	Middle part	Infraorbital nerve, middle superior alveolar branch	Middle	Buccal nerve
	posterior part	Infraorbital nerve, posterior superior alveolar branch	Posterior	
Palatal or lingual mucosa, gingiva	Anterior part	Nasopalatine nerve	Anterior part	Inferior alveolar nerve
	Middle part	greater palatine nerve (hard palate)	Middle part	
	Posterior part		Posterior part	

superior alveolar nerve. The lower teeth are innervated by the inferior alveolar nerve arising from the mandibular nerve. Both the upper and lower teeth are supplied by branches of the maxillary artery. The upper teeth are supplied by the anterior, middle, and posterior superior alveolar arteries, and the lower teeth are supplied by the inferior alveolar artery. The veins accompanying the maxillary artery drain the upper and lower jaw into the pterygoid venous plexus and collect the maxillary vein, deep facial vein, and buccal vein and then drain into the retromandibular vein and facial vein.

Gingiva/Alveolar Mucosa

The immobile and keratinized mucosa that surrounds the alveolar bone and coheres to the periosteum is called gingiva (**Table 20.1**). The mobile mucosa between the gingiva and the gingivobuccal fold is known as the alveolar mucosa and is not normally keratinized. The gingiva is further subdivided into free gingiva and attached gingiva by the free gingival groove (**Fig. 20.6**). Innervation of the lower gingiva and alveolar mucosa comes from the lingual, buccal, and mental nerves; innervation of the upper gingiva and alveolar mucosa comes from the nasopalatine, greater palatine, and buccal nerves (**Fig. 20.8a,b**).

Palate

The hard palate forms the roof of the oral cavity and is lined by bone (**Fig. 20.8b, Table 20.1**). The posterior soft part of the palate lacks bone, is called the soft palate, and consists of striated muscles. The border between the hard and soft palates is easy to visualize by having the patient say "Ah"; then only the soft palate vibrates. The posterior end of the soft palate is the palatine velum, in the middle of which the uvula hangs. The bony palate is formed by the maxillary bone in its anterior two-thirds and by the palatine bone in its posterior one-third. On the surface of the palatine mucosa are incisive papilla, transverse palatine folds, palatine raphe, and palatine foveolae. The mucosa of the hard palate is composed of the epithelium, proper lamina and submucosal tissue. The epithelium is keratinized, and the proper lamina is thick and filled with connective tissue in the anterior part of the hard palate. The submucosal tissue of the incisive papilla and the transverse palatine folds are filled with fat tissue, but the palatine raphe lacks submucosal tissue. If the palatine torus exists, the palatine mucosa is so thin that it is easily injured and may form ulcers caused by physical and chemical damage. Palatine glands are present at the posterior surface of the soft palate. Many taste buds are also located in the soft palate. The incisive fossa is just under the incisive papilla and ascends to the incisive canal. The nasopalatine artery, vein, and nerve run through the incisive canal; so care needs to be taken when incising over the incisive papilla. The greater palatine foramen is located 15 mm lateral to the palatine raphe, between the second and third molar. The greater palatine artery and nerve run to the anterior part of the hard palate from the greater palatine foramen, so it is risky to incise the palate transversely. Many clinicians have reported cases in which repair of an oroantral fistula was undertaken using the palatine mucosa for the axial pattern flap and using the greater palatine artery as a feeding vessel.[5] The muscles that form the soft palate are described in the section on swallowing.

Tongue

The tongue is a muscular organ, arising from the oral floor and spreading into the oral cavity proper (**Fig. 20.9**). The intrinsic muscles change the shape of the tongue, and the extrinsic muscles move the tongue and intersect and play important roles in mastication, swallowing, and speech. In addition, one of the most important functions of the tongue is as a taste receptor. Three cranial nerves convey the taste fibers: CN VII (facial nerve, chorda tympani branch), CN IX (glossopharyngeal nerve),

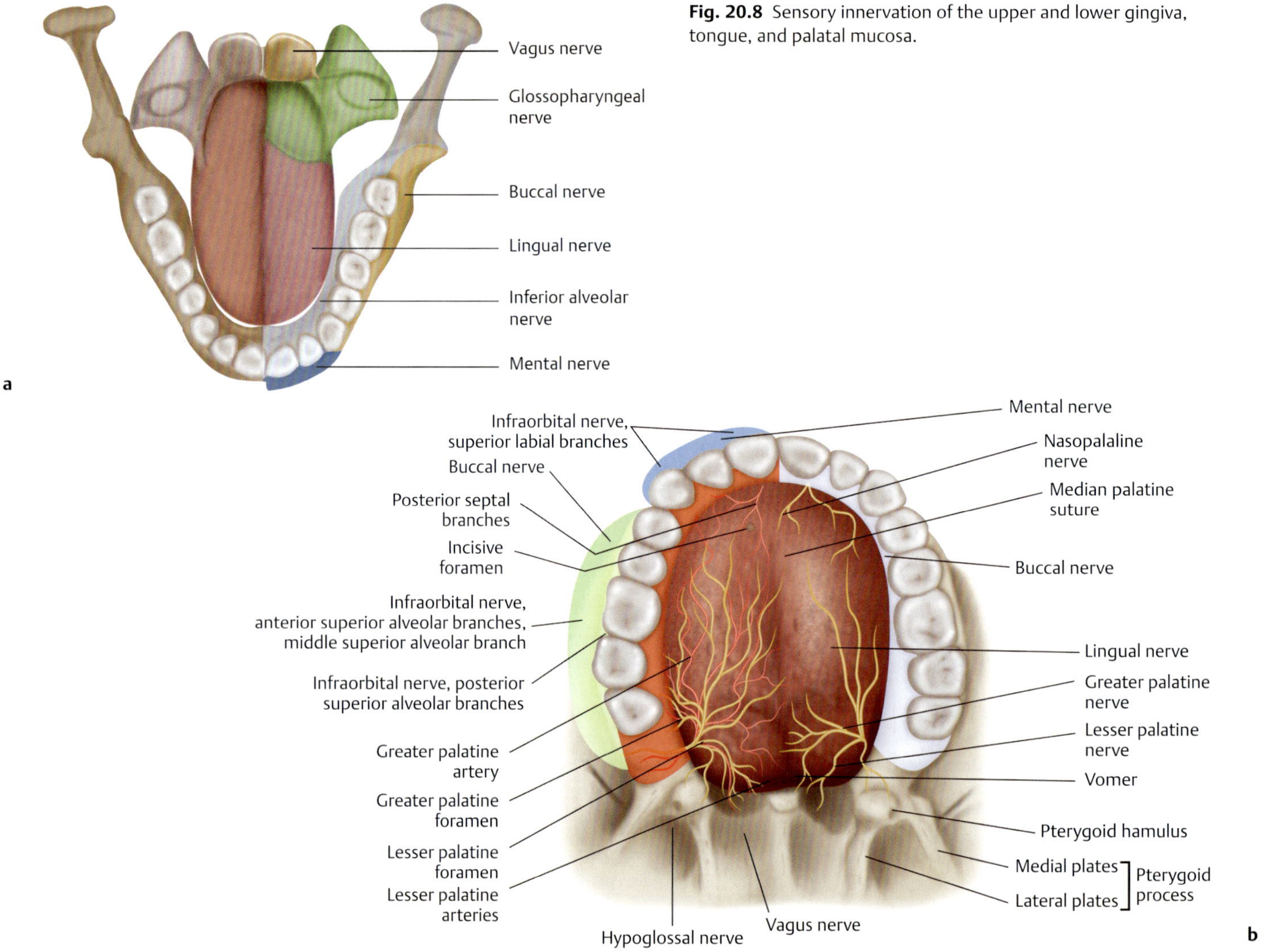

Fig. 20.8 Sensory innervation of the upper and lower gingiva, tongue, and palatal mucosa.

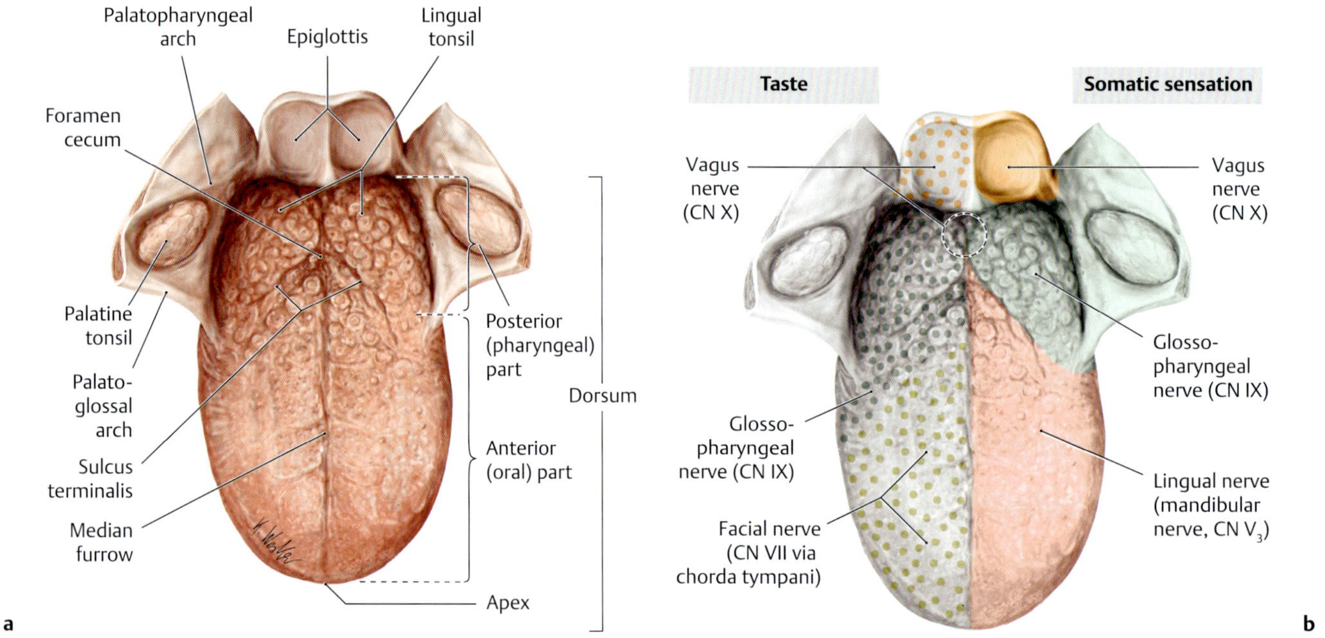

Fig. 20.9 **(a)** Surface anatomy of the lingual mucosa. **(b)** Somatosensory innervation (left side) and taste innervation (right side) of the tongue. (Modified from THIEME Head and Neck Anatomy for Dental Medicine. © Thieme 2010, Illustrations by Karl Wesker.)

and CN X (vagus nerve). Thus, a disturbance in taste sensation involving the anterior two-thirds of the tongue indicates the presence of a facial nerve (chorda tympani) lesion, whereas a disturbance of somatic sensation indicates a lingual nerve lesion.

On the dorsal mucosa of the tongue are four kinds of papillae: filiform papillae, fungiform papillae, foliate papillae, and circumvallate papillae (**Fig. 20.10**). Filiform papillae are the smallest and are distributed over the whole anterior two-thirds of the tongue; they are the only papillae that have no taste buds. They are keratinized and white. Fungiform papillae exist predominantly at the lingual apex and sometimes have taste buds. They are not keratinized, so they take on the red color of the capillary vessels. Foliate papillae are the four to seven folds located on the posterolateral region of the tongue. In adults, the taste buds in the foliate papillae degenerate. Serous glands lie under the foliate papillae for the purpose of cleaning the taste buds. Approximately 10 circumvallate papillae are positioned in front of the terminal sulcus and form a V-shaped line. They are the largest tongue papillae (3 mm in diameter) and are surrounded by a deep groove in which there are taste buds in the epithelium. In adults, approximately two-thirds of the taste buds are on the tongue. The soft palate also has many taste buds. Innervation of the anterior two-thirds of the tongue comes from the chorda tympani, and the posterior third is innervated by the glossopharyngeal and vagus nerves. Therefore, it is known that if these nerves are injured by surgical procedures, chemotherapy, or radiotherapy, dysgeusia may occur. It is difficult to examine the root of the tongue when the mouth is open. In cases of ankyloglossia, in which the lingual frenulum is too rigid to allow movement of the tongue and speech is hampered, lingual frenoplasty might be necessary. The deep lingual artery and vein and the lingual nerve are situated on the inferior surface of the tongue, so sensory paralysis and bleeding may occur if they are injured. In particular, care should be taken not to injure the deep lingual vein because of its position directly under the mucosa (**Fig. 20.11**). If the tongue is extended, the border between

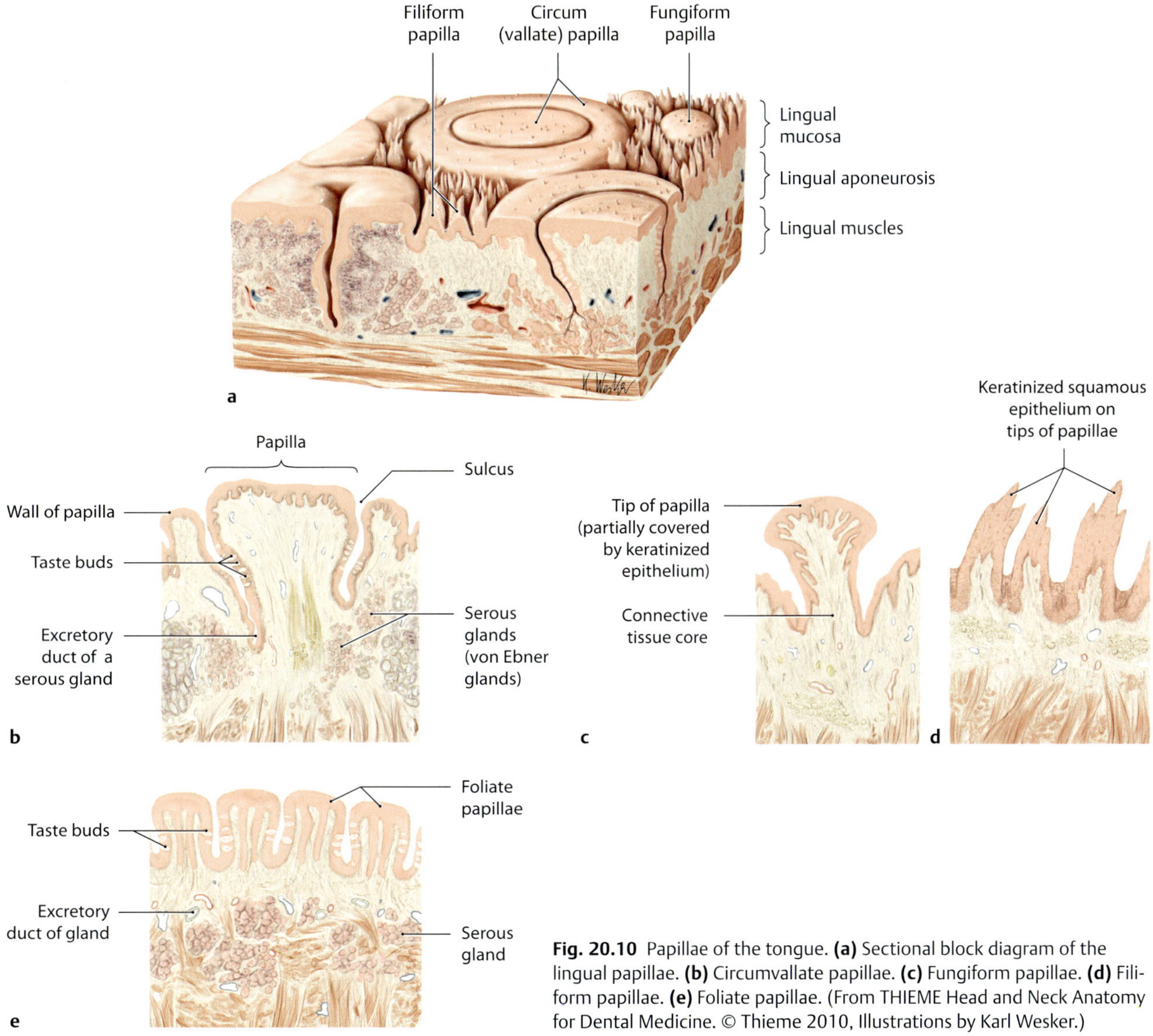

Fig. 20.10 Papillae of the tongue. **(a)** Sectional block diagram of the lingual papillae. **(b)** Circumvallate papillae. **(c)** Fungiform papillae. **(d)** Filiform papillae. **(e)** Foliate papillae. (From THIEME Head and Neck Anatomy for Dental Medicine. © Thieme 2010, Illustrations by Karl Wesker.)

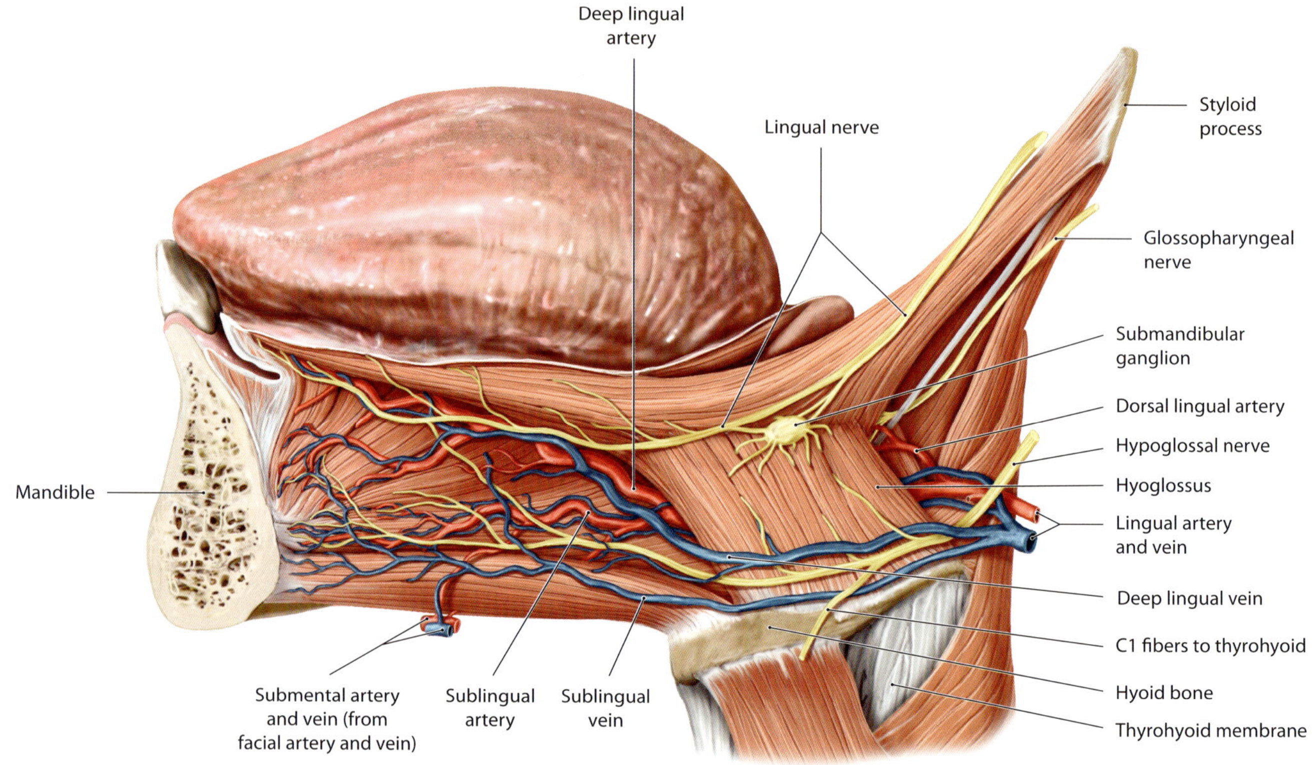

a

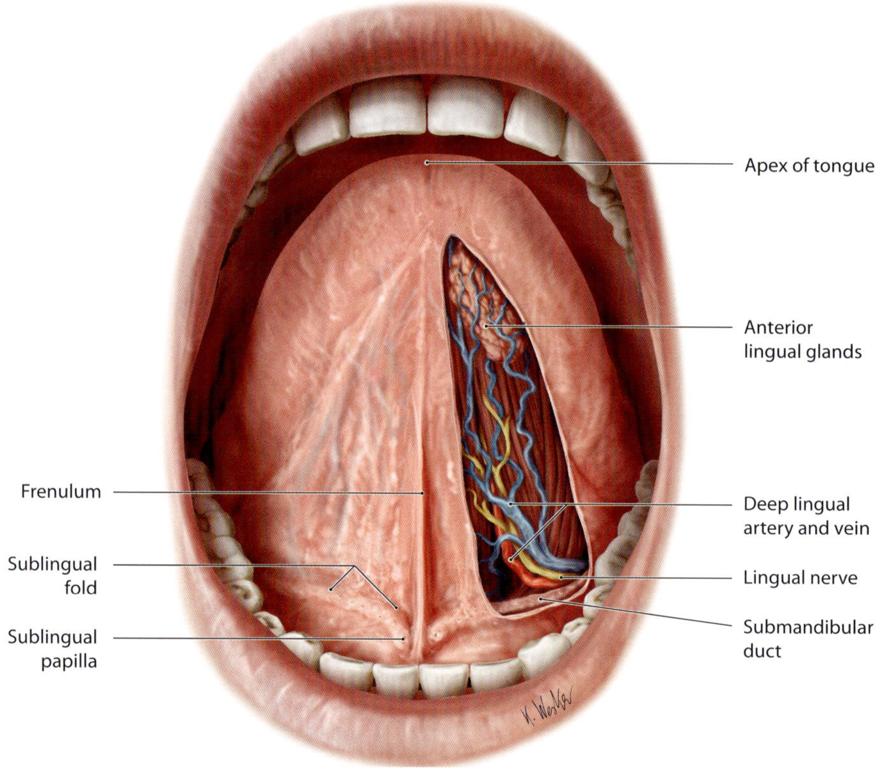

b

Fig. 20.11 Nerves and vessels of the tongue. **(a)** Left lateral view. **(b)** View of the inferior surface of the tongue. (From THIEME Head and Neck Anatomy for Dental Medicine. © Thieme 2010, Illustrations by Karl Wesker.)

the inferior surface of the tongue and the oral floor is hard to see. It is well known that there are communicating branches between the lingual and hypoglossal nerves in the body and apex of tongue; however, their physiologic function is not fully understood.[6]

Buccal Fat Pad

The buccal fat pad (anatomically, the corpus adiposum buccae) is the fat located deep in the cheek region (**Fig. 20.12**). This fat is also called Bichat's fat pad and is named after the French anatomist who first recognized the nature of this tissue. The buccal fat pad is located between the muscles of mastication in what is called the masticatory space and has a role in facilitating the smooth gliding of the masticatory muscles. It also forms the shape of the bulge of the cheek.

According to Stuzin et al, the buccal fat pad consists of a main body and three extensions: buccal, pterygoid, and temporal.[7] The main body is the part above the parotid duct and is located superficial to the buccinator and anterior to the anterior edge of the masseter. It also extends medially to the posterior part of the maxilla. At the superior and medial section, it touches the maxillary artery and the maxillary nerve (a branch of the trigeminal nerve). The buccal extension is the superficial segment located along the anterior edge of the masseter and beneath the parotid duct. The buccal branches of the facial nerve run over this extension. At the anterior border, the facial artery and vein run obliquely. The pterygoid extension is in the area between the ramus of mandible and the pterygoid muscles. The temporal extension passes beneath the anterior part of

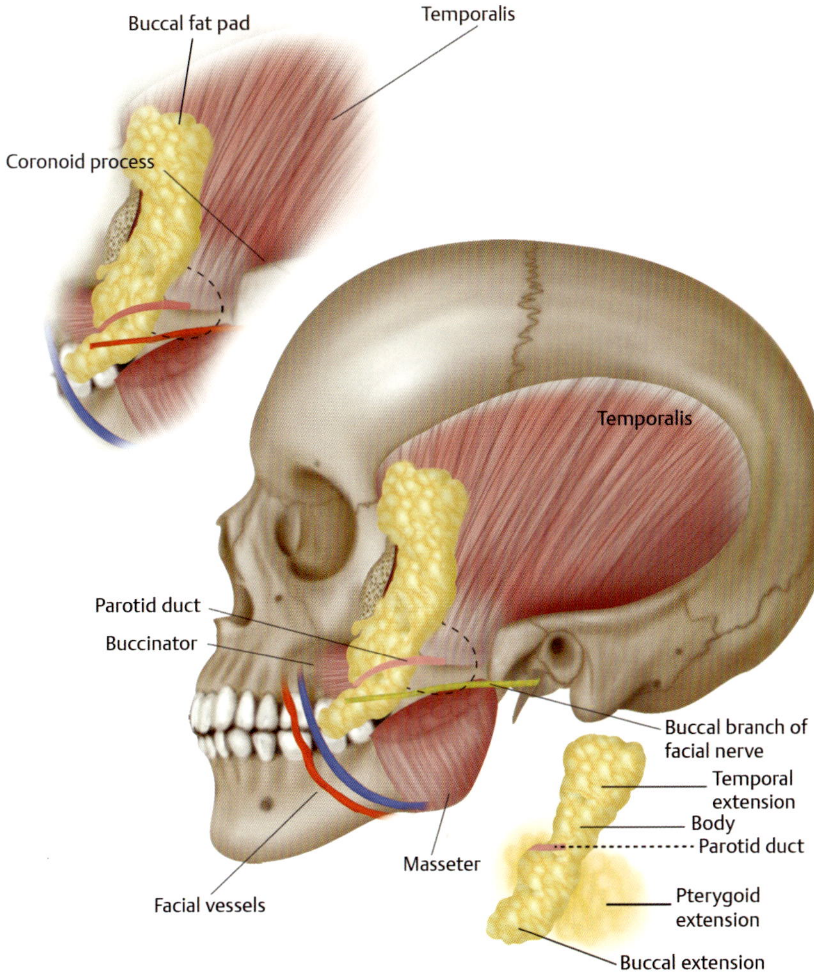

Fig. 20.12 Buccal fat pad. The buccal fat pad consists of a main body and three extensions: buccal, pterygoid, and temporal. The main body is the part above the parotid duct and is located superficial to the buccinator and anterior to the anterior edge of the masseter. The buccal extension is the superficial segment located along the anterior edge of the masseter and beneath the parotid duct. The pterygoid extension is in the area between the ramus of mandible and the pterygoid muscles. The temporal extension passes beneath the anterior part of the zygomatic arch and lies between the temporalis muscle and the deep temporal fascia.

the zygomatic arch and lies between the temporalis muscle and the deep temporal fascia.

The buccal fat pad is used in free grafts and pedicle flaps for various tissue defects, most commonly for the repair of oroantral fistulae and also for the treatment of other oral cavity tissue defects, ranging from the angle of mouth to the retromolar trigone and palate.[8]

Floor of Mouth and Sublingual Space

The floor of the mouth is the region surrounded by the lower alveolus and the tongue. The submucosal tissue of the floor of the mouth is composed of sparse connective tissue and is highly mobile. The floor of the mouth is divided into two parts by the lingual frenulum. The submandibular duct (Wharton's duct) opens at the sublingual caruncle after joining the greater sublingual duct, and many lesser sublingual ducts open at the sublingual fold posterior to the sublingual caruncle. Beneath the floor of the mouth is a sublingual space located superior to the mylohyoid muscle and on the lateral side of the genioglossus and geniohyoid muscle. The contents of this space are the sublingual gland; the submandibular duct; the greater and lesser sublingual ducts; the lingual nerve, artery, and vein; and the hypoglossal nerve. This space is therefore quite important in clinical situations. The submandibular duct arises from the submandibular gland, which is located posterior to the end of the mylohyoid muscle and runs to the sublingual caruncle. On the proximal part of the submandibular duct, the lingual nerve traverses inferior to the submandibular duct and is then distributed to the tongue. The reported incidence of sublingual gland protrusion through defects in the mylohyoid muscle is approximately 25 to 40%.[9] Care should be taken around this area, as the submental artery (a branch of the facial artery) and the sublingual artery (a branch of the lingual artery) travel into the dorsal side of the midline of the mandible at the lingual foramen. There are many variations of anastomoses of the submental and sublingual arteries.[10]

Oropharyngeal Isthmus

The oropharyngeal isthmus forms the border of the oral cavity and the pharynx and is the posterior end of the oral vestibule (**Fig. 20.2**). The posterior end of the soft palate forms the palatine velum with a median process known as the uvula. Two folds run laterally downward from the palatine velum. The anterior fold is the palatoglossal arch, and the posterior fold is the palatopharyngeal arch. The palatine tonsils are situated between these two folds on both sides.

Pharynx

The pharynx is the digestive tube located between oral cavity and the esophagus, posterior to the oral and nasal cavity. The pharyngeal cavity is the intersection of the digestive tract and the respiratory system. The pharynx is composed of the epi(naso)pharynx, oropharynx, and hypopharynx. The epipharynx is positioned dorsal to the posterior nasal apertures at the back end of the nose; the pharyngeal opening of the auditory tube, which is connected with the tympanum opens in the lateral wall; and the pharyngeal tonsil is located in the posterior wall. Waldeyer's ring is composed of the palatine tonsil, the lingual tonsil, and the pharyngeal tonsil, and it comprises immunocompetent lymphatic tissue. This is the first biophylaxis against foreign invasion. The oropharynx is located posterior to the oral cavity, and the hypopharynx communicates with the laryngeal cavity through the laryngeal aperture.

Swallowing

The act of eating and swallowing, which is required for the intake of food, can be easily explained by dividing it into five stages: the awareness phase (preliminary phase), the preparatory phase (chewing phase), the oral cavity phase, the pharyngeal phase, and the esophageal phase. In the awareness phase, the body becomes aware of food and creates a natural eating pace. During the preparatory phase, food placed in the mouth is chewed and mixed to create a food bolus in a condition that can be swallowed. During the oral cavity phase, the bolus thus created is transferred from the mouth to the throat, after which it moves from the throat to the esophagus during the pharyngeal phase. During the esophageal phase, it is transferred from the esophagus to the stomach in a process of continual movement (**Fig. 20.13**).[11] Reports note cases in which food is transferred into the oropharynx during chewing, before the swallowing reflex begins,[12–15] and in which repeated swallowing results in a pattern in which the larynx is elevated.[16,17] During swallowing, many muscle groups, including the mimetic muscles surrounding the oral cavity, masticatory muscles, tongue muscles, palate

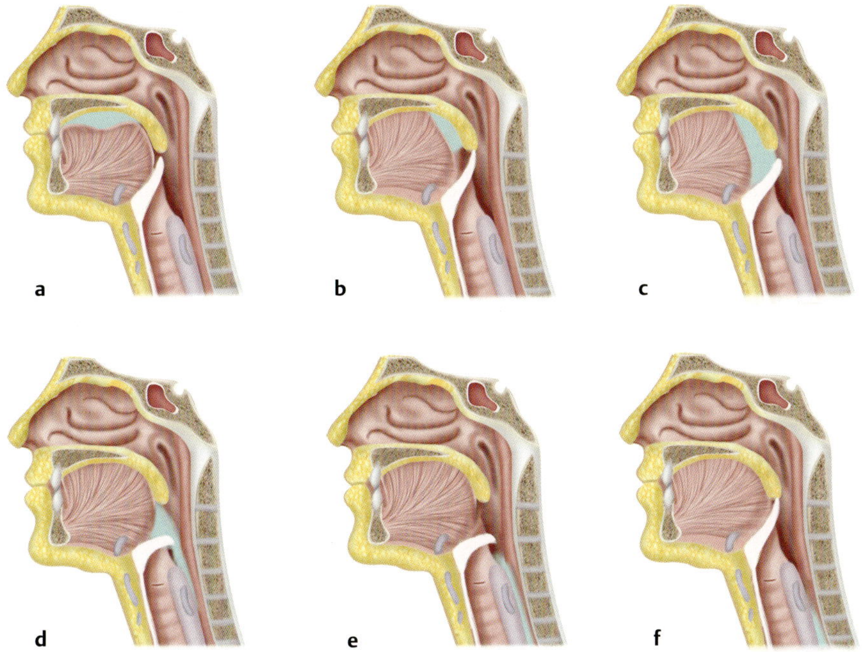

Fig. 20.13 Schematic diagram of swallowing. **(a)** Retention of the food bolus in the oral cavity. **(b)** Immediately before the beginning of the swallowing reflex. **(c)** Food bolus moves to the oropharynx. **(d)** Food bolus moves from the lower pharynx to the esophageal entrance. **(e)** Food bolus passes through the esophageal entrance. **(f)** Food bolus moves from the esophagus to the stomach.

muscles, upper and lower hyoid muscles, the pharyngeal muscle, and laryngeal muscle, all work together, with these muscles controlled by the trigeminal nerve, facial nerves, glossopharyngeal/vagus nerve, hypoglossal nerve, and cervical nerves, which receive instructions from the mastication and swallowing center. In this section, we present an explanation of swallowing movement from the preparatory phase onward, based mainly on the muscles related to swallowing.

Mechanism of Swallowing and the Involved Muscles

Preparatory Phase (Chewing and Food Bolus Formation)

The food taken into the oral cavity is formed into a food bolus by the tongue if it does not require chewing (**Fig. 20.13a, Fig. 20.14e**).[11] Food that requires chewing is broken down by the action not only of the tongue but also of the jaw and cheeks, and then it is mixed with saliva. When chewing begins, the food is swiftly positioned on the molars and chewed by the subsequent raising action of the jaw while being held in place by the expression muscles, mimetic muscles such as the cheek and tongue muscles (**Fig. 20.14b–e, Fig. 20.15**). The lower jaw closes when the masseter muscle, temporalis muscles, and medial pterygoid muscles on both sides contract; moves forward when the anterior lateral pterygoid muscle contracts; and rotates when the lateral pterygoid muscle on one side contracts (**Fig. 20.14b, Fig. 20.16**). It opens as a result of the movement of the lateral pterygoid muscle and suprahyoid muscle. The tongue contains intrinsic and extrinsic muscles (**Fig. 20.14e**), with movement of the intrinsic muscles causing it to contract or become long and thin or wide and flat. Of the extrinsic muscles, the genioglossus muscle protrudes the tongue; the styloglossus muscle raises the posterior aspect of the tongue, along with the palatoglossal muscle. The genioglossus muscle and the styloglossus muscle move together to retract the tongue. The hyoglossus muscle works to move the sides of the tongue downward; the tongue is lowered by the genioglossus muscle and hyoglossus muscle. When a food bolus is formed within the oral cavity, a depression is created in the center of the tongue, which “holds” the food bolus, requiring the soft palate and the tongue to be close

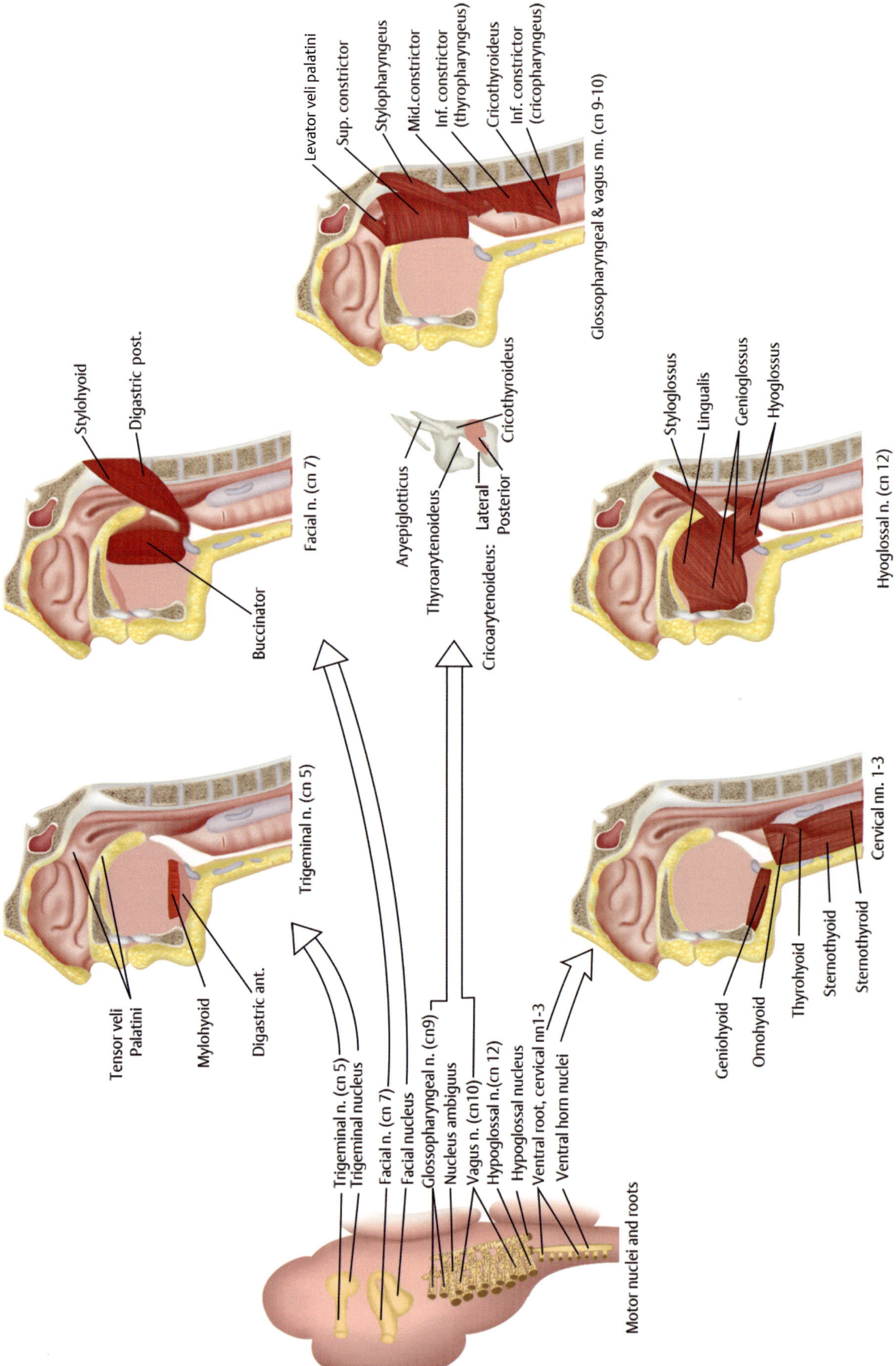

Fig. 20.14 Oropharyngeal muscles and nerve innervation.

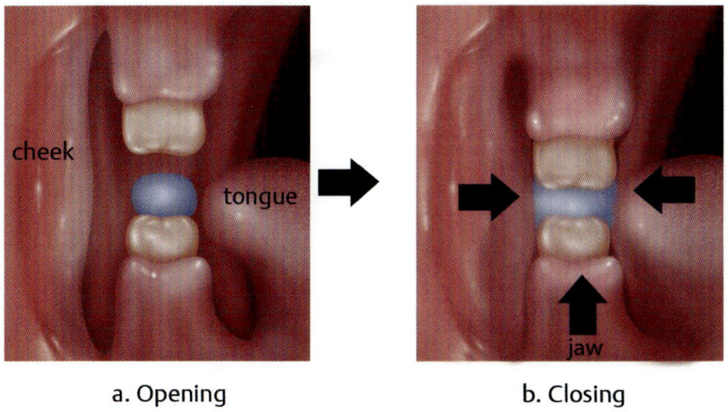

Fig. 20.15 Schematic diagram of the movement of the cheeks, tongue, and lower jaw during chewing.

to one another. To facilitate this action, the tongue takes on the formation of a spoon and is elevated at the back by the styloglossus muscle; the soft palate is drawn toward the tongue by the palatoglossal and palatopharyngeal muscles (**Fig. 20.14d, Fig. 20.17**).[18]

End of the Oral Cavity Phase and Beginning of the Pharyngeal Phase

The food bolus in the oral cavity is transferred to the pharynx; immediately before the pharyngeal phase begins, the intrinsic and extrinsic tongue muscles cause the tongue to adhere to the palate, gripping the food bolus so that it is moved towards the pharynx (**Fig. 20.13b**). From the start of the transfer (oral cavity phase), the action becomes reflexive, and voluntary control becomes impossible. When the transfer is finally implemented, the lower jaw and the lips are usually closed. At the same time, to prevent the food bolus from passing into the nasopharynx, the soft palate is elevated by the tensor and levator muscles of the palatine velum (**Fig. 20.14b,d, Fig. 20.17**); furthermore, contraction of the pharyngeal contractor causes the formation of Passavant's ridge, resulting in the upper pharynx being firmly closed (**Fig. 20.14d, Fig. 20.17**).

The food then begins to be passed into the pharynx, and the swallowing reflex begins, at which point the hyoid bone begins to be elevated (**Fig. 20.18**). The hyoid bone moves slightly backward at first, after which it begins to move upward, and then finally strongly forward and downward. The rearward movement of the hyoid bone at the start is furthermore believed to be caused by contraction of the stylohyoid muscle and the posterior belly of the digastric muscle (**Fig. 20.14c, Fig. 20.18**).

Pharyngeal Phase (Food Bolus Moves to the Oropharynx)

With the soft palate still elevated, the food bolus is pushed out from the base of the tongue to the oropharynx (**Fig. 20.13c, Fig. 20.14b,c**), at which point the upper pharyngeal and oropharyngeal contractors begin to contract (**Fig. 20.14d**), causing the hyoid bone and larynx to move toward their highest position (**Fig. 20.14d, Fig. 20.18**). Once the hyoid bone is elevated, the mylohyoid muscle and the anterior belly of the digastric muscle move the hyoid bone upward while the geniohyoid muscle moves the hyoid bone forwards (**Fig. 20.14b,f**). It is believed that these actions together cause elevation of the hyoid bone (**Fig. 20.14f**). Next, the thyrohyoid muscle contracts to elevate the larynx. At the same time as the elevation of the larynx, the pharyngeal constrictor muscles implement peristaltic constriction from the upper to the lower pharynx to transfer the food from the pharynx into the esophagus. Contraction in the oropharynx is caused not only by the pharyngeal constrictor action but also by the base of the tongue, which forms the pharyngeal anterior wall, moving toward the rear (**Fig. 20.14e**).

Furthermore, during the swallowing reaction, the glottis is closed by the action of the laryngeal intrinsic muscles, inhibiting the airway (**Fig. 20.14d, Fig. 20.19**). The laryngeal muscles and lateral thyroarytenoid muscles both act to adduct the vocal cords; however, the thyroarytenoid muscle shortens the vocal cords by contracting inward, and the lateral thyroarytenoid

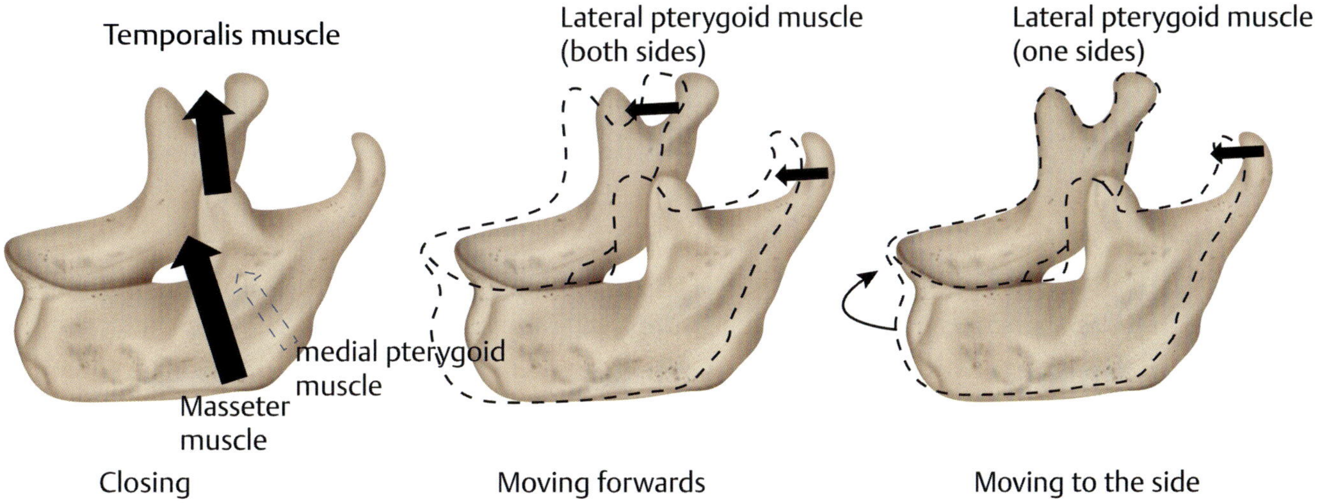

Fig. 20.16 Movements of the mandible by attached muscles.

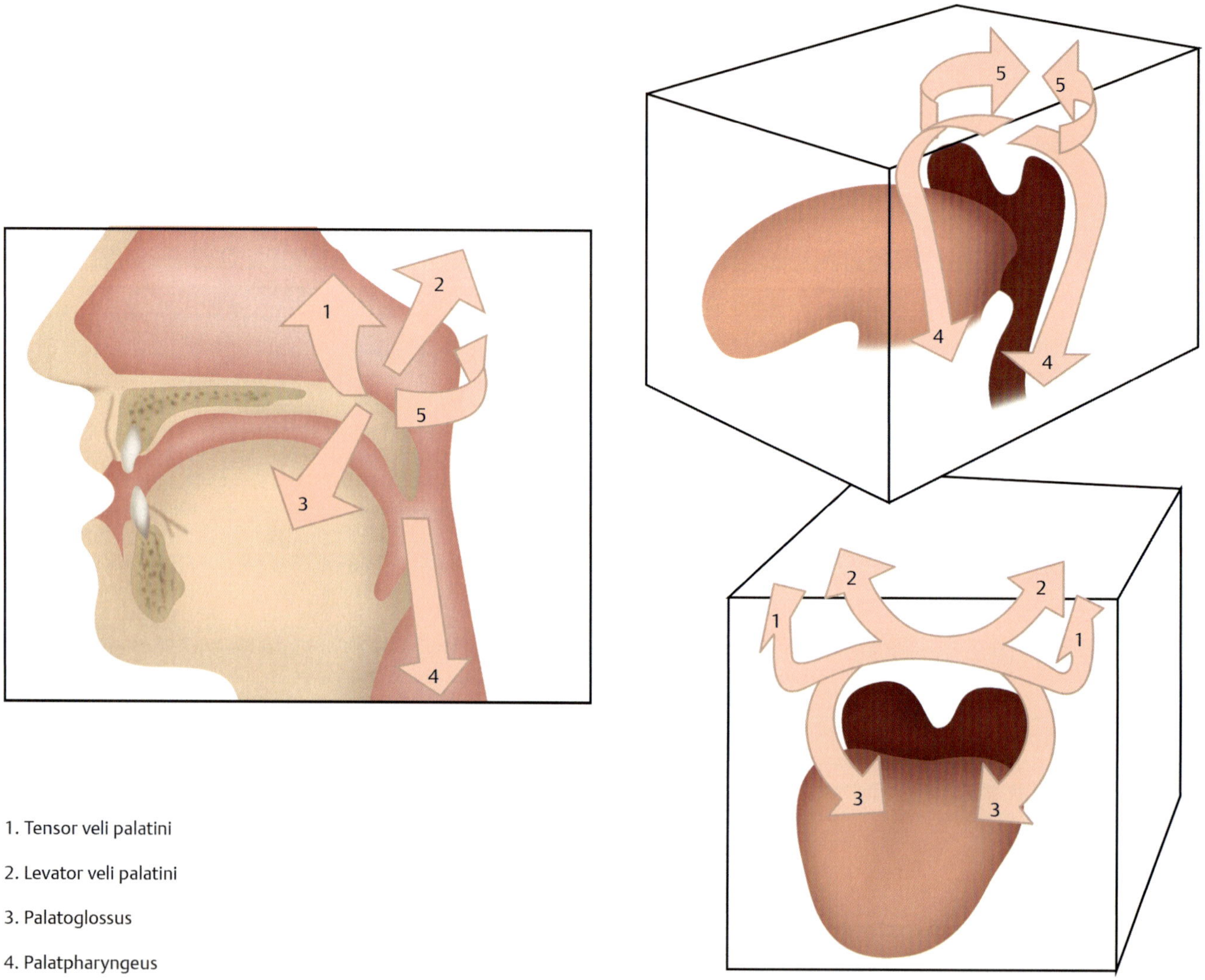

1. Tensor veli palatini
2. Levator veli palatini
3. Palatoglossus
4. Palatpharyngeus
5. Superior constrictor

Fig. 20.17 Schematic diagram of velopharyngeal muscles action during speech. 1, Tensor veli palatini; 2, levator veli palatini; 3, palatoglossus; 4, palatpharyngeus; 5, superior constrictor.

muscle lengthens the vocal cords by contracting outward. Because the interarytenoid muscles also adduct the vocal cords, the posterior cricoarytenoid muscle is the only muscle that abducts the vocal cords. In addition, the cricothyroid muscle causes the thyroid cartilage and cricoid cartilage to approach one another, stretching the vocal cords and raising the pitch of the voice (**Fig. 20.14d**).

Pharyngeal Phase (Food Bolus Moves from the Lower Pharynx to the Esophageal Entrance)

The action of the suprahyoid and infrahyoid muscles results in the hyoid bone being moved as far upward and forward as possible, bringing the hyoid bone close to the larynx (**Fig. 20.20**). Pharyngeal contraction reaches the oropharynx, and the action of the palatopharyngeal and palatoglossal muscles lowers the soft palate (**Fig. 20.13d, Fig. 20.14d,f, Fig. 20.18**). The glottis remains closed, and contraction of the aryepiglottic muscle results in the epiglottis and arytenoid cartilage being brought close together, narrowing the entrance to the larynx (**Fig. 20.14d**). The further rearward movement of the base of the tongue and the downward pressure from above on the food that has been swallowed result in the epiglottis collapsing inward, closing the larynx and preventing foreign bodies from entering the airway during swallowing and temporarily stopping breathing (swallowing apnea). With the larynx closed, the food bolus passes through the lower pharynx on the side of the larynx. The base of the lower pharynx features depressions to the left and right

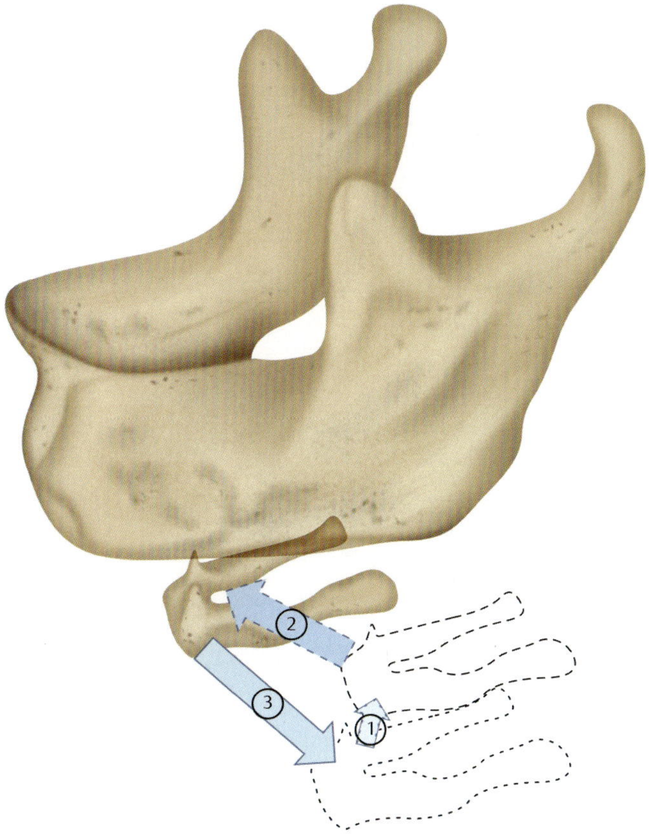

Fig. 20.18 Elevation patterns of the hyoid bone during swallowing 1. Moving backward; 2. moving forward; 3. to a lowered resting position.

known as the piriform recesses, which are in the form of an inverted cone. Their bases are closed by the contraction of the cricopharyngeus muscle, the sphincter muscle that forms the entrance to the esophagus. The cricopharyngeus muscle is part of the lower pharyngeal constrictor muscles; when the cricopharyngeus muscle relaxes and the larynx is elevated (moved forward), the esophageal entrance is opened, allowing the food bolus to pass through (**Fig. 20.14d**). Once the food bolus passes through the esophageal entrance, it is compressed by the larynx and the cervical vertebrae and passes, separately, to the left and right piriform recesses, avoiding the center.

End of the Pharyngeal Phase to the Esophageal Phase

When the food bolus is transferred to the esophagus, the soft palate, tongue, hyoid bone, and larynx return to their original positions (**Fig. 20.13f**). The glottis is opened wide and the cricopharyngeus muscle constricts, closing the entrance to the esophagus. The food bolus that has entered the esophagus is carried to the stomach by peristalsis, at a transfer speed of approximately 40 cm per second in the upper esophagus and 4 cm per second in the lower part, passing through the esophagus in

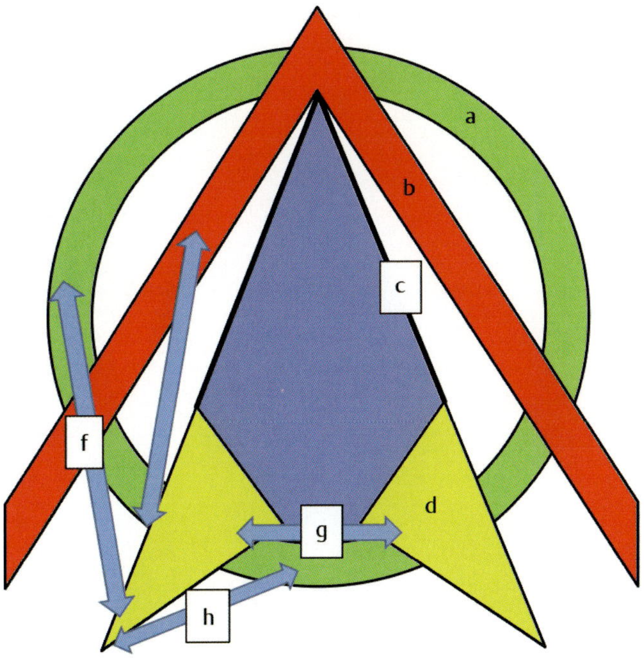

Fig. 20.19 Schematic diagram of laryngeal muscle actions. **(a)** Cricoid cartilage. **(b)** Thyroid cartilage. **(c)** Vocal cord membranous part. **(d)** Arytenoid cartilage. **(e)** Thyroarytenoid muscle. **(f)** Lateral cricoarytenoid muscle. **(g)** Interarytenoid muscles. **(h)** Posterior cricoarytenoid muscle.

around 10 seconds. In a healthy esophagus, peristalsis occurs after swallowing via a first contraction, occurring at the same time that the food bolus enters the upper esophagus, and a second contraction that occurs in response to the stimulation of the esophagus being widened by the food bolus.

Occlusion

Concepts about occlusion between the upper and lower teeth have changed over time; however, the theory relating to occlusion in the treatment of facial fractures is simple and unchanging. In this subchapter, we describe occlusion in relation to jaw fracture treatment. During surgery after facial trauma, the aim is to set the occlusion in the intercuspal position with the teeth in maximum intercuspation and then tighten the bones with screws. For simple fractures, it is easy to find the intercuspal position; however, in cases of complicated and multiple fractures, it is difficult for the surgeon to determine the correct occlusal position. One method for determining the intercuspal position is to look for occlusal facets in the upper and lower teeth. According to Schyler, these facets are present on the occlusal surfaces of the teeth as a result of functional or sometimes secondary movement of the mandible. This is regarded as a natural and inevitable process of occlusal equilibration. The facets also guide the mandible during the occlusal phase of mastication.[19]

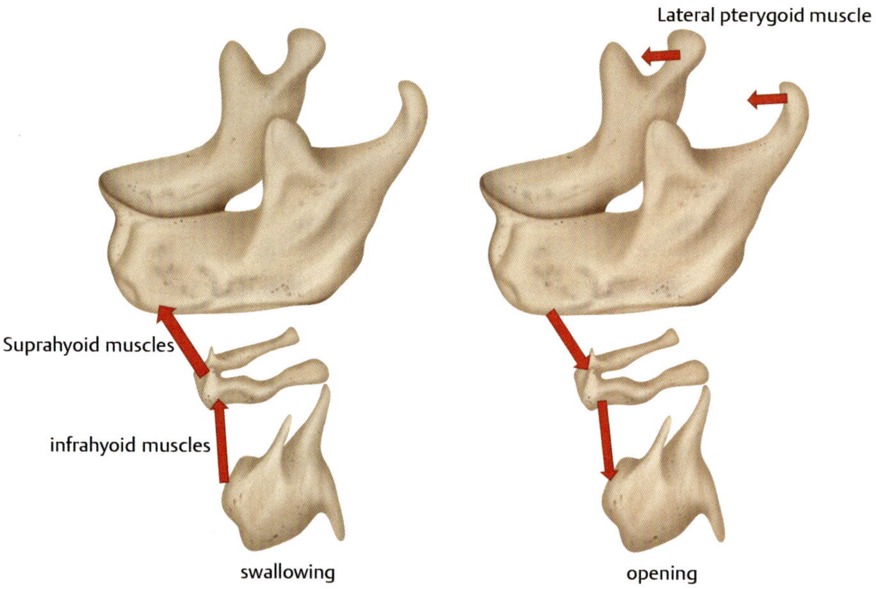

Fig. 20.20 Schematic diagram of the action of the muscles during swallowing and opening of the mouth.

Aesthetic Region

When considering the maxillofacial region as an aesthetic zone, we should think about many factors, such as face, eyes, lips, gingiva, and teeth.[20] In this section, we have made slight mention of the lips, gingiva, and teeth, which are closely related to the oral cavity. According to Lombardi, the facial midline is located at the center of the face and perpendicular to the interpupillary line.[21] Magne et al described the importance of the relationship between the edge of the incisor teeth and the lower lip line (**Fig. 20.21**). They also mentioned that the "golden proportion" and the "golden percentage," which apply to the apparent size of the teeth when viewed directly from the front (lateral incisor in a proportion of 1:1.618 to the central incisor and 1:0.618 to the canine) are too rigid for dentistry.[20] In 2012, Tsukiyama et al undertook a study comparing the morphology of the central incisor, lateral incisor, canine, and first premolar between white and Asian populations. They concluded that the central incisors of Asian subjects were narrower and more slender than those of white subjects (**Fig. 20.22**).[22] This study confirms that there is racial variation between white and Asian populations in terms of the morphology of the maxillary central incisor teeth and the facial skeleton. When thinking about the ideals of the aesthetic region, including the oral cavity, we should acknowledge the existence of different ideals among the races.

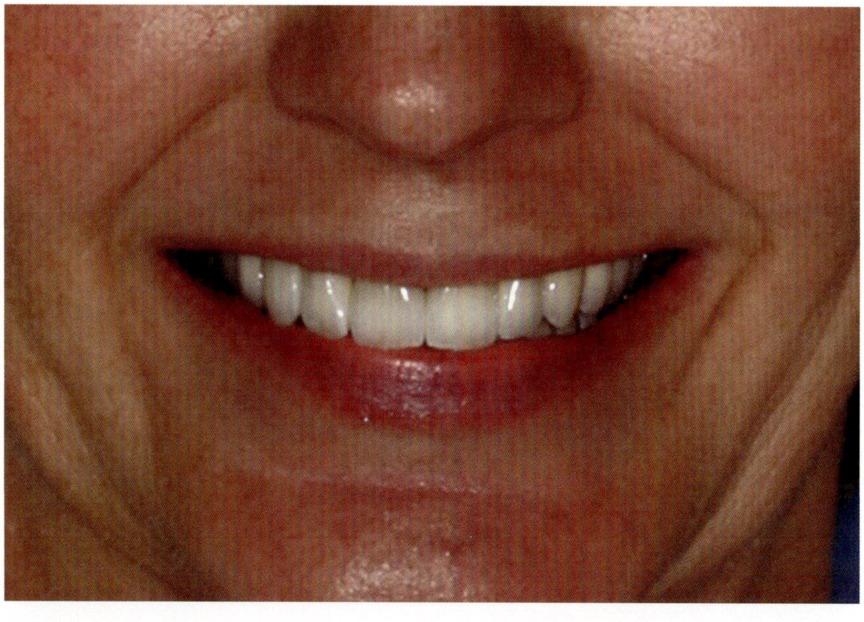

Fig. 20.21 Relationship between the edge of the incisor teeth and the lower lip line. (Picture provided by Dr. T. Tsukiyama with permission from Elsevier.)

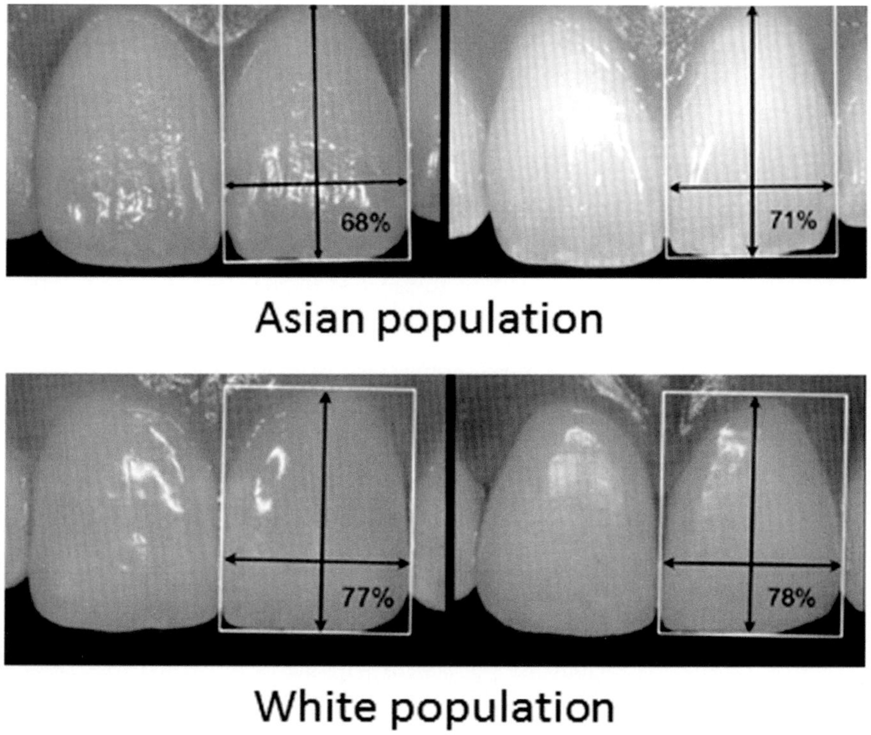

Fig. 20.22 Comparison of central incisors between Asian and white subjects. The numbers on the surface of the teeth show the width-to-length ratio of the central incisors (%). (Picture provided by Dr. T. Tsukiyama, with permission from Elsevier.)

References

1. Behnia H, Kheradvar A, Shahrokhi M. An anatomic study of the lingual nerve in the third molar region. J Oral Maxillofac Surg 2000;58(6):649–653
2. Udhaya K, Saraladevi KV, Sridhar J. The morphometric analysis of the mental foramen in adult dry human mandibles: a study on the South Indian population. J Clin Diagn Res 2013;7(8):1547–1551
3. Kalender A, Orhan K, Aksoy U. Evaluation of the mental foramen and accessory mental foramen in Turkish patients using cone-beam computed tomography images reconstructed from a volumetric rendering program. Clin Anat 2012;25(5):584–592
4. Naitoh M, Yoshida K, Nakahara K, Gotoh K, Ariji E. Demonstration of the accessory mental foramen using rotational panoramic radiography compared with cone-beam computed tomography. Clin Oral Implants Res 2011;22(12):1415–1419
5. Anavi Y, Gal G, Silfen R, Calderon S. Palatal rotation-advancement flap for delayed repair of oroantral fistula: a retrospective evaluation of 63 cases. Oral Surg Oral Med Oral Pathol Oral Radiol Endod 2003;96(5):527–534
6. Fitzgerald MJT, Law ME. The peripheral connexions between the lingual and hypoglossal nerves. J Anat 1958;92(2):178–188
7. Stuzin JM, Wagstrom L, Kawamoto HK, Baker TJ, Wolfe SA. The anatomy and clinical applications of the buccal fat pad. Plast Reconstr Surg 1990;85(1):29–37
8. Alkan A, Dolanmaz D, Uzun E, Erdem E. The reconstruction of oral defects with buccal fat pad. Swiss Med Wkly 2003;133(33-34): 465–470
9. Otonari-Yamamoto M, Nakajima K, Tsuji Y, et al. Mylohyoid muscle defects: comparison of CT findings and dissected specimens. Oral Radiol 2011;27:50–56
10. Loukas M, Kinsella CR Jr, Kapos T, Tubbs RS, Ramachandra S. Anatomical variation in arterial supply of the mandible with special regard to implant placement. Int J Oral Maxillofac Surg 2008; 37(4):367–371
11. Donner MW, Bosma JF, Robertson DL. Anatomy and physiology of the pharynx. Gastrointest Radiol 1985;10(3):196–212
12. Palmer JB, Rudin NJ, Lara G, Crompton AW. Coordination of mastication and swallowing. Dysphagia 1992;7(4):187–200
13. Palmer JB, Hiiemae KM, Liu J. Tongue-jaw linkages in human feeding: a preliminary videofluorographic study. Arch Oral Biol 1997; 42(6):429–441
14. Palmer JB. Bolus aggregation in the oropharynx does not depend on gravity. Arch Phys Med Rehabil 1998;79(6):691–696
15. Hiiemae KM, Palmer JB. Food transport and bolus formation during complete feeding sequences on foods of different initial consistency. Dysphagia 1999;14(1):31–42
16. Chi-Fishman G, Sonies BC. Motor strategy in rapid sequential swallowing: new insights. J Speech Lang Hear Res 2000;43(6):1481–1492
17. Daniels SK, Foundas AL. Swallowing physiology of sequential straw drinking. Dysphagia 2001;16(3):176–182
18. Fritzell B. The velopharyngeal muscles in speech. An electromyographic and cinéradiographic study. Acta Otolaryngol 1969;250: 250, 1
19. Schuyler CH. Factors contributing to traumatic occlusion. J Prosthet Dent 1961;11:708–715
20. Magne P, Gallucci GO, Belser UC. Anatomic crown width/length ratios of unworn and worn maxillary teeth in white subjects. J Prosthet Dent 2003;89(5):453–461
21. Lombardi RE. The principles of visual perception and their clinical application to denture esthetics. J Prosthet Dent 1973;29(4):358–382
22. Tsukiyama T, Marcushamer E, Griffin TJ, Arguello E, Magne P, Gallucci GO. Comparison of the anatomic crown width/length ratios of unworn and worn maxillary teeth in Asian and white subjects. J Prosthet Dent 2012;107(1):11–16

21 Neck

Sherine S. Raveendran and Lucian Ion

Introduction

The neck is a cylindrical structure that extends from the base of the skull to the thoracic inlet (**Fig. 21.1**). The neck encloses many vital structures and acts as a conduit between the cranium superiorly and the thorax and upper limb inferiorly. Anatomically, the neck is organized into three basic compartments:

- Posterior compartment: musculoskeletal (support and movement of the head and neck)
- Anterior compartment: visceral (glandular, respiratory, and gastrointestinal)
- Lateral compartment: large blood vessels and nerves

Skeletal Support

Cervical Spine

The cervical spine consists of seven vertebrae with some common characteristics and specific features for C1, C2, and C7 (**Fig. 21.2**). In the cervical region, the bodies of the vertebrae are relatively small, and wider transversely than anteroposteriorly, the pedicles are directed laterally and posteriorly, and the laminae are relatively narrow. The transverse processes are pierced by foramen transversaria, through which pass the vertebral artery from usually C1 to C6 vertebrae (**Fig. 21.3**).

The atlas (C1) is the uppermost of the vertebrae; it articulates with the base of the skull and allows anteroposterior movement. It does not have a vertebral body. The axis (C2) is the second vertebra and articulates with the atlas as a pivot that allows rotation. It has a characteristic odontoid process, rising perpendicular from the superior surface of the body. A strong transverse ligament completes the articulation between the atlas and the odontoid process posteriorly. C7 is known as the vertebra prominens and has a characteristic prominent spinous process that can be palpated; it represents the external landmark for the lower part of the cervical spine. In some individuals, C7 is associated with an abnormal extra rib (cervical rib), which can produce symptoms of compression of blood vessels at the root of the neck or of the brachial plexus. When symptomatic, it is referred to as thoracic outlet syndrome.

Surgical Annotation

In a number of genetic syndromes, including Down's syndrome, after infections of the spine and in patients with a history of rheumatoid arthritis, the atlantoaxial joint can be unstable, and in hyperextension, it leads to compression of the spine, which may be fatal. Patients who have a history of rheumatoid or predisposing genetic syndromes are at greater risk for a general anesthetic as a result of the need to hyperextend the neck during intubation.

Hyoid Bone

The hyoid takes support only from the muscles and ligaments associated with mobility of the gastroesophageal and respiratory visceral structures in the neck and floor of mouth (**Fig. 21.4**). The bone has a U-shape contour and is divided into three components: the body, positioned anterior and horizontally, and laterally paired projections, the greater and lesser horns or cornua. The greater horns project posteriorly and superiorly, and the lesser horns project superiorly. The hyoid bone provides attachment to muscles that move the tongue, depresses the mandible, and moves the larynx. The superior attachments are for the middle pharyngeal constrictor, hyoglossus, mylohyoid, geniohyoid, stylohyoid, and digastric muscles. The inferior attachments are for the thyrohyoid, stylohyoid, and omohyoid muscles.

Skin, Adipose Tissue, Fascia

Skin

The skin on the neck is thin and drapes along the contour of the deeper structures anteriorly. The skin on the posterior neck has thicker dermis, with stronger stabilizing fibrous septae, and has limited mobility. In the submental and submandibular areas, the skin is less adherent. In the postauricular and mastoid regions, it is closely attached to the underlying tissues.

Adipose Tissue

The adipose tissue in the neck is distributed in the supraplatysmal, interplatysmal, and subplatysmal planes (**Fig. 21.5**). The anatomical studies reveal that the fat in the subcutaneous plane ranges from 8.4 to 15 g (**Fig. 21.5a**). The total amount of fat in this region can vary in the presence of weight excess. The fat in the subplatysmal plane averages 3.7 g (**Fig. 21.5b**). In clinical settings, it appears to be less influenced by weight variations. The fat is compartmentalized in the submental region.[1–3]

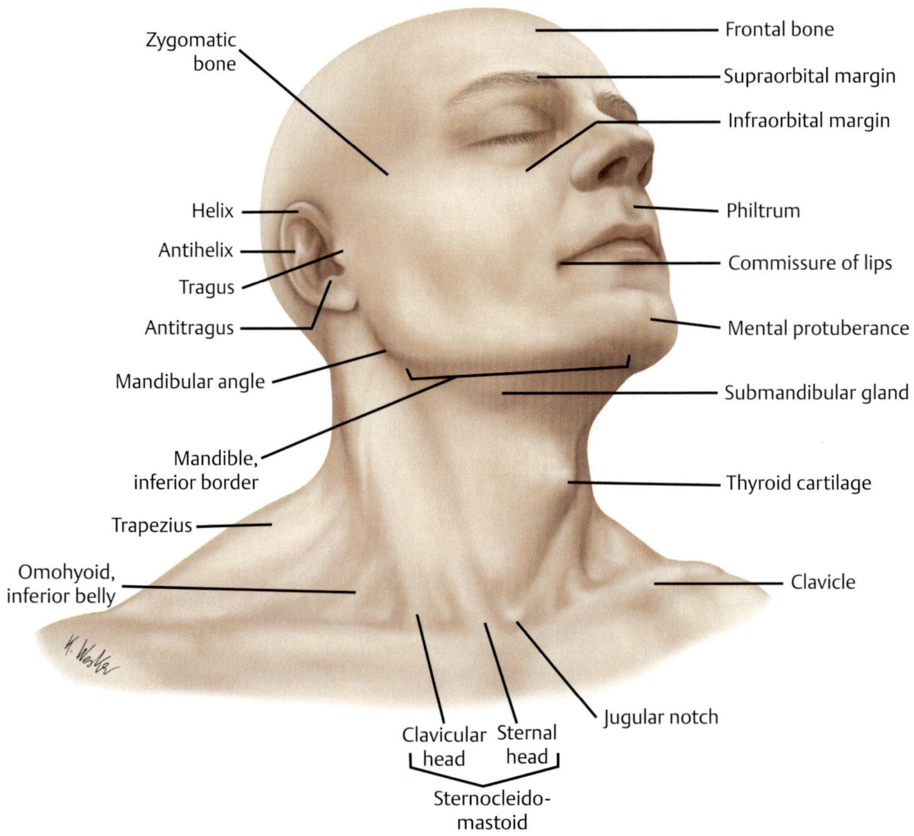

Fig. 21.1 Surface anatomy and external landmarks of the neck. (From THIEME Atlas of Anatomy, General Anatomy and Musculoskeltal System. © Thieme 2005, Illustration by Karl Wesker.)

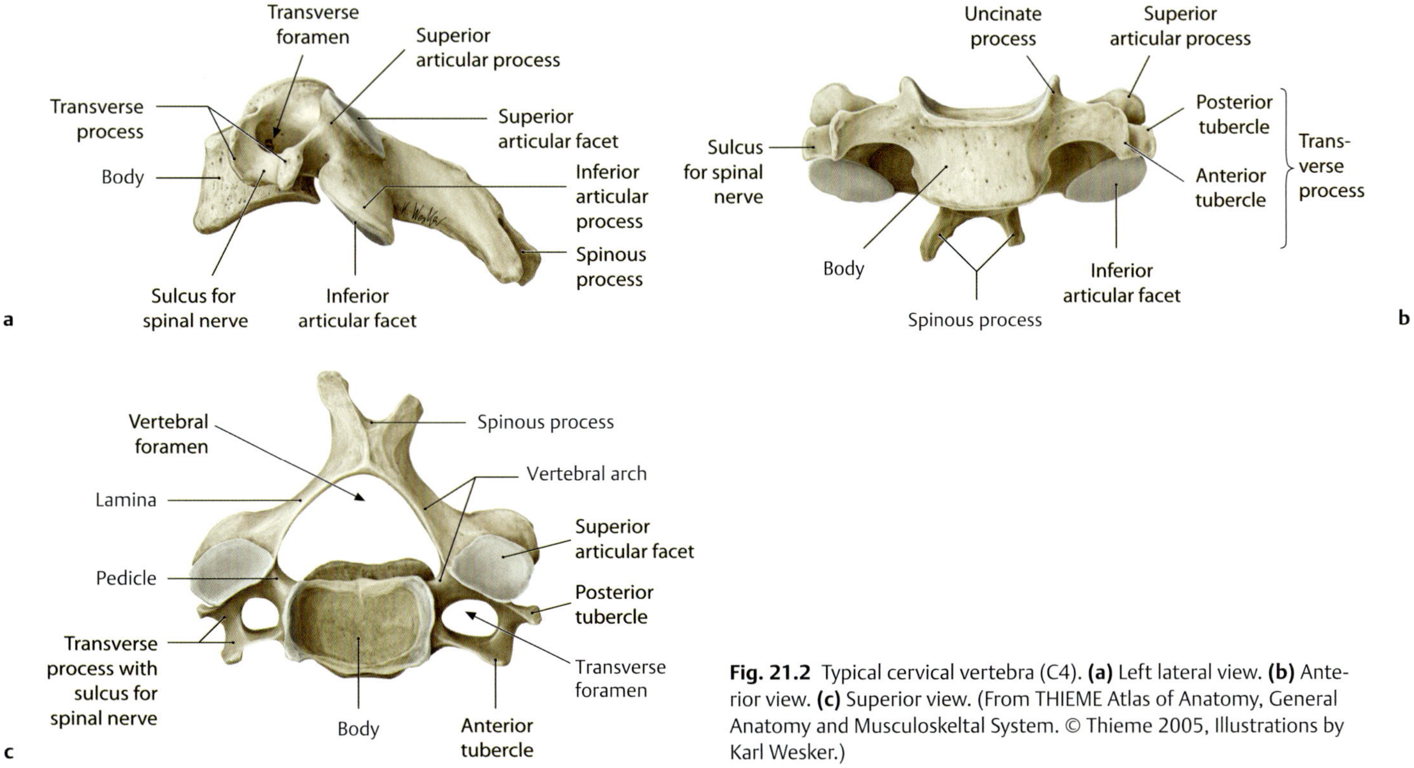

Fig. 21.2 Typical cervical vertebra (C4). **(a)** Left lateral view. **(b)** Anterior view. **(c)** Superior view. (From THIEME Atlas of Anatomy, General Anatomy and Musculoskeltal System. © Thieme 2005, Illustrations by Karl Wesker.)

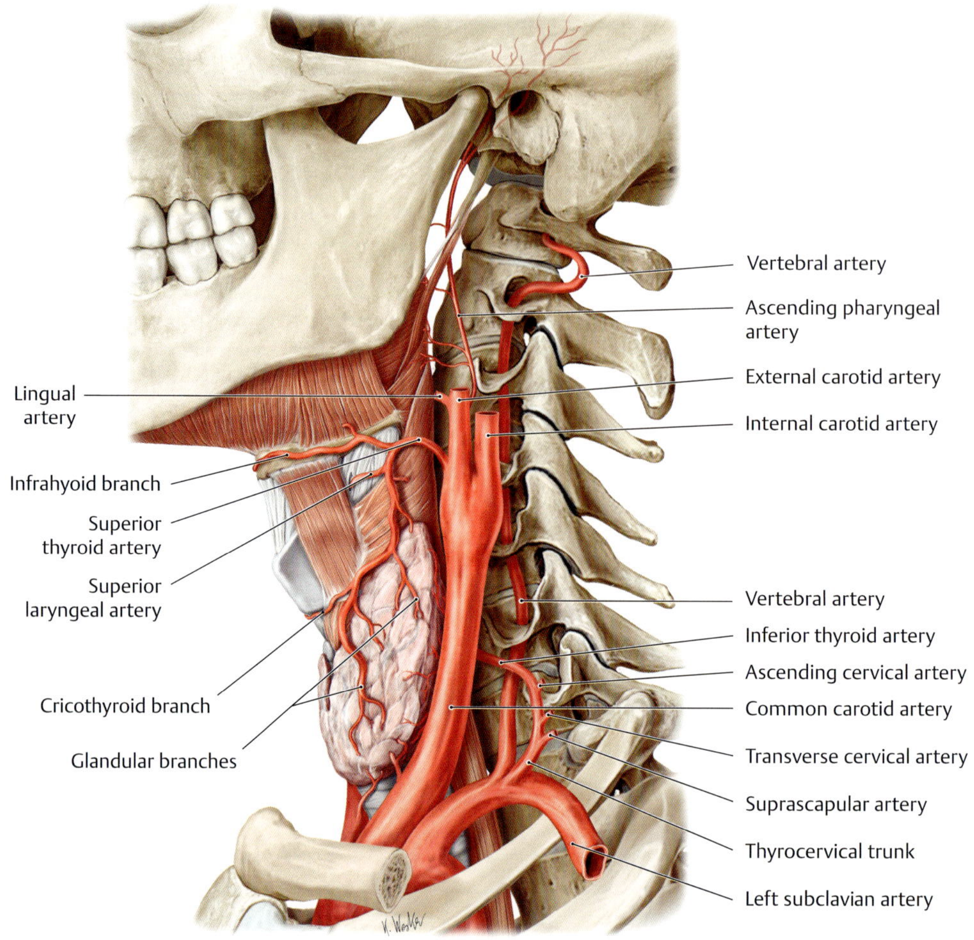

Fig. 21.3 Passage of the vertebral artery through the foramen transversarium of the cervical vertebra. (From THIEME Atlas of Anatomy, General Anatomy and Musculoskeltal System. © Thieme 2005, Illustration by Karl Wesker.)

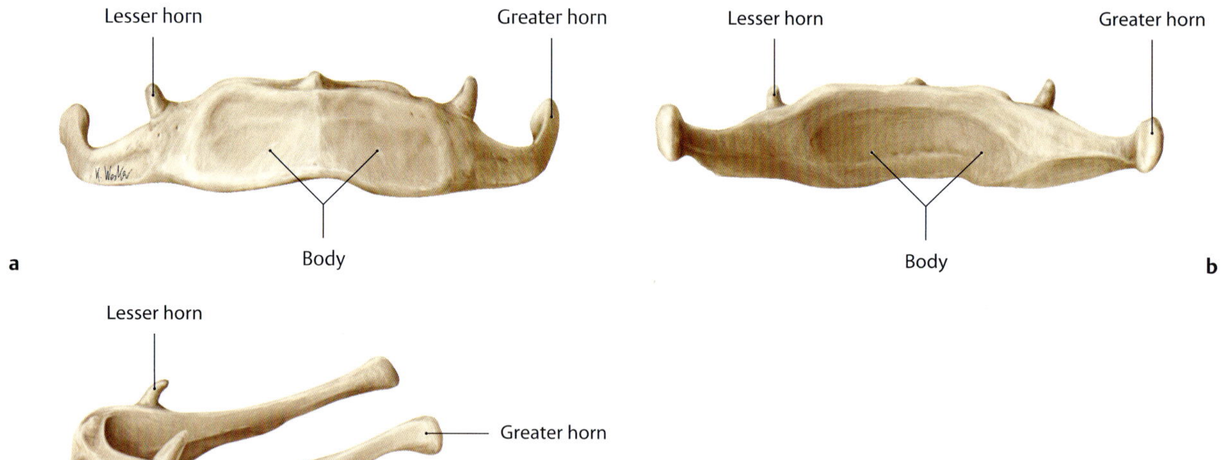

Fig. 21.4 The hyoid bone. **(a)** Anterior view. **(b)** Posterior view. **(c)** Left lateral view. (From THIEME Atlas of Anatomy, General Anatomy and Musculoskeltal System. © Thieme 2005, Illustrations by Karl Wesker.)

a

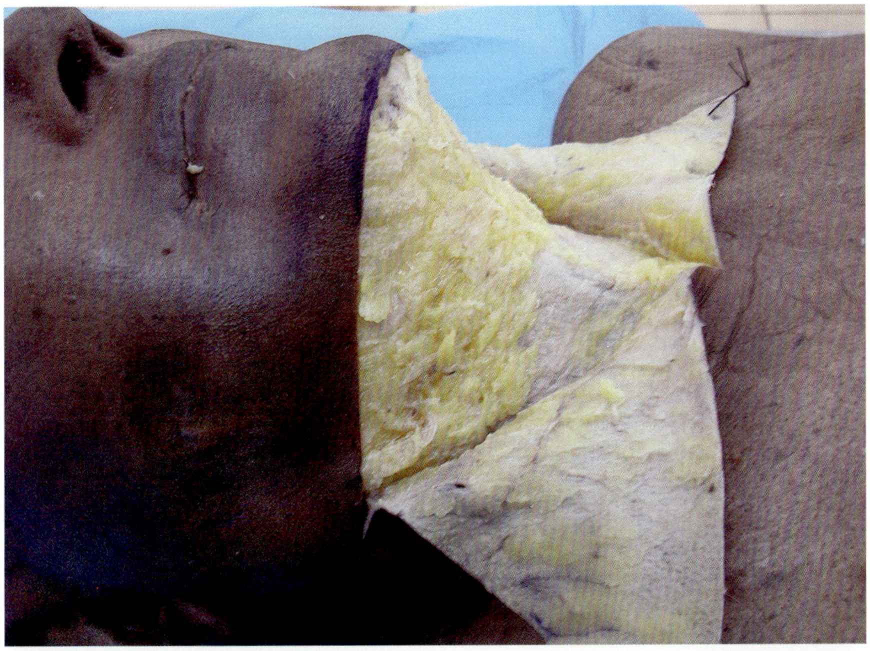

b

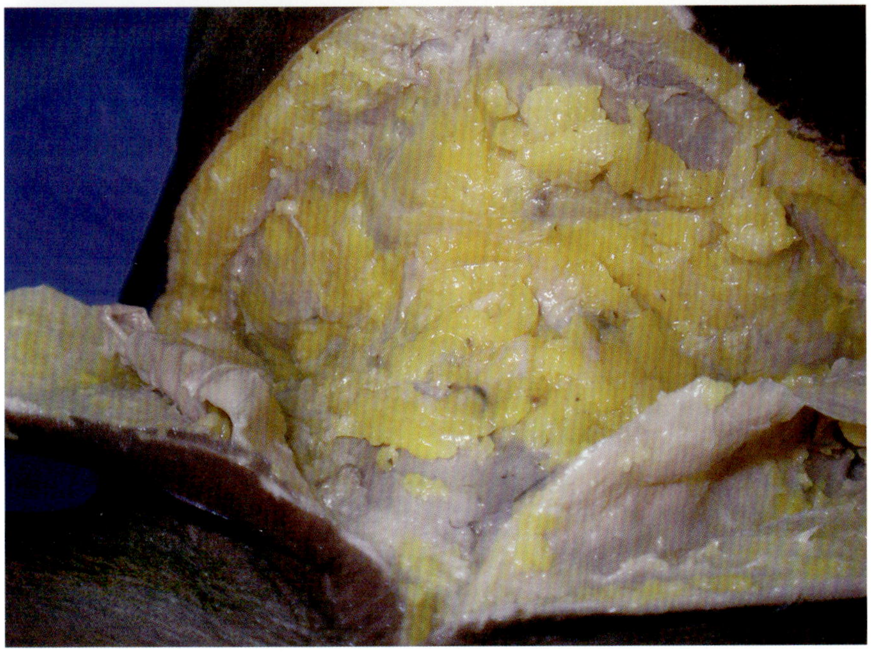

Fig. 21.5 Adipose tissue distribution in the superficial and deep planes of the neck **(a)** superficial fat and **(b)** deep fat.

Surgical Annotation

The volume of the neck is determined by the extent of fat deposition, which in turn determines the girth of the neck. In the fatty neck, there is fat deposition in the superficial and the deeper layers, generating a less defined or even convex shape of the cervicomental angle. Volume reduction during neck contouring can incorporate volume reduction in all fat compartments of the anterior neck to reduce girth and to improve contours. In slim necks, there is minimal fat and the skin drapes over the platysma causing visible bands in older subjects.

Cervical Fascia

The cervical fascia is broadly divided into superficial and deep layers (**Fig. 21.6**).

Superficial Cervical Fascia

Superficial cervical fascia is the continuation of the superficial musculoaponeurotic system (SMAS), also referred to as the SMAS layer. It contains cutaneous nerves, blood vessels, lymphatics, and variable amounts of fat. The platysma is found

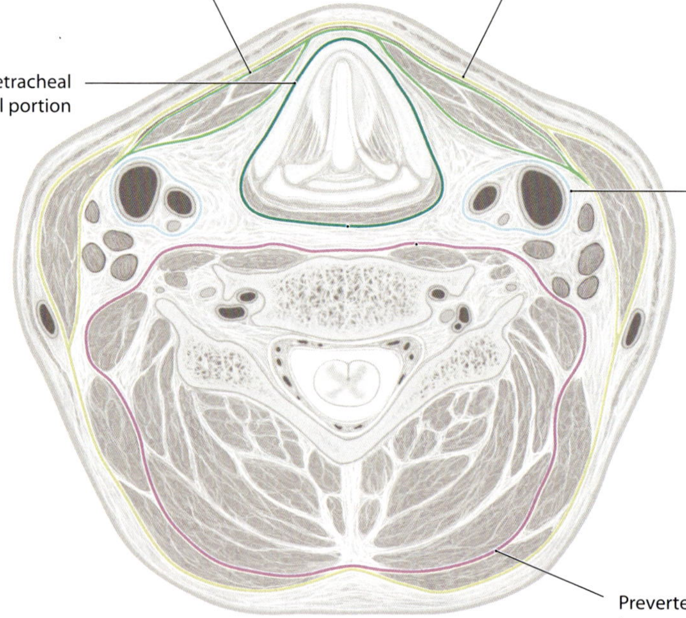

a

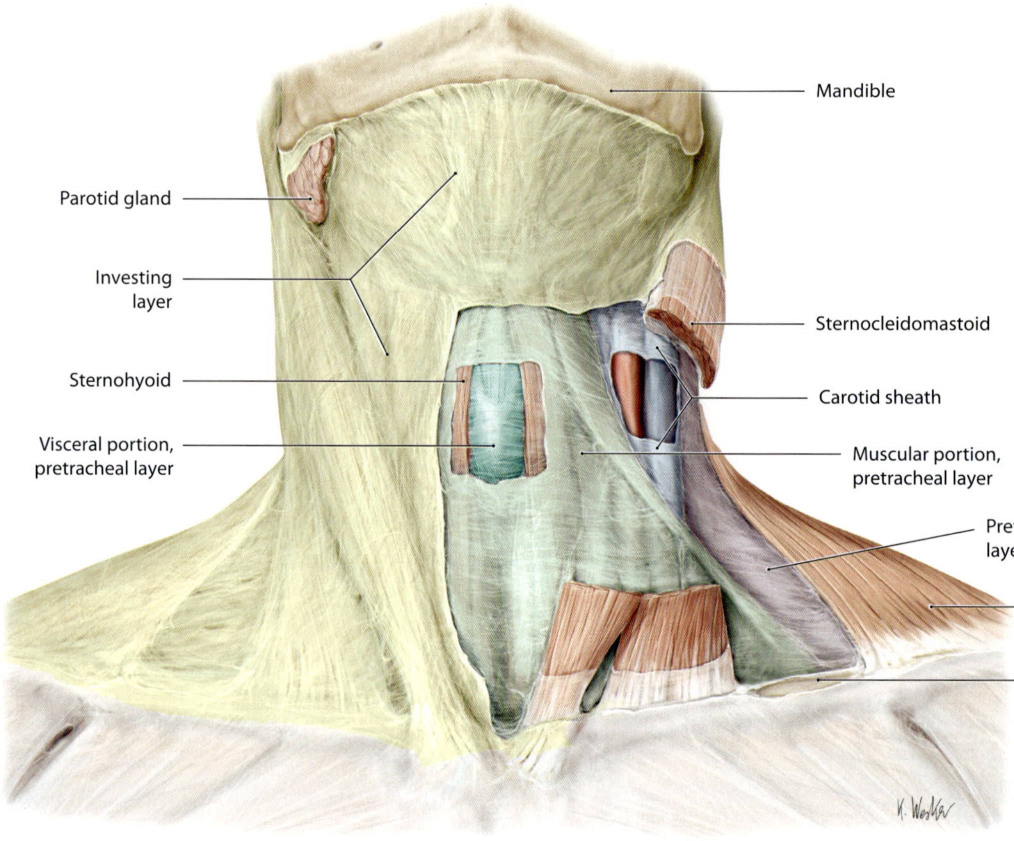

b

Fig. 21.6 Cervical fascia layers. **(a)** Transverse section of the neck. **(b)** Anterior view with skin, superficial fascia, and platysma removed. (From THIEME Atlas of Anatomy, General Anatomy and Musculoskeltal System. © Thieme 2005, Illustrations **(a)** by Markus Voll and **(b)** by Karl Wesker.)

anterolaterally and is adherent to the skin via multiple connective tissues bands. It is a paired muscle found lateral to the midline.

Platysma

The platysma muscle is a thin, wide superficial muscle, originating from the superficial fascia over the upper thorax (**Fig. 21.7a**). The muscle fibers fan out superiorly and inserted into the lower border of the mandible and skin and intermingle with the muscles of facial expression on the lower face. Its innervation is provided by the cervical branch of the facial nerve, and the blood supply is provided by the facial artery, superior thyroid artery, and branches of the posterior auricular and occipital arteries. Its main action in humans is as an accessory depressor of the oral commissure. The platysma muscle courses over the concave contours of the neck and does not have any retention ligaments or pulleys superficial to it. Its deep attachments, the cervical retaining ligaments, adherent to the superficial layer of the deep fascia, are responsible limiting the anterior displacement of the muscle belly during contraction. Later in life, the muscle is responsible for the appearance of vertical dynamic bands, labelled as platysma bands.

Surgical Annotation

The platysma is classified into three types, depending on the extent of decussation[4]:

- Type 1: Limited decussation of the platysma muscles, extending 1 to 2 cm below the mandibular symphysis (75%)
- Type 2: Decussation of the platysma from the mandibular symphysis to the thyroid cartilage (15%)
- Type 3: No decussation of the platysma muscles in the midline (10%)

Isolated platysmal bands associated with ageing can be successfully treated with neurotoxins. Correction of extensive laxity and divarication requires open procedures with interventions on the platysma muscles; plication, excision, and myotomy, and so forth.[5–7] The superiorly and posteriorly based platysma muscle myocutaneous flaps are supplied primarily by the submental artery and secondarily by the superior thyroid, postauricular, and occipital arteries. The external jugular and submental veins provide the venous drainage. The platysma skin flap can be used to reconstruct defects in the orofacial region.[8,9]

Deep Cervical Fascia

The deep fascia can be divided into three layers: the investing layer of the deep cervical fascia, prevertebral fascia, and pretracheal fascia.

Investing Layer of the Deep Cervical Fascia

The investing layer completely encircles the neck and splits to enclose the trapezius and sternocleidomastoid muscles. The investing layer of the deep cervical fascia is attached superiorly to the external occipital protuberance and superior nuchal line and inferiorly to the sternum, clavicle, and acromion of the scapula. The posterior attachments are on the spines of the cervical vertebrae and ligamentum nuchae, and the anterior attachments are on the mandibular midline, body of the hyoid, and manubrium sterni. The fascia splits to enclose the suprasternal space and the attachments of the trapezius and sternocleidomastoid muscles.

In the mastoid region, the investing layer of the fascia is referred to as the parotid fascia, which splits into two layers to enclose the parotid gland. The parotid fascia is attached to the tip of the mastoid process, cartilaginous part of the external acoustic meatus, and lower border of the zygomatic arch. The deep layer extends along the base of the skull and merges with the carotid sheath. The fascia between the styloid process and the angle of the mandible forms the stylomandibular ligament.

Pretracheal Fascia

The pretracheal fascia extends from the hyoid to the thorax. The visceral layer envelops the trachea, esophagus, and thyroid gland and the muscular part encloses the infrathyroid muscles.

It is attached superiorly to the larynx, and inferiorly it extends along the superior mediastinum and merges with the fibrous pericardium.

Prevertebral Fascia

The prevetebral fascia encloses the cervical spine and the prevetebral and postvertebral muscles. It also forms the floor of the posterior triangle of the neck. The fascia extends superiorly to the skull base in front of the longus capitis and rectus capitis lateralis muscles and inferiorly into the thorax, where it merges with the anterior longitudinal ligament of the third thoracic vertebra. The fascia inserts posteriorly on the transverse and spinous processes of the cervical vertebrae and ligamentum nuchae. Inferiorly, the fascia covers the scalene muscles and extends laterally as axillary sheath.

Carotid Sheath

The carotid sheath receives contributions from prevetebral and pretracheal fasciae. It encloses the carotid artery, vagus nerve, lymph nodes, and internal jugular vein. The attachments of the carotid sheath are superiorly to the skull base, and inferiorly the fascia merges with the connective tissue surrounding the aortic arch.

Attachments

- Superior: Base of the skull
- Inferior: The fascia merges with the connective tissue around the arch of the aorta

Surgical Annotation

The arrangements of the fascial layers of the neck determine the spread of infection in the neck. They form important barriers to infection; once infection is established, the fascial layers play a part in directing its spread. The infection may travel through paths of least resistance from one space to another. The investing layer limits the spread of superficial infection. Deeper infections can spread to the thorax and retropharyngeal spaces.[10,11]

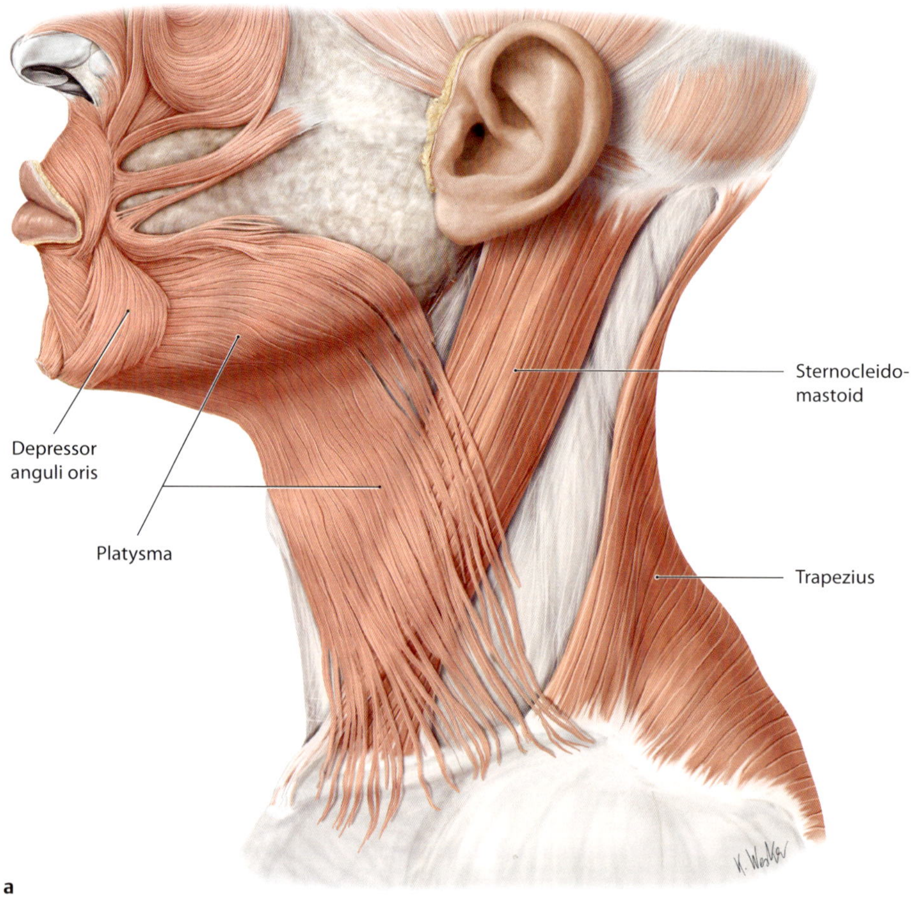

a

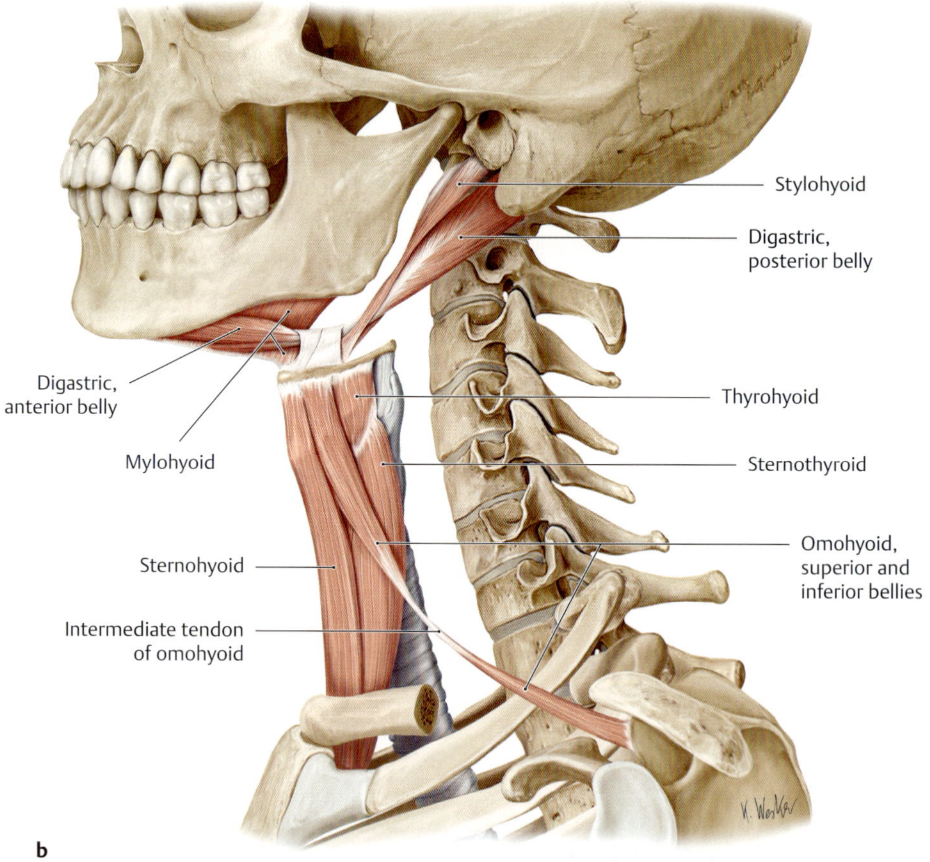

b

Fig. 21.7 Neck muscles. **(a)** The platysma muscle. **(b)** The superficial and middle layers of the muscle in the neck.

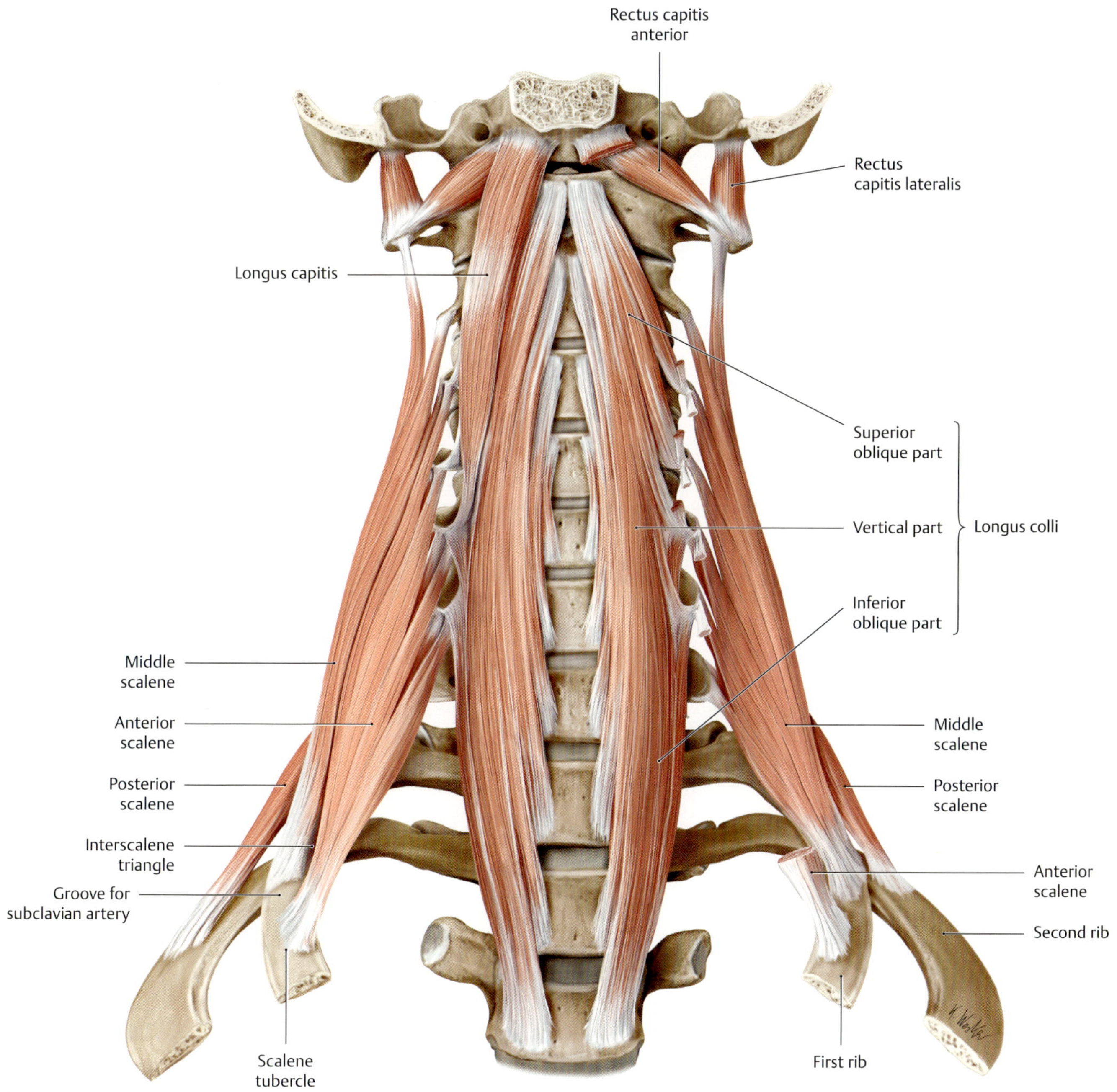

Fig. 21.7 (*continued*) **(c)** The deep muscle layers of the neck. (From THIEME Atlas of Anatomy, General Anatomy and Musculoskeltal System. ©Thieme 2005, Illustrations by Karl Wesker.)

Muscular Anatomy

Lateral Compartment

Sternocleidomastoid

This muscle is an important landmark of the neck as it defines the triangles of the neck and is closely related to the deeper neurovascular structures (**Fig. 21.7b**):

- Origin: It arises from two heads, tendinous (sternal) head from the manubrium sterni and muscular (clavicular) head from the upper surface of the medial third of the clavicle.
- Insertion: The muscle passes upward and outward and is inserted onto the mastoid process and the superior nuchal line.
- Blood supply: The blood supply is through the superior thyroid, occipital, posterior auricular, and suprascapular arteries.
- Nerve supply: The spinal accessory nerve is the nerve supply.

- Action: When one muscle contracts, the head is tipped toward the shoulder on the same side to rotate the face to the opposite side. When acting together, the head is moved forward.

The muscle is sacrificed in radical neck dissection along with other structures of the neck.

Surgical Annotation

In congenital unilateral hypoplasia of the sternocleidomastoid muscle, the muscle belly is shortened and tight, leading to a condition called torticollis. If left untreated, it leads to progressive mandibular and facial asymmetry through the growth period.

Anterior Compartment

Strap Muscles of the Neck

- Superficial layer: Omohyoid, sternohyoid
- Deep layer: Sternothyroid, thyrohyoid
- Nerve supply: Ansa cervicalis, thyrohyoid by the first cervical nerve
- Blood supply: Superior thyroid and lingual arteries

The omohyoid has superior and inferior bellies that are joined by an intermediate tendon. The superior belly is attached to the hyoid bone, and the inferior belly is attached to the scapula. The intermediate tendon is attached to the clavicle and first rib. The omohyoid depresses the hyoid bone from the elevated position. The sternohyoid and sternothyroid muscles originate from the posterior surface of the manubrium sterni. Sternohyoid has additional attachment on the clavicle and is inserted into the inferior border of the body of the hyoid bone. The sternothyroid is attached to the oblique line of the thyroid cartilage. The thyrohyoid muscle arises from the oblique line of the thyroid cartilage and is attached to the body and grater horn of the hyoid. The strap muscles act on the hyoid bone and larynx and assist in swallowing. The digastric, stylohyoid, mylohyoid, geniohyoid, hyoglossus, and genioglossus are classified together as muscles of the floor of the mouth.

Digastric Muscle

The digastric muscle consists of two bellies: the anterior belly and the posterior belly. Both bellies are connected by an intermediate tendon anchored to the hyoid.

Posterior Belly

- Origin: The mastoid notch is posterior to the mastoid process.
- The posterior belly of the digastric muscle runs forward and downward and passes through the stylohyoid muscle.
- Insertion: Insertion is to the greater horn of the hyoid bone by a fibrous loop.
- Blood supply: The blood supply is through the posterior auricular and occipital arteries.
- Nerve supply: The posterior belly is supplied by the facial nerve.

Anterior Belly

- Origin: The digastric fossa on the inferior border of the mandible is the origin.
- Insertion: The muscle runs downward and backward and is connected to the posterior belly via the intermediate tendon.
- Blood supply: Blood supply is through the submental branch of the fascial artery.
- Nerve supply: The mandibular division of the trigeminal nerve provides the nerve supply.
- Action: The digastric muscle helps to raise the hyoid bone and base of the tongue and assists in depressing and retracting the mandible.

Surgical Annotation

Excision of the anterior belly of digastric muscles is carried out as part of some neck dissections, as well as during some cosmetic interventions on the neck. The hypoglossal nerve courses deep to the anterior belly of the digastric muscle and mylohyoid muscles, transversely over the hypoglossus, and needs to be protected during surgery. Blunt dissection with hemostat clamps can be used to elevate the muscle belly from the underlying structures, and once the hypoglossal nerve has been visualized, superior and inferior transection of the muscle belly can be carried out safely.

Posterior Compartment

Posterior Neck Muscles: Trapezius

- Origin: External occipital protuberance, superior nuchal line, ligamentum nuchae, and the spine of the seventh cervical vertebra and spines of the all the thoracic vertebrae.
- Insertion: Spine and acromion of the scapula, lateral third of the clavicle
- Nerve supply: Accessory nerve, cervical plexus
- Blood supply: Superficial cervical, transverse cervical arteries
- Action: Elevates, rotates, and retracts the scapula with other muscles. When scapula is fixed, the trapezius moves the head backward and lateral.

Surgical Annotation

The trapezius myocutaneous flap is used for most of the head and neck reconstruction. It is classified as type V in the Mathes and Nahai classification and can be used as pedicled-islanded flap, free flap, and turnover flap. The flap is a popular choice for reconstruction of the defects over the occipital, parotid gland, cervical spine, and anterior neck. The superior fibers are designed mainly for head and neck reconstruction, but the arc of rotation is limited; however, it is possible to use the middle and inferior fibers of the trapezius for myocutaneous flaps.[12,13]

Paravertebral Muscles

The paravertebral muscles are located in front of the bodies of the cervical vertebrae, deep to the prevertebral fascia (**Fig. 21.7c**). The muscles are longus colli, longus capitis, rectus capitis anterior and lateralis, scalene muscles, and the levator scapulae.

- Blood supply: Vertebral arteries, ascending pharyngeal, and inferior thyroid arteries
- Nerve supply: Cervical spinal nerves
- Action: Scalene muscles are flexors and rotators of the vertebral column. The scalenus anterior and medius elevate the first rib and scalenus posterior elevates the second rib.

Postvertebral Muscles

The post vertebral muscles lie deep to the trapezius, behind the vertebral column, and are arranged in three layers: superficial layer (splenius cervicis and capitis muscles); middle layer (the erector spinae muscles); and deep layer (transversospinalis muscles). When acting on both sides of the splenius capitis, they cause extension of the head. The splenius cervicis is involved in the extension of the cervical spine. When acting on one side, they cause tilting of the head with slight rotation to one side.

Peripheral Nerves of the Neck

The ventral and dorsal rami of the second and third cervical nerves innervate the anterior and posterior skin of the neck, respectively.

Cervical Plexus

The cervical plexus is formed from the ventral rami of the first cervical nerves (C1–C4) and also receives anastomoses from the accessory nerve, hypoglossal nerve, and sympathetic trunk. Its cutaneous branches emerge from the posterior border of the sternocleidomastoid approximately midpoint along the muscle; the motor divisions remain posterior to the sternocleidomastoid. The cutaneous branches of the cervical plexus include the lesser occipital nerve, greater auricular nerve, and the supraclavicular nerves (**Fig 21.8**). The motor branches are the ansa cervicalis and the segmental branches to the anterior and middle scalene nerves (**Fig 21.9**). The phrenic nerve arises from the cervical plexus and has both the sensory and motor components.

The dorsal rami of the first, sixth, seventh, and eighth cervical nerves have no cutaneous branches. The ansa cervicalis is part of cervical plexus, which mainly innervates the infrahyoid muscles. The brachial plexus is derived from the ventral rami of the cervical spinal nerves and lies deep in the posterior triangle of the neck. The cervical sympathetic trunk lies behind the carotid sheath on the prevertebral fascia. The main cutaneous branches of the cervical plexus are the lesser occipital, the great auricular, the transverse cervical, and the supraclavicular nerves. The lesser occipital nerve arises from the ventral ramus of the second and third cervical nerves and supplies the lateral part of the scalp. The greater occipital nerve is a branch of dorsal ramus of the second cervical nerve. This nerve is found in the suboccipital triangle; it pierces the trapezius and supplies the posterior scalp. The transverse cervical nerve arises from the second and third cervical nerves and passes across the sternocleidomastoid muscle to supply the skin on the anterior neck. The supraclavicular nerve receives fibers from the third and fourth cervical nerves. The nerve runs downward toward the clavicle and divides into three branches. These are the medial, intermediate, and lateral supraclavicular nerves, and they supply the skin over the lower neck and upper thorax.

The great auricular nerve arises from the second and third nerves of the cervical plexus and travels from a deep to superficial plane. The nerve reaches the posterior border of the sternocleidomastoid muscle at the junction of the superior and middle thirds of the muscle.[14]

Surgical Annotation

The surface landmark of the great auricular nerve is referred to as the nerve point, located 6.5 cm inferior to the external auditory meatus. The nerve takes an oblique path toward the earlobe following the course of the external jugular vein. The vein lies about 0.5 cm medial to the nerve. Because the nerve is covered only by the SMAS superiorly, this layer should be identified to protect the nerve during dissection. Damage to the nerve leads to numbness of the lower two-thirds of the ear, preauricular skin, and postauricular skin and may result in neuroma formation.

The phrenic nerves arise from C3, C4, and C5 and descend over the anterior scalene muscle deep to the prevertebral fascia.

Cranial Nerves in the Neck

The cranial nerves in the neck are anatomically related to the carotid sheath. The vagus nerve runs within the carotid sheath, and the glossopharyngeal, accessory, and hypoglossal nerves are closely related to these structures.

The glossopharyngeal nerve exits the skull through the jugular foramen. The superior and inferior ganglia are found within the foramen. The nerve is found anterior to the vagus and accessory nerves and runs between the internal jugular vein and carotid artery. It winds around the stylopharyngeus muscle and passes between the superior and middle constrictors. The main branches include the tympanic, lesser petrosal, carotid, pharyngeal, tonsillar, lingual, and a branch to the stylopharyngeus muscle.

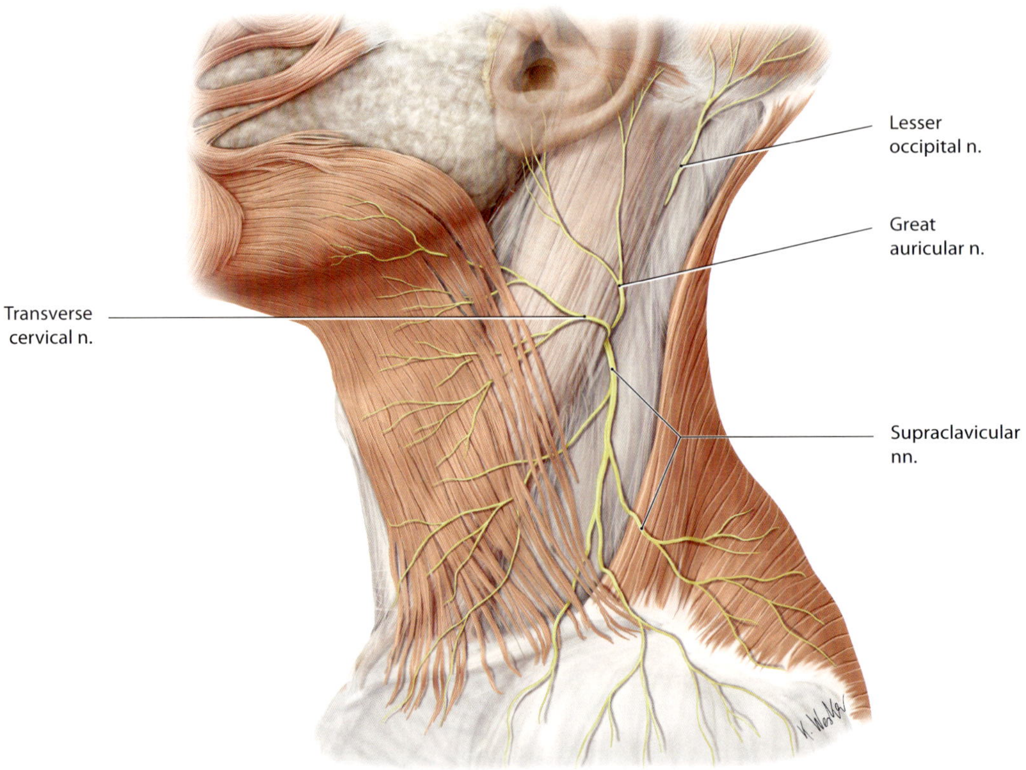

Fig. 21.8 Cutaneous branches of the cervical plexus. (From THIEME Atlas of Anatomy, General Anatomy and Musculoskeltal System. © Thieme 2005, Illustration by Karl Wesker.)

The accessory nerve has cranial and spinal parts. The cranial part joins the vagus nerve. The spinal part of the nerve is derived from the upper five cervical segments. The main trunk passes through the foramen magnum, crosses the internal jugular vein, and runs downward toward the sternocleidomastoid muscle and supplies the muscle. It then crosses the posterior triangle and supplies the trapezius muscle. The spinal and cranial parts of the accessory nerves unite in the jugular foramen and soon separate as they emerge through the cranium.

The vagus nerve exits the jugular foramen and is joined by the cranial part of the accessory nerve. The nerve passes within the carotid sheath and gives rise to the right recurrent laryngeal

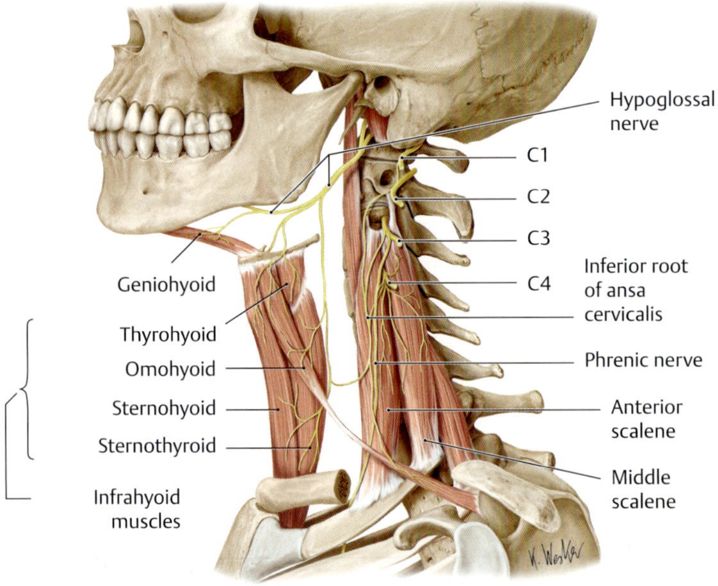

Fig. 21.9 The motor innervations of the neck muscles. (From THIEME Atlas of Anatomy, General Anatomy and Musculoskeltal System. © Thieme 2005, Illustration by Karl Wesker.)

nerve in the root of the neck. The left recurrent laryngeal nerve arises in the thorax, and both nerves course upwards between the trachea and esophagus. The other branches of the vagus nerve include the meningeal, auricular, pharyngeal, carotid body, superior laryngeal, and cardiac nerves.

Surgical Annotation

The nerves that are closely related to the carotid sheath can be damaged during neck dissection. The accessory nerve emerges at the posterior border of the sternocleidomastoid and takes a posterior and inferior course toward the trapezius muscle. It runs superficially, under the cervical fascia, and can be easily injured during neck dissection. Dissection in the posterior region of the posterior border of the sternocleidomastoid needs to take into account the superficial position of the nerve. At this point, the nerve emerges approximately at the midportion of the sternocleidomastoid and courses posteriorly. The accessory nerve is removed in radical neck clearance and is preserved in modified radical dissections. Removal of this nerve causes weakness and chronic shoulder pain.[15,16]

Facial Nerve Branches in the Neck

The marginal mandibular nerve is a branch of facial nerve and is one of the most common nerves to be damaged during neck surgery (**Fig. 21.10**). The nerve follows the mandibular border anteriorly and lies 2 cm below the inferior border before crossing the facial artery and vein. It supplies the depressor labii inferioris, depressor anguli oris, and the mentalis muscles (**Fig. 21.11**).

Surgical Annotation

The nerve is vulnerable during liposuction, neck lift, neck dissection, and mandibular implant placement. Surgical techniques, such as staying deep to the superficial cervical fascia and elevation of the deep fascia with the periosteum of the mandible, will help to protect the nerve.[17]

The cervical branch of the facial nerve innervates the platysma muscle and enters the deeper surface of the muscle superolaterally. Damage to this nerve is reported at 1.7% during rhytidectomy.[18] Injury to this nerve can mimic marginal mandibular nerve damage; however, the patient will still be able to evert the lower lip due to an intact mentalis muscle. In the lower face, the facial nerve runs deep to the platysma and SMAS and innervates the muscles on their under surfaces except for the buccinator, levator anguli oris, and mentalis muscles.

Surgical Annotation

Identification of the facial nerve during parotidectomy can be carried out in the neck. Dissection starts with the posterior border of the platysma approximately 5 cm below the gonial angle and extends inferiorly and superiorly. The parotid fascia and parotid gland are exposed, and the dissection can progress to the anterior border of the gland for a retrograde identification of the facial nerve branches and dissection or to the posterior border of the gland for identification of the nerve trunk with an antegrade

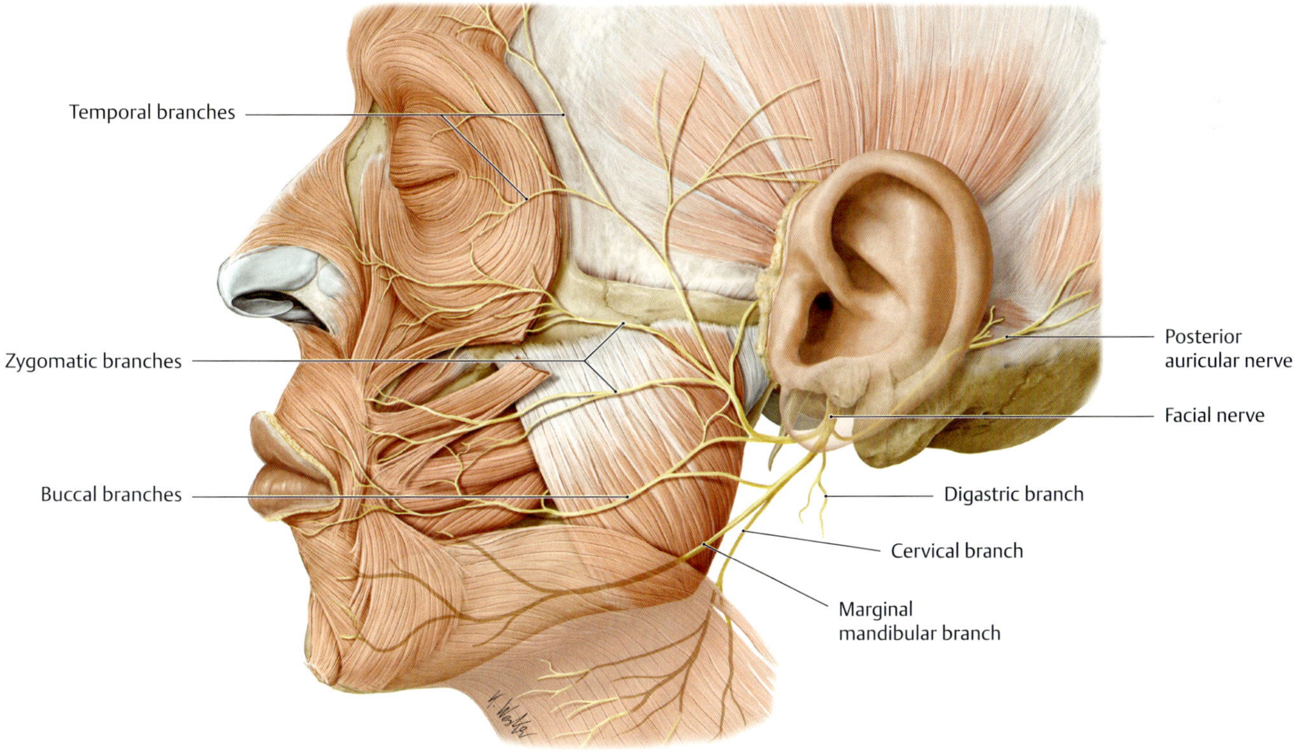

Fig. 21.10 Branches of facial nerve. (From THIEME Atlas of Anatomy, General Anatomy and Musculoskeltal System. © Thieme 2005, Illustration by Karl Wesker.)

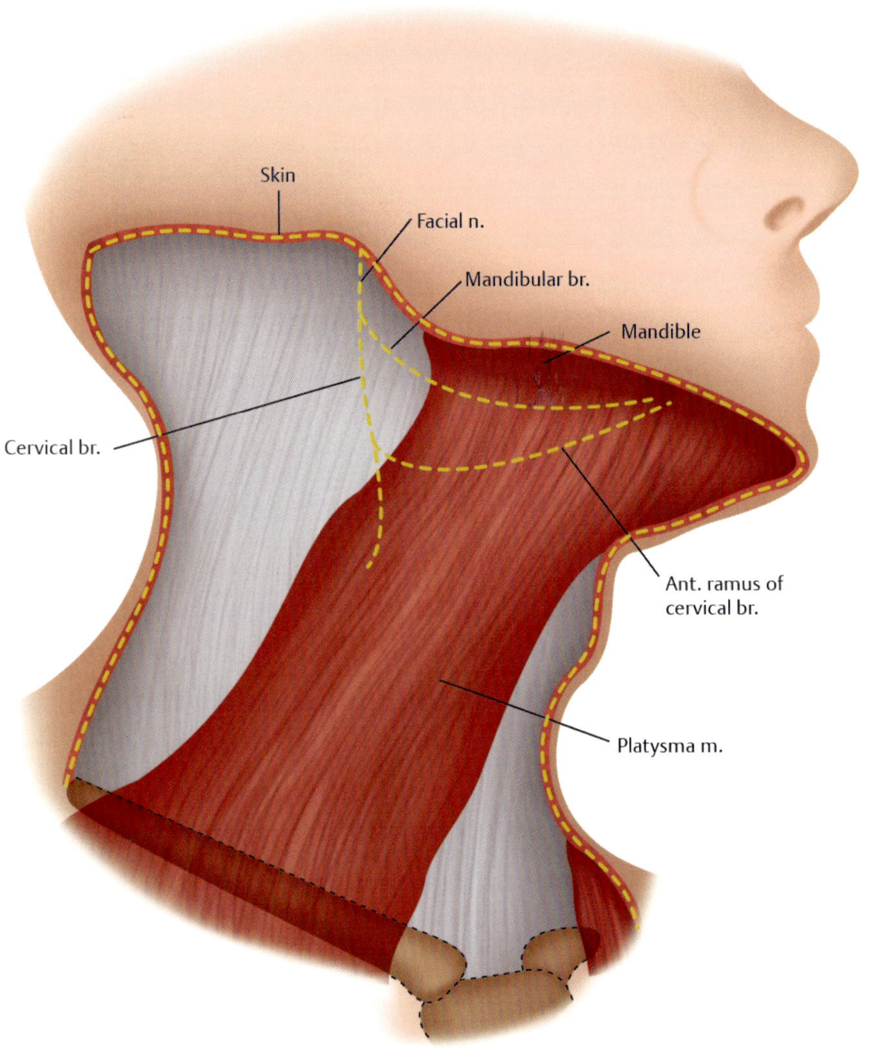

Fig. 21.11 Course of the marginal mandibular nerve.

dissection. During facelift surgery, dissection under the platysma starts superiorly and progresses inferiorly along the posterior border of the muscle. The marginal mandibular branch exits the parotid above the junction between the lower border and anterior aspect of the gland, and the cervical branch exits at the lower border; they need to be protected. Blunt dissection with a small cotton ball is commonly used to provide safe dissection.

Vascular Anatomy of the Neck

Arteries

The carotid arteries are the main arterial structures of the neck (**Fig. 21.12**). The right common carotid artery arises from the brachiocephalic artery, and the left arises from the arch of the aorta. They bifurcate at the level of the upper border of the thyroid cartilage into the internal and external carotid arteries. The internal carotid artery usually does not have any branches in the neck and passes through the carotid canal to the cranium. Branches of the external carotid artery are the superior thyroid, ascending pharyngeal, lingual, facial, occipital, posterior auricular, maxillary, and superficial temporal arteries. The first branch of the external carotid artery is the superior thyroid artery. It arises just below the grater horn of the hyoid bone and runs downward toward the upper pole of the thyroid gland. The artery supplies the thyroid, sternocleidomastoid muscle, infrahyoid muscles, and laryngeal musculature. The facial artery arises from the external carotid artery and runs forward and upward to enter the digastric triangle. It courses deep to the digastric muscle and posterior to the submandibular gland, where it gives rise to the branches to the gland. The artery exits from the superior part of the gland, winding around the inferior border of the mandible, and enters the face along the anterior border of the masseter muscle. In the neck, it gives rise to the ascending palatine, tonsillar, and submental arteries.

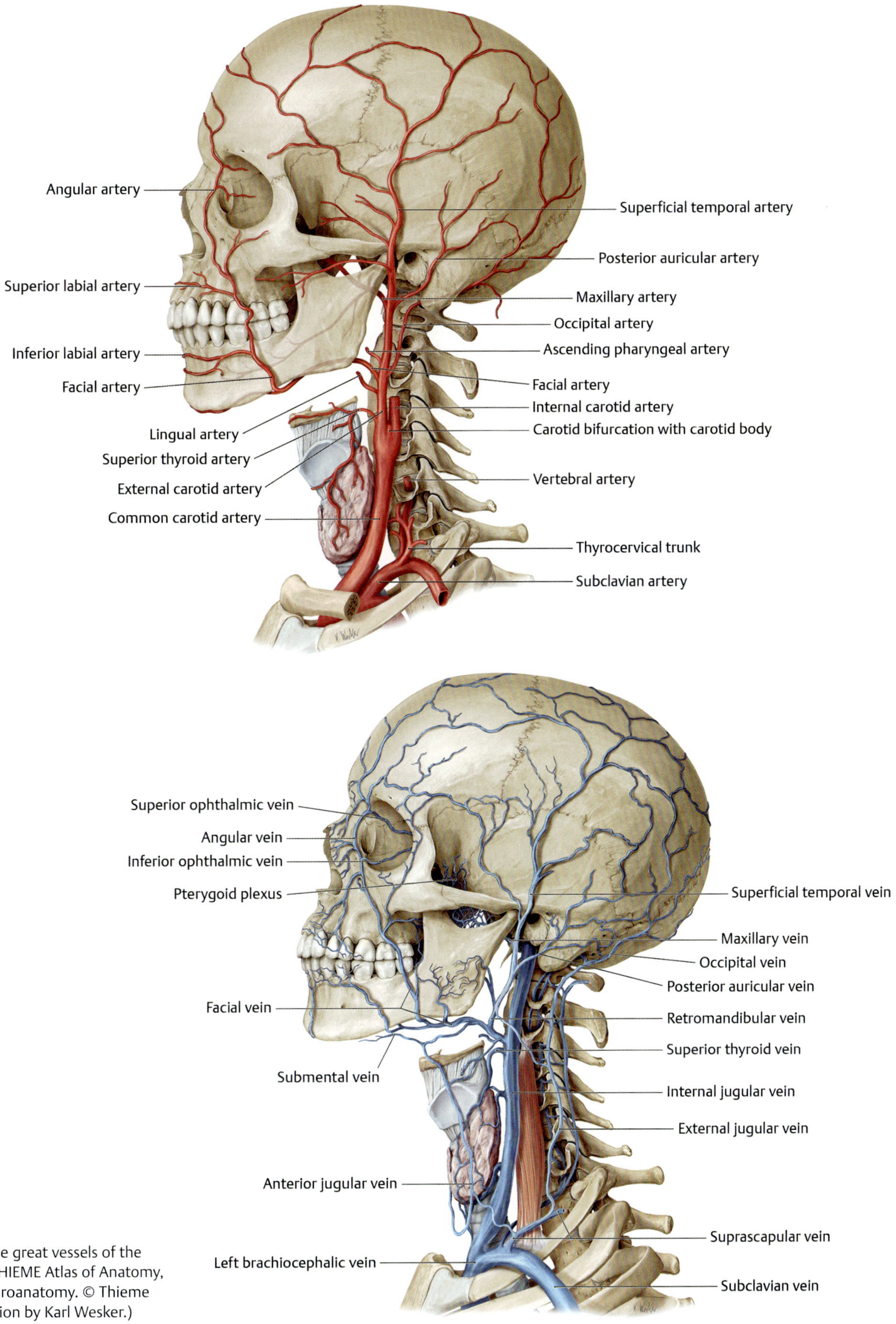

Fig. 21.12 The great vessels of the neck. (From THIEME Atlas of Anatomy, Head and Neuroanatomy. © Thieme 2010, Illustration by Karl Wesker.)

Surgical Annotation

Carotid body tumors arise from the adventitia of the carotid artery bifurcation medially. They often manifest as an asymptomatic lump in the anterior neck, with cranial nerve palsies, or with paroxysmal hypertension and palpitations. The carotid arteries are in imminent danger during neck dissection, and carotid artery blowout can occur in patients who undergo neck dissection and radiotherapy, which can be fatal.[19–21]

Veins

The main veins in the neck are the external and internal jugulars (**Fig. 21.13**). The internal jugular vein emerges from the base of the skull through the jugular foramen, and accompanies the carotid artery within the carotid sheath. It joins the subclavian vein to form the brachiocephalic vein. The important tributaries include the facial, lingual, pharyngeal, superior, and inferior thyroid veins. The external jugular vein originates at the apex of the parotid gland and passes along the lateral border of the sternocleidomastoid muscle, pierces the deep cervical fascia, and drains into the subclavian vein. The tributaries are occipital, posterior external jugular, superficial cervical, suprascapular, and anterior jugular veins. The anterior jugular vein receives veins from the submandibular region and the facial and parotid veins, passes anteriorly in the neck, and drains into the external jugular or subclavian veins. The union of superficial temporal and maxillary veins forms the retromandibular vein. The vein enters the parotid gland superficial to the external carotid artery, between the mandibular ramus and sternocleidomastoid muscle. It divides into anterior and posterior branches. The anterior branch joins the facial vein and become the common facial vein. The posterior branch joins the posterior auricular vein and become the external jugular vein. The relationship of the vein to the facial nerve is important during parotidectomy. In most situations, the vein lies medial to the upper and lower trunks of the facial nerve.

Surgical Annotation

The lower platysma myotomy is sometimes carried out during neck lift surgery. When dissecting along the posterior border of the muscle, care must be taken to avoid injury to the greater auricular nerve. This nerve emerges at the posterior border of the sternocleidomastoid approximately 6 cm below the mastoid and courses anterior and superior. The external jugular vein can be identified under the superficial cervical fascia and below the posterior fibers of the platysma approximately at the level of

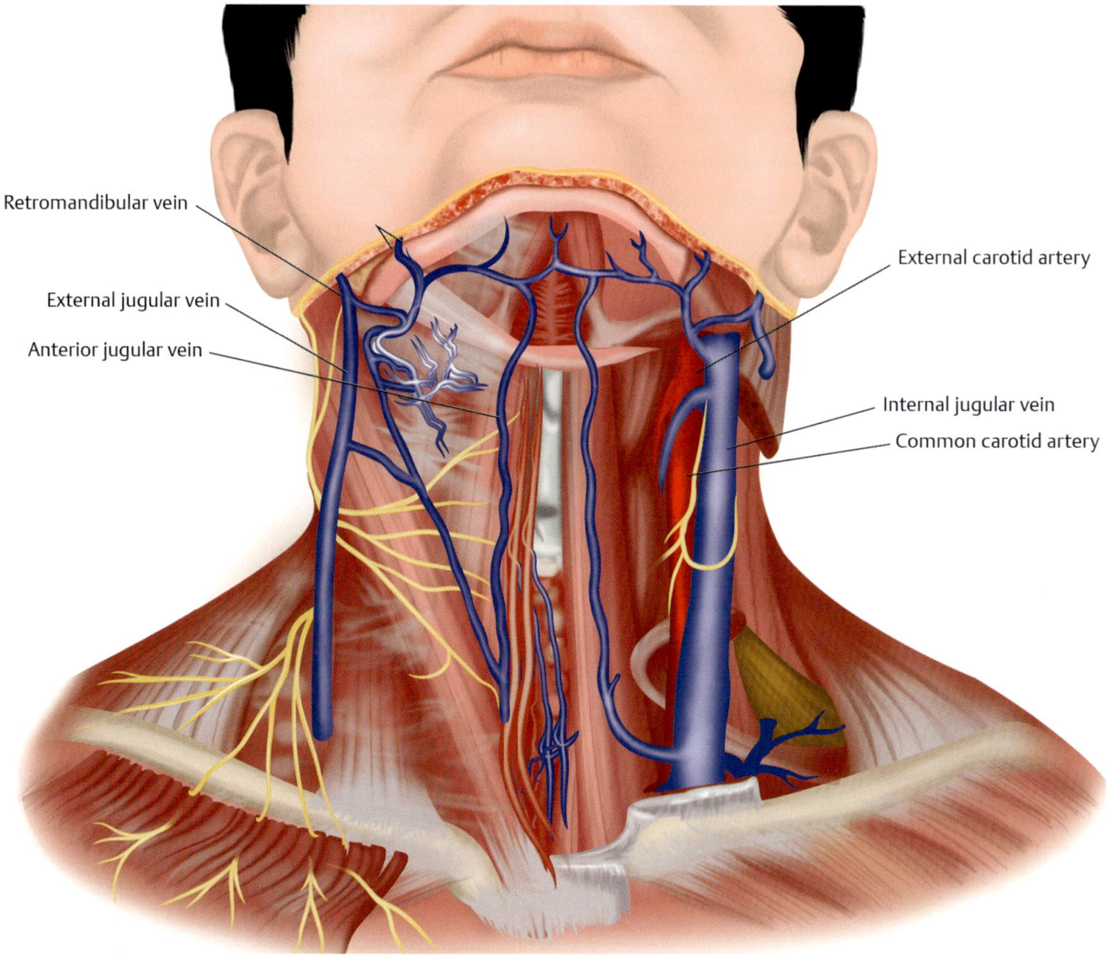

Fig. 21.13 The triangles of the neck.

the cricoid cartilage. Dissection of the posterior platysma fibers with gentle elevation reduces the risk of injury to the vein, which is restrained by the fascia. During radical dissection of the neck, the internal jugular vein is removed along with other structures, which may lead to facial edema as a long-term complication.[22,23]

Lymphatics

The lymph nodes in the neck are broadly classified into superficial and deep groups, and the lymph nodes are found to be in relation to the triangles of the neck. The superficial group consists of submental, submandibular, anterior cervical, and superficial cervical lymph nodes. The deep group consists of infrahyoid, prelaryngeal, pretracheal, retropharyngeal, and deep cervical nodes.

Superficial group drain into the deep group and deep group in turn drain into the jugular trunk. On the left side, the left jugular trunk drains into the thoracic duct. The thoracic duct is the main lymphatic trunk in the body, collecting from all areas except the right side of the head, neck, thorax, and arm. The thoracic duct enters the neck through the thoracic inlet behind the left carotid artery and left vagus nerve. It passes between the left common carotid artery and subclavian arteries and enters the left subclavian trunk. At this point, the duct receives the left subclavian trunk. On the right side, the jugular trunk and subclavian trunk drain into the right lymphatic duct. The right lymphatic duct passes along the medical border of the scalenus muscle to drain into the subclavian vein.

Classification of the Lymph Nodes

- Level 1: Submental (1a), submandibular (1b) (**Fig. 21.14**)
  - Boundaries: The body of the mandible, stylohyoid muscle, anterior belly of the digastric muscle
- Levels 2, 3, and 4: The upper, middle, and lower jugular nodes
  - Level 2 is divided in to 2a and 2b by the spinal accessory nerve.
  - Level 3 nodes boundaries: The hyoid bone and a horizontal plane defined by the inferior border of the cricoid cartilage, sternohyoid muscle, and posterior border of the sternocleidomastoid muscle.
  - Level 4 refers to the group of nodes related to the lower third of the jugular vein.
    Boundaries: Inferior border of the cricoid cartilage, clavicle, sternohyoid muscle, and posterior border of the sternocleidomastoid muscle.
- Level 5 nodes are located in the posterior triangle of the neck.
  - Boundaries: The posterior border of the sternocleidomastoid, anterior border of the trapezius muscle and clavicle. This level is subdivided by a plane defined by the inferior border of the cricoid cartilage into level 5a superiorly and level 5b inferiorly.
- Level 6 nodes are in the anterior, or central, compartment of the neck.
  - Boundaries: Carotid arteries, hyoid bone, suprasternal notch

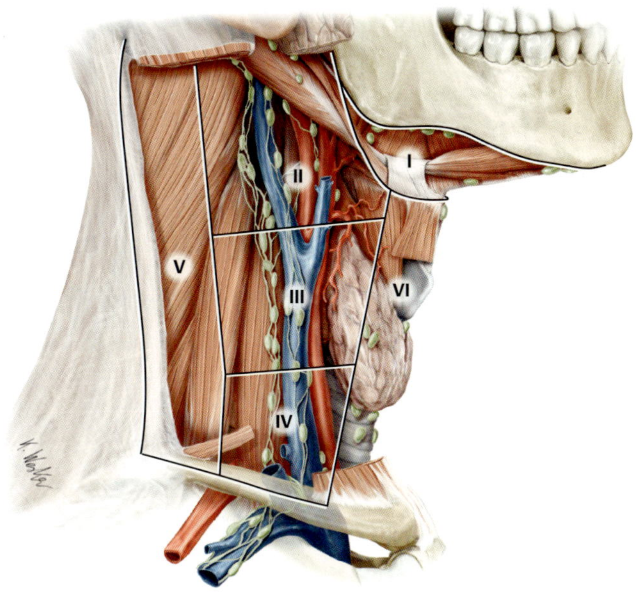

Fig. 21.14 The lymph node of the neck. (From THIEME Atlas of Anatomy, General Anatomy and Musculoskeltal System. © Thieme 2005, Illustration by Karl Wesker.)

Lymph nodes in this compartment are located in the tracheoesophageal groove (paratracheal nodes), in front of the trachea (pretracheal nodes), around the thyroid gland (parathyroidal nodes), and on the cricothyroid membrane (precricoid).

Surgical Annotation

- Metastasis: Level 1a from the floor of the mouth, anterior tongue, anterior mandibular alveolar ridge, and lower lip. Level Ib receives metastases from cancers of the oral cavity, anterior nasal cavity, soft tissue structures of the midface, and submandibular gland.
- Level 2 nodes may be involved in cancers of the oral cavity, nasal cavity, nasopharynx, oropharynx, hypopharynx, larynx, and parotid gland may involve these nodes.
- Level 3 receives metastasis from cancers that originate in the oral cavity, nasopharynx, oropharynx, hypopharynx, and larynx. The nodes of level 4 commonly harbor metastasis from cancer that originates in the larynx, hypopharynx, thyroid, and cervical esophagus.
- Level 5 may harbor metastasis from cancers that arises in the nasopharynx, oropharynx, or skin of the posterior scalp and neck. Lymph nodes in the central compartment are not routinely excised in radical neck dissection; most commonly, they are removed during surgery for thyroid, laryngeal, and hypopharyngeal cancers.[24–27]

Triangles of the Neck

The neck is broadly divided in to anterior and posterior triangles (**Fig. 21.15**).

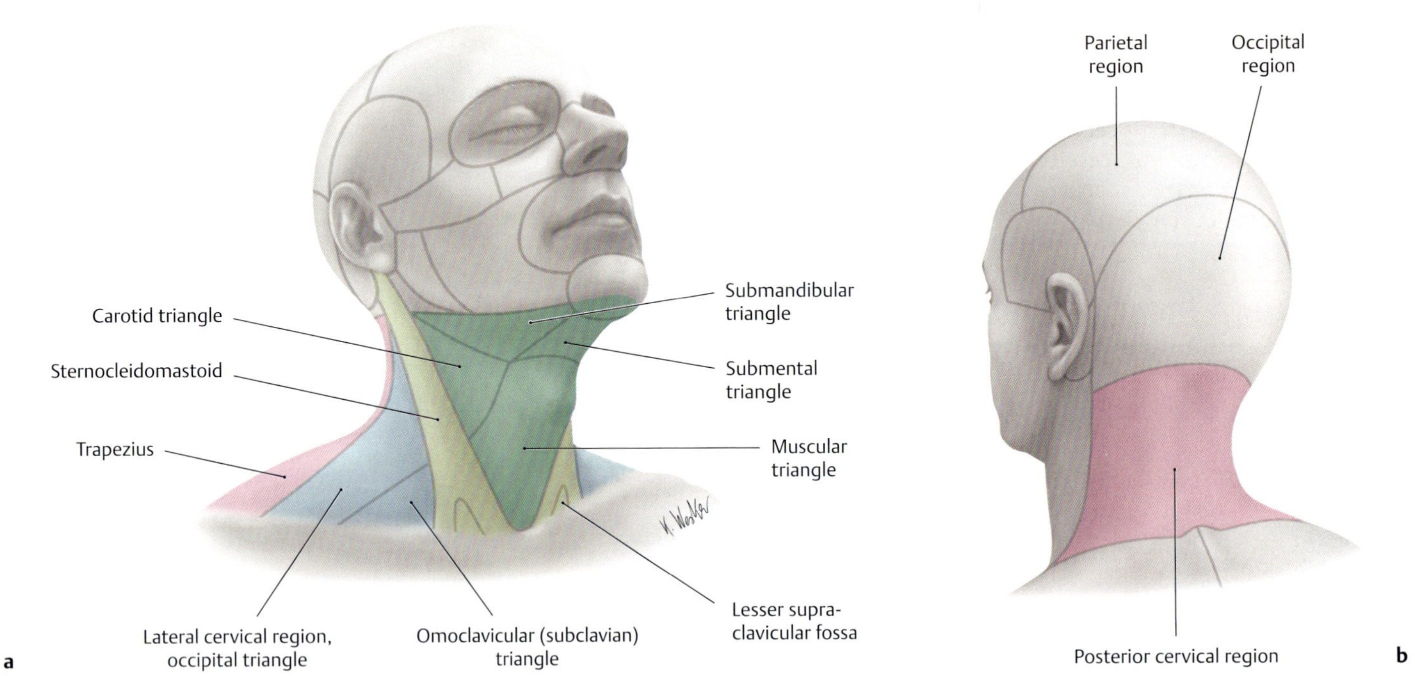

Fig. 21.15 Regions of the neck (cervical regions), right lateral view. For descriptive purposes, the anterior and lateral neck are divided into two triangles which share the sternocleidomastoid as a boundary. (From THIEME Atlas of Anatomy, Neck and Internal Organs. © Thieme 2010, Illustrations by Karl Wesker.)

Anterior Triangle

The anatomical boundaries of the two anterior triangles of the neck commence from the midline of the neck, extending from the sternal notch to the chin. They are bordered posteriorly by the anterior margin of the sternocleidomastoid muscle and superiorly by the inferior border of the mandible. The space can be further divided into submental, submandibular carotid and muscular triangles.

Submental Triangle/Suprahyoid Triangle

The submental triangle, also referred to as the suprahyoid triangle, is bound anteriorly by the anterior belly of the digastric muscle. The hyoid bone forms the inferior border, and the mylohyoid forms the floor of the triangle. The medial border extends up to the midline of the neck. The submental triangle contains the submental lymph nodes and the veins.

Submandibular Triangle/Digastric Triangle

The submandibular triangle is bordered anteroinferiorly and posteroinferiorly by the anterior and posterior belly of the digastric muscle respectively. The lower border of the mandible forms the superior border. The important contents include the submandibular salivary gland, facial artery and vein, and the marginal mandibular nerve.

Carotid Triangle

The carotid triangles contain some of the important structures of the neck. These include the hypoglossal, accessory and vagus nerves, superior laryngeal nerve and branches of the facial nerve, sympathetic trunk, carotid vessels, and the branches of the jugular veins. The anterior border of the carotid triangle is formed by the omohyoid muscle. Posteriorly, it is lined by the sternocleidomastoid muscle and superiorly by the posterior belly of the digastric and stylohyoid muscles. The floor is formed by the middle and inferior pharyngeal constrictors, hyoglossus, and the thyrohyoid muscles.

Muscular Triangle/Inferior Carotid Triangle

The muscular triangle is also referred to as the inferior carotid triangle and contains the sternothyroid and sternohyoid muscles, oesophagus, thyroid gland, and trachea. The space is bordered posteriorly by the anterior border of the sternocleidomastoid muscle. The superior belly of the omohyoid forms the postero superior border, and the space extends up to the midline of the neck from the hyoid bone to the sternum.

Posterior Triangle

The posterior triangle is bounded anteriorly by the posterior border of the sternocleidomastoid muscle. The posterior border is formed by the anterior border of the trapezius, and the inferior border is formed by the middle third of the clavicle. The triangle is further divided into the occipital and subclavican triangle by the inferior belly of the omohyoid. The contents include the spinal accessory nerve, branches of the cervical plexus, roots and trunks of the cervical plexus and phrenic nerve, subclavian and transverse cervical artery, external jugular vein, inferior belly of the omohyoid muscle, scalene, splenius and levator scapulae muscles.

Surgical Annotation

Lymph node status is one of the important prognostic factors for head and neck cancers. Appropriate management of the regional lymphatics, therefore, plays a central role in the treatment of the head and neck cancer patients. The triangles of the neck have oncologic significance related to the surgical management of the regional metastasis.

The neck dissection can be broadly divided into comprehensive or selective. The comprehensive neck dissection is further divided into radical, modified radical, and extended radical dissection. The selective neck dissection includes supraomohyoid, anterolateral, anterior, and posterior dissections. The classification is mainly based on the surgical management of regional lymph nodes and preservation or removal of structures in relation to these nodes.[28,29]

Submandibular Gland

The submandibular gland is located in the submandibular triangle (**Fig. 21.16**). The gland is enveloped by a capsule and has two portions. The superficial lobe is large and is found superficial to the mylohyoid muscle. The gland parenchyma extends along the posterior border of the muscle to form the smaller deep lobe. Wharton's duct arises from the deeper lobe, crosses the sublingual space, and opens near the frenulum of the tongue.

Many important structures are closely related to the submandibular gland and have significant clinical relevance. The marginal mandibular branch of the facial nerve passes along the anteroinferior part of the gland, crosses the mandible, and supplies the muscles of the lower lip and chin. The cervical branches of the facial nerve and the facial vein are related to the anteroinferior part of the gland. The facial artery courses superolaterally, and the deep lobe is closely related to the glossopharyngeal, lingual, and hypoglossal nerves and the submandibular ganglion. The deep surface of the gland overlies the mylohyoid, hyoglossus, styloglossus, stylohyoid, and the posterior belly of the digastric muscle. The lingual nerve lies above and lateral to the duct of the submandibular gland.

Surgical Annotation

Dissection of the gland is often performed in oncologic neck surgery and neck lift procedures, and it is important to acknowledge the close relationship of these structures to the gland.[30] Direct access to the gland in neck and oncologic procedures is through the submandibular approach, whereas the aesthetic resection is carried out via submental approach. With the aging process, there may be pseudoptosis rather than actual descent of the gland in the neck. Anatomical studies have revealed that about 40% of the gland represents the cervical part of the submandibular gland. Partial resection of the prominent gland during neck contouring carries a risk of damage to the facial artery, vein, and marginal mandibular nerve. Dissecting the gland in the subcapsular plane may prevent injury to the nerve.[3,30–32] Submandibular gland excision involves direct access, during which it is important to protect the marginal mandibular branch of the facial nerve. The skin incision is therefore placed approximately 4 cm below the mandibular border, and the platysma muscle needs to be elevated carefully. Intracapsular dissection allows protection of the pericapsular structures as in reduction of the gland. At the upper segment of the dissection, the lingual nerve should be identified superior to Wharton's duct and protected, and the nerve fibers passing to the gland are divided. Intracapsular dissection provides protection to the hypoglossal nerve, which courses over the hyoglossus. When the submandibular gland is reduced during neck lift surgery, access is through the anteroinferior segment of the capsule. To avoid damage to surrounding structures, the dissection needs to remain intra capsular. The relationships of the capsule are the facial nerve and facial artery posterior and superior, the facial vein posterior, and the lingual nerve at the superior border of the gland. The hypoglossal nerve lies to the medial side in the lower two-thirds; depending on the size of the submandibular gland, it takes a transverse course over hyoglossus and passes superior to the mylohyoid muscle.[33,34]

Visceral Structures

The important visceral structures are the pharynx, larynx, trachea, and esophagus. The thyroid, parathyroid, and thymus glands are closely related to these structures. The cervical esophagus begins at the lower border of the cricoid cartilage and takes a curved course down the neck. The recurrent laryngeal nerves, thyroid gland, carotid sheath, and branches of the arteries are related anterolaterally. The thyroid gland consists of two lobes, which may be connected by the isthmus.

Surgical Annotation

Tracheostomy is one of the most common surgical procedures performed in intensive care units. The most common indication for tracheostomy is for prolonged airway access in impaired respiratory function. During tracheostomy, the structures anterior to the second to fourth rings are addressed such as the isthmus of the thyroid. During primary and reoperations of the thyroid glands, it is crucial to appreciate the relationship between the important landmarks, such as the recurrent and superior laryngeal nerves, brachiocephalic artery, and parathyroid glands.[35–37]

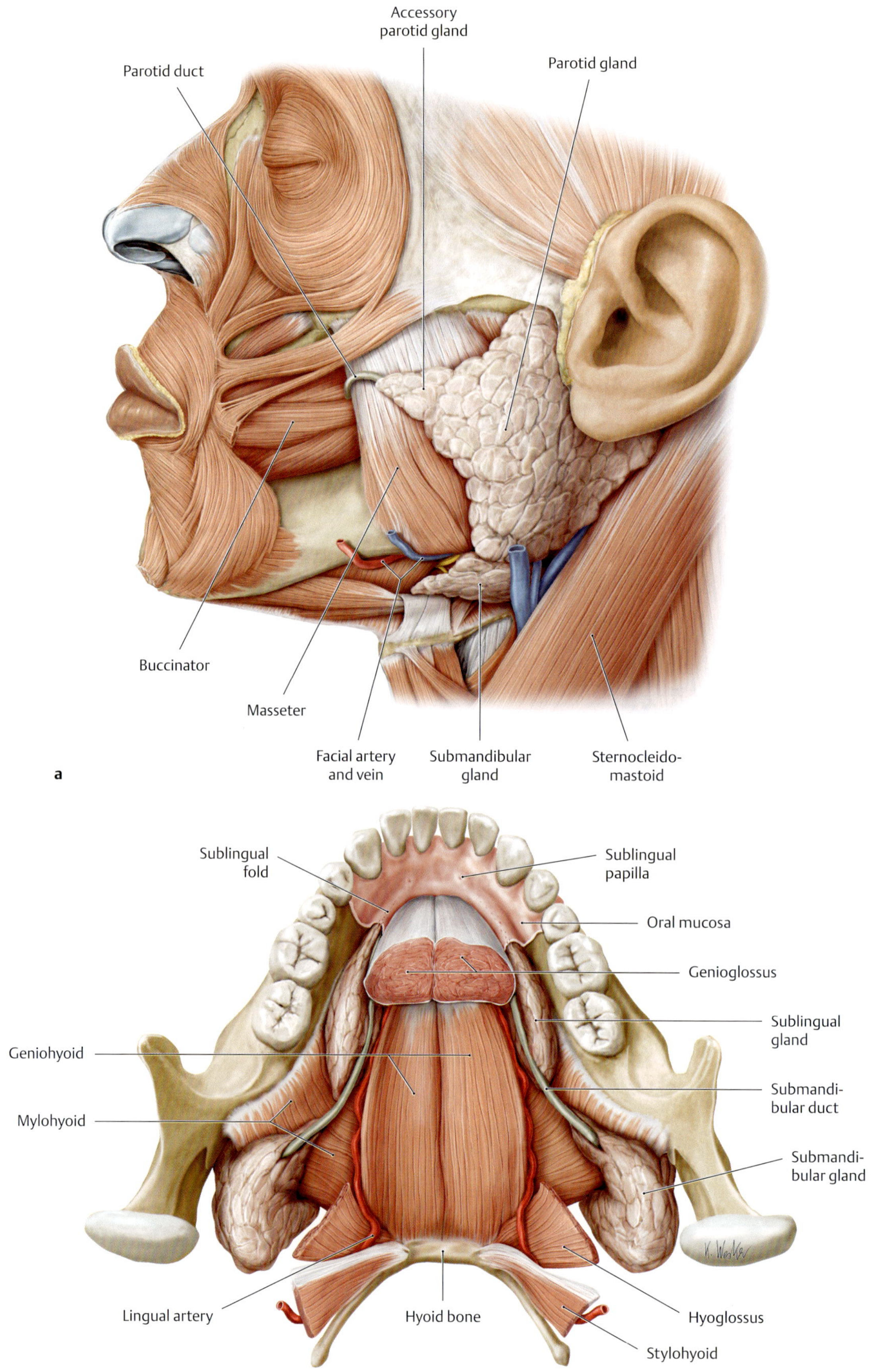

Fig. 21.16 Major salivary glands. **(a)** Lateral view and **(b)** superior view. Three large, paired sets of glads are distinguished: 1. Parotid glands 2. Submandibular glands 3. Sublingual glands. (From THIEME Atlas of Anatomy, Head and Neuroanatomy. © Thieme 2010, Illustrations by Karl Wesker.)

References

1. Renaut A, Orlin W, Ammar A, Pogrel MA. Distribution of submental fat in relationship to the platysma muscle. Oral Surg Oral Med Oral Pathol 1994;77(5):442–445
2. Hatef DA, Koshy JC, Sandoval SE, Echo AP, Izaddoost SA, Hollier LH. The submental fat compartment of the neck. Semin Plast Surg 2009;23(4):288–291
3. Raveendran SS, Anthony DJ, Ion L. An anatomic basis for volumetric evaluation of the neck. Aesthet Surg J 2012;32(6):685–691
4. de Castro CC. The anatomy of the platysma muscle. Plast Reconstr Surg 1980;66(5):680–683
5. Mejia JD, Nahai FR, Nahai F, Momoh AO. Isolated management of the aging neck. Semin Plast Surg 2009;23(4):264–273
6. Rohrich RJ, Rios JL, Smith PD, Gutowski KA. Neck rejuvenation revisited. Plast Reconstr Surg 2006;118(5):1251–1263
7. Caplin DA, Perlyn CA. Rejuvenation of the aging neck: current principles, techniques, and newer modifications. Facial Plast Surg Clin North Am 2009;17(4):589–601, vi–vii
8. Uehara M, Helman JI, Lillie JH, Brooks SL. Blood supply to the platysma muscle flap: an anatomic study with clinical correlation. J Oral Maxillofac Surg 2001;59(6):642–646
9. Hurwitz DJ, Rabson JA, Futrell JW. The anatomic basis for the platysma skin flap. Plast Reconstr Surg 1983;72(3):302–314
10. Vieira F, Allen SM, Stocks RM, Thompson JW. Deep neck infection. Otolaryngol Clin North Am 2008;41(3):459–483, vii
11. Osborn TM, Assael LA, Bell RB. Deep space neck infection: principles of surgical management. Oral Maxillofac Surg Clin North Am 2008;20(3):353–365
12. Ramirez CA, Fernandes RP. The supraclavicular artery island and trapezius myocutaneous flaps in head and neck reconstruction. Oral Maxillofac Surg Clin North Am 2014;26(3):411–420
13. Haas F, Weiglein A, Schwarzl F, Scharnagl E. The lower trapezius musculocutaneous flap from pedicled to free flap: anatomical basis and clinical applications based on the dorsal scapular artery. Plast Reconstr Surg 2004;113(6):1580–1590
14. McKinney P, Katrana DJ. Prevention of injury to the great auricular nerve during rhytidectomy. Plast Reconstr Surg 1980;66(5):675–679
15. Cappiello J, Piazza C, Giudice M, De Maria G, Nicolai P. Shoulder disability after different selective neck dissections (levels II-IV versus levels II-V): a comparative study. Laryngoscope 2005;115(2): 259–263
16. Cappiello J, Piazza C, Nicolai P. The spinal accessory nerve in head and neck surgery. Curr Opin Otolaryngol Head Neck Surg 2007; 15(2):107–111
17. Dingman RO, Grabb WC. Surgical anatomy of the mandibular ramus of the facial nerve based on the dissection of 100 facial halves. Plast Reconstr Surg Transplant Bull 1962;29:266–272
18. Daane SP, Owsley JQ. Incidence of cervical branch injury with "marginal mandibular nerve pseudo-paralysis" in patients undergoing face lift. Plast Reconstr Surg 2003;111(7):2414–2418
19. Makeieff M, Raingeard I, Alric P, Bonafe A, Guerrier B, Marty-Ane Ch. Surgical management of carotid body tumors. Ann Surg Oncol 2008;15(8):2180–2186
20. Luna-Ortiz K, Rascon-Ortiz M. Villavicencio-Valencia V etal. Carotid body tumors: review of a 20-year experience. Oral Oncol 2005; 41:56–61
21. Cohen J, Rad I. Contemporary management of carotid blowout. Curr Opin Otolaryngol Head Neck Surg 2004;12(2):110–115
21. Ahn C, Sindelar WF. Bilateral radical neck dissection: report of results in 55 patients. J Surg Oncol 1989;40(4):252–255
23. Dulguerov P, Soulier C, Maurice J, Faidutti B, Allai AS, Lehmann W. Bilateral radical dissection with unilateral internal jugular vein reconstruction. Laryngoscope 1998;108:1692–1696
24. Cohan DM, Popat S, Kaplan SE, Rigual N, Loree T, Hicks WL Jr. Oropharyngeal cancer: current understanding and management. Curr Opin Otolaryngol Head Neck Surg 2009;17(2):88–94
25. Sixth edition of the American Joint Committee on Cancer (AJCC) 2010 staging system for oropharygeal cancer. 2010. (https://cancer staging.org/referencestools/ deskreferences/Documents/AJCC6thEd CancerStagingManualPart1.pdf)
26. Belcher R, Hayes K, Fedewa S, Chen AY. Current treatment of head and neck squamous cell cancer. J Surg Oncol 2014;110(5):551–574
27. Ferlito A, Silver CE, Rinaldo A. Elective management of the neck in oral cavity squamous carcinoma: current concepts supported by prospective studies. Br J Oral Maxillofac Surg 2009;47(1):5–9
28. Robbins KT, Clayman G, Levine PA, et al; American Head and Neck Society; American Academy of Otolaryngology--Head and Neck Surgery. Neck dissection classification update: revisions proposed by the American Head and Neck Society and the American Academy of Otolaryngology-Head and Neck Surgery. Arch Otolaryngol Head Neck Surg 2002;128(7):751–758
29. Robbins KT, Shaha AR, Medina JE, et al; Committee for Neck Dissection Classification, American Head and Neck Society. Consensus statement on the classification and terminology of neck dissection. Arch Otolaryngol Head Neck Surg 2008;134(5):536–538
30. Singer DP, Sullivan PK. Submandibular gland I: an anatomic evaluation and surgical approach to submandibular gland resection for facial rejuvenation. Plast Reconstr Surg 2003;112(4):1150–1156
31. Hamilton MM, Chan D. Adjunctive procedures to neck rejuvenation. Facial Plast Surg Clin North Am 2014;22(2):231–242
32. Preuss SF, Klussmann JP, Wittekindt C, Drebber U, Beutner D, Guntinas-Lichius O. Submandibular gland excision: 15 years of experience. J Oral Maxillofac Surg 2007;65(5):953–957
33. Roh JL. Removal of the submandibular gland by a submental approach: a prospective, randomized, controlled study. Oral Oncol 2008;44(3):295–300
34. Berini-Aytes L, Gay-Escoda C. Morbidity associated with removal of the submandibular gland. J Craniomaxillofac Surg 1992;20(5): 216–219
35. Salgarelli AC, Collini M, Bellini P, Capparè P. Tracheostomy in maxillofacial surgery: a simple and safe technique for residents in training. J Craniofac Surg 2011;22(1):243–246
36. Haspel AC, Coviello VF, Stevens M. Retrospective study of tracheostomy indications and perioperative complications on oral and maxillofacial surgery service. J Oral Maxillofac Surg 2012;70(4): 890–895
37. Thiruchelvam JK, Cheng LH, Drewery H. How to do a safe tracheostomy. Int J Oral Maxillofac Surg 2008;37(5):484–486

Index